# THE HEART

Seventh Edition

## Companion Handbook

D0756066

Presented as a service to medicine by

Merck Frosst Canada Inc.

A leader in cardiovascular therapy

RNIT-90-CDN-3558-BK

# NOTICE

To our wives,
Maria Ellingsen-Schlant
and
Nelie Wiley Hurst.

# CONTENTS

# CONTRIBUTORS

**Subodh K. Agrawal, M.D.,** Fellow in Cardiology, Emory University School of Medicine, Atlanta, Georgia

**James K. Alexander, M.D.,** Professor of Medicine, Baylor College of Medicine, Houston, Texas

**Michael E. Assey, M.D.,** Associate Professor of Medicine (Cardiology), Director, Adult Cardiac Catheterization Laboratory, Medical University of South Carolina, Charleston, South Carolina

**Hisham A. Ba'albaki, M.D.,** Associate, Interventional Cardiology, Emory University School of Medicine, Atlanta, Georgia

**Harisios Boudoulas, M.D.,** Professor of Medicine and Pharmacy, Division of Cardiology, Department of Internal Medicine, Colleges of Medicine and Pharmacy, The Ohio State University, Columbus, Ohio

**Edmund Bourke, M.D.,** Professor and Vice Chairman, Department of Medicine, State University of New York Health Science Center at Brooklyn; Chief, Medical Service, VA Medical Center, Brooklyn, New York

**W. Scott Brooks, M.D.,** Formerly Associate Professor of Medicine (Digestive Diseases), Emory University School of Medicine, Atlanta, Georgia

**Peter M. Buttrick, M.D.,** Assistant Professor of Medicine, Physiology and Biophysics, Division of Cardiology, Montefiore Medical Center, Albert Einstein College of Medicine, Bronx, New York

**Marilyn Cox, M.D.,** Cardiology Fellow, University of Miami School of Medicine, Miami, Florida

**Vera B. Delaney, M.D., Ph.D.,** Assistant Professor of Medicine, State University of New York, Health Science Center at Brooklyn, New York

**Samuel J. De Maio, Jr., M.D.,** Associate, Interventional Cardiology, Emory University School of Medicine, Atlanta, Georgia

**David T. Durack, M.B., D. Phil.,** Professor of Medicine, Microbiology and Immunology; Chief, Division of Infectious Diseases, Duke University Medical Center, Durham, North Carolina

**Frederick S. Fein, M.D.,** Associate Professor of Medicine, Division of Cardiology, Albert Einstein College of Medicine, Bronx, New York

**David W. Ferguson, M.D.,** Associate Professor of Medicine, University of Iowa College of Medicine; Director, Cardiovascular Intensive Care Unit and Clinical Cardiovascular Physiology Laboratory, University of Iowa Hospitals and Clinics, Iowa City, Iowa

**Charles Fisch, M.D.,** Distinguished Professor of Medicine, Indiana University School of Medicine; Director, Cardiovascular Division and Krannert Institute of Cardiology, Indianapolis, Indiana

**William H. Frishman, M.D.,** Professor of Medicine, Epidemiology and Social Medicine, Albert Einstein College of Medicine; Director of the Department of Medicine, Hospital of the Albert Einstein College of Medicine, Bronx, New York

**Peter C. Gazes, M.D.,** Professor of Medicine, Distinguished University Professor of Cardiology, Medical University of South Carolina, Charleston, South Carolina

**Scott M. Grundy, M.D., Ph.D.,** Professor of Internal Medicine and Biochemistry, Director, Center for Human Nutrition, Chairman, Department of Clinical Nutrition, The University of Texas Southwestern Medical Center at Dallas, Dallas, Texas

**Robert J. Hall, M.D.,** Clinical Professor of Medicine, Baylor College of Medicine and the University of Texas Medical School at Houston, Medical Director, Texas Heart Institute; Chief of Cardiology, St. Luke's Episcopal Hospital, Houston, Texas

**W. Dallas Hall, Jr., M.D.,** Professor of Medicine (Hypertension), Director, Division of Hypertension, Emory University School of Medicine and Grady Memorial Hospital, Atlanta, Georgia

**Kenneth M. Kessler, M.D.,** Professor of Medicine, University of Miami School of Medicine; Chief, Cardiology Section, Veterans Administration Medical Center, Miami, Florida

**Hiroshi Kuida, M.D.,** Professor of Internal Medicine, Professor of Physiology, University of Utah School of Medicine, Salt Lake City, Utah

**Eliot J. Lazar, M.D.,** Associate Director, Medical Service, Co-Director, Intensive Care Unit, Hospital of the Albert Einstein College of Medicine, Bronx, New York

**Thierry H. LeJemtel, M.D.,** Associate Professor of Medicine, Division of Cardiology, Albert Einstein College of Medicine, Bronx, New York

**Angel R. Leon, M.D.,** Fellow in Cardiology, Emory University School of Medicine, Atlanta, Georgia

**Richard P. Lewis, M.D.,** Professor of Medicine, Division of Cardiology, Department of Internal Medicine, College of Medicine, The Ohio State University, Columbus, Ohio

**Joseph Lindsay, Jr., M.D.,** Professor of Medicine, The George Washington University; Chairman, Section of Cardiology, The Washington Hospital Center, Washington, D.C.

**Frank I. Marcus, M.D.,** Professor of Medicine, Cardiology Section, University of Arizona College of Medicine, Tucson, Arizona

**John H. McAnulty, M.D.,** Professor of Medicine, Division of Cardiology, Oregon Health Sciences University, Portland, Oregon

**James Metcalfe, M.D.,** Assistant Chief of Staff, Veterans Administration Medical Center, Vancouver Division; Professor of Medicine, Oregon Health Sciences University, Portland, Oregon

**Harry G. Mond, M.D.,** Physician to Pacemaker Clinic, Department of Cardiology, The Royal Melbourne Hospital, Victoria, Australia

**Douglas C. Morris, M.D.,** Associate Professor of Medicine (Cardiology), Emory University School of Medicine; Director, Carlyle Fraser Heart Center, Crawford Long Memorial Hospital, Atlanta, Georgia

**Kari E. Murros, M.D.,** Neurologist, Department of Neurology, Central Hospital of Central Finland, Jyvaskyla, Finland

**Robert J. Myerburg, M.D.,** Professor of Medicine and Physiology, Director, Division of Cardiology, University of Miami School of Medicine, Miami, Florida

**Elizabeth W. Nugent, M.D.,** Associate Professor of Pediatrics, Cardiology Division, Emory University School of Medicine, Atlanta, Georgia

**David P. Rardon, M.D.,** Assistant Professor of Medicine, Indiana University School of Medicine, Indianapolis, Indiana

**Timothy J. Regan, M.D.,** Professor of Medicine, Director, Division of Cardiovascular Diseases, University of Medicine and Dentistry of New Jersey, New Jersey Medical School, Newark, New Jersey

**James Scheuer, M.D.,** Professor of Medicine, Physiology and Biophysics; Chairman, Department of Medicine, Montefiore Medical Center and Albert Einstein College of Medicine, Bronx, New York

**Ralph Shabetai, M.D.,** Professor of Medicine, University of California San Diego; Chief of Cardiology, San Diego Veterans Administration Medical Center, San Diego, California

**Robert B. Smith III, M.D.,** Professor of Surgery, Head of General Vascular Surgery, Emory University School of Medicine; Attending Surgeon, Veterans Medical Center, Atlanta, Georgia

**Edmund H. Sonnenblick, M.D.,** Olson Professor of Medicine, Chief, Division of Cardiology, Albert Einstein College of Medicine, Bronx, New York

**James F. Spann, Jr., M.D.,** Professor of Medicine, Director, Cardiology Division, Director, Gazes Cardiac Research Institute, Medical University of South Carolina, Charleston, South Carolina

**Mark T. Stewart, M.D.,** Thoracic and Cardiovascular Associates of Austin, Austin, Texas

**Panagiotis N. Symbas, M.D.,** Professor of Surgery, Thoracic and Cardiovascular Surgery Division, Emory University School of Medicine; Director, Thoracic and Cardiovascular Surgery, Grady Memorial Hospital, Atlanta, Georgia

**James F. Toole, M.D.,** Walter Teagle Professor of Neurology, Professor of Public Health Sciences, Bowman Gray School of Medicine, Winston-Salem, North Carolina

**Kent Ueland, M.D.,** Professor Emeritus, Department of Gynecology and Obstetrics, Stanford University School of Medicine, Stanford, California

**R. Verhaeghe, M.D., Ph.D.,** Professor of Medicine, University of Leuven, Leuven, Belgium

**Marc Verstraete, M.D., Ph.D.,** Professor of Medicine, University of Leuven, Leuven, Belgium

**James V. Warren, M.D.,** Professor of Medicine (Emeritus), College of Medicine, The Ohio State University, Columbus, Ohio

**Arnold M. Weissler, M.D.,** Professor of Medicine, Mayo Medical School, Rochester, Minnesota

**Nanette Kass Wenger, M.D.,** Professor of Medicine (Cardiology), Emory University School of Medicine; Director, Cardiac Clinics, Grady Memorial Hospital, Atlanta, Georgia

**Raymond L. Woosley, M.D., Ph.D.,** Chairman, Department of Pharmacology, Director, Clinical Pharmacology Center, Georgetown University School of Medicine, Washington, D.C.

# PREFACE

The first *Handbook of the Heart* evolved from a perceived need of our students and house officers for a concise, portable book that they could use in the middle of the night or in instances when they did not have access to a larger reference textbook. It was not intended to be used in place of more specialized books of cardiology or larger textbooks of medicine or cardiology. Based on the enthusiastic response to the first *Handbook*, we have continued with these objectives in this second *Handbook*, which is designed to be used in conjunction with the Seventh Edition of *The Heart*. Most of the contributions were prepared by one or more of the authors of the corresponding chapters in *The Heart*. We express our deep appreciation to them. We also ask our readers to assist us by letting us know their suggestions of ways to improve and make more useful future efforts.

# ACKNOWLEDGMENTS

The editors would like to express their sincere appreciation to each of the authors who contributed to this *Handbook*. In particular, we would like to thank them for their efforts to complete this *Handbook* so soon after the publication of the seventh edition of *The Heart*.

We would also like to thank Ms. Catherine DeVries for the invaluable time and extra efforts she devoted to bringing this book to a successful completion. In addition, we wish to recognize the skill and resourcefulness that the editorial and production staffs at McGraw-Hill displayed in preparing and producing this book, particularly Mr. Peter McCurdy and Mr. Dereck Jeffers.

R.C.S.
J.W.H.

# The Recognition and Management of Congestive Heart Failure

*Michael E. Assey, M.D.*
*James F. Spann, Jr., M.D.*

All house officers and practicing physicians should be competent in the diagnosis and in the early management (at least) of congestive heart failure. Indeed, this syndrome—which is not a specific disease entity—is responsible for over one million admissions annually. The prevalence is estimated at between two and three million (1 percent of the U.S. population), but the syndrome may affect as many as 10 percent of patients over 75 years of age. Approximately 400,000 new cases are diagnosed each year.

Prognosis for those patients with moderate and severe heart failure remains poor even now. The 5-year mortality approaches 50 percent when heart failures from all causes are considered. For those with the most severe degree of heart failure—manifested by symptoms occurring at rest—the 1-year mortality may be as high as 50 percent. Many of these deaths are sudden, implicating ventricular arrhythmias as the cause.

## DEFINITION

Traditionally, heart failure has been defined as the inability of the heart to pump enough blood to meet the demands of the metabolizing tissues. This definition is not useful clinically, and incorrectly suggests that cardiac output in heart failure is always low. Moreover, it fails to mention the prominent circulatory congestion that reflects the hemodynamic derangement of elevated cardiac filling pressures. Symptoms of low cardiac output (fatigue) and congestion (dyspnea) occur most prominently during exercise. This has led many authors to define heart failure in terms of exercise tolerance, emphasizing the abnormal distribution of blood flow and inappropriate vasoconstrictive circulatory response. While left ventricular systolic dysfunction (defined as a low ejection fraction) is often present in heart failure, a low ejection fraction *per se* may cause no symptoms. Following treatment, patients may be asymptomatic at rest; such patients are said to have *compensated congestive heart failure*. Regardless of the specific definition used, from an operational standpoint heart failure is a syndrome with multiple etiologies in which low output and congestive symptoms are prominent. Exercise capacity is generally decreased, and life expectancy may be significantly reduced.

## PATHOPHYSIOLOGY

Cardiac pump function should be viewed within the framework of the total cardiovascular system. Arterial blood pressure is the product of cardiac output and systemic vascular resistance. The major determinants of cardiac output are heart rate and stroke volume. Stroke volume is determined by preload (ventricular volume at the end of diastole), contractility, and afterload (those forces resisting ventricular ejection). The basic lesion in many forms of heart failure is a depression of myocardial contractility. This may be due to a chronic volume or pressure overload (as in valvular heart disease) or a primary reduction in contractility (cardiomyopathy or ischemic heart disease). When reduced contractility reduces stroke volume, several compensatory mechanisms are activated in an attempt to normalize cardiac output and maintain blood flow to critical organs. In fact, it is the "overshoot" of these expected compensatory phenomena that causes many of the symptoms, and most signs, of heart failure. One of these is the Frank-Starling mechanism. This cardiac dilatation during diastole increases the subsequent force and volume of systolic contraction and ejection. Unfortunately, the resulting elevation in left ventricular filling pressure may cause dyspnea and other congestive symptoms. A chronically dilated left ventricle increases wall stress. This can be minimized by an appropriate degree of ventricular hypertrophy, as described by Laplace.

Enhanced sympathetic nervous system activity supports contractility and raises the heart rate by producing a higher level of circulating catecholamines. Angiotensin release raises systemic vascular resistance and maintains blood flow to critical organs. Aldosterone provides sodium and water retention, increasing central blood volume and maximizing the Frank-Starling mechanism. Unfortunately, these compensations generally overshoot and result in further depression of ventricular contractility and cardiac performance. The increased arteriolar tone limits ventricular emptying, reducing ejection fraction and cardiac output. Increased venous tone contributes to an already congested venous circulation, thus worsening dyspnea and other congestive symptoms.

These physiological events characterize the heart as it functions during systole. Many patients with congestive heart failure may have normal left ventricular size and systolic function but, with them, a diastolic dysfunction wherein left ventricular filling is impaired. This results in suboptimal cardiac pump function with elevated cardiac filling pressures and reduced cardiac output.

Diastolic dysfunction may result from hypertrophy of any cause, infiltrative diseases of the myocardium, or pericardial disease. Systolic and diastolic dysfunction may coexist, and often do. Some patients with low ejection fraction have good exercise tolerance, while others with only a modest reduction in ejection fraction have very poor exercise tolerance. This paradox may be explained by the coexistence of diastolic dysfunction.

## CLINICAL MANIFESTATIONS

### History

Symptoms of heart failure vary in severity and type. A thorough history may uncover a patient who has maintained his asymptomatic status and level of exercise tolerance only by reducing his activity. Traditionally, symptoms are classified as *congestive* (reflecting elevated diastolic intracardiac pressures) and as *low-output* (reflecting a relatively reduced cardiac output with exertion, if not also at rest).

Dyspnea, orthopnea, and paroxysmal nocturnal dyspnea are common congestive symptoms of left-sided heart failure. Anxiety and chronic obstructive lung disease may produce similar symptoms. In the latter case an accumulation of bronchial secretions in the recumbent position causes these symptoms, and often a productive cough; a nonproductive cough is more typical of heart failure. Peripheral edema is well known as a sign of heart failure. However, it occurs relatively late—usually requiring up to 10 pounds of excess body water before becoming noticeable. Edema may also be due to noncardiac conditions, including venous insufficiency, renal disease, hepatic insufficiency, and nutritional hypoalbuminemia. Low-output symptoms include weakness, fatigue, and decreased exercise tolerance.

### Physical Examination

The findings on physical examination depend on the etiology and acuteness of onset. The skin is typically cool and clammy, and the peripheral pulse is rapid in rate and low in amplitude. Pulsus alternans is relatively uncommon, but when present is usually a strong indicator of left-sided heart failure and severe underlying ventricular dysfunction. The quality of the peripheral pulse may be a clue to the underlying etiology, as with the parvus et tardus pulse of aortic stenosis. When the neck veins can be clearly seen, the right-sided filling pressure can be estimated. It is often elevated. Subtle right-heart volume overload may be uncovered by compression of the right upper quadrant (hepatojugular reflux test). Examination of the lungs may reveal an assortment of abnormalities, including moist rales, wheezing (from interstitial pulmonary edema), and decreased breath sounds from overlying pleural fluid (usually bilateral, or on the right side if unilateral).

Examination of the heart itself may demonstrate abnormalities of palpation and auscultation. If enough time has elapsed for the Frank-Starling mechanism to be used, the PMI will be displaced to the left and inferiorly. Pressure and volume overloads may cause displacements of the PMI even in the absence of heart failure. The most important auscultatory indicators of heart failure are a reduced intensity of $S_1$ and the presence of an $S_3$ gallop. The $S_4$ gallop indicates a change in left ventricular compliance, but occurs commonly in patients without heart failure, particularly in the elderly. Any cardiac murmur may be an important clue to the cause of the heart failure. However, systolic murmurs of tricuspid and mitral insufficiency may also be functional, indicating advanced cardiac enlargement with dilatation of the annuli.

The patient with acute pulmonary edema appears in distress, is difficult to interview, and is comfortable only in the upright position.

### Ancillary Tests

The *chest x-ray* may demonstrate an assortment of abnormalities in heart failure, including cardiomegaly, redistribution of pulmonary venous flow to the superior veins in an upright chest x-ray, dilatation of the pulmonary arteries, interstitial pulmonary edema (perivascular haziness, peribronchial cuffing), alveolar infiltrates, excessive lung water (pseudotumors, Kerley lines), and pleural effusions.

The *ECG* may show acute myocardial ischemia or injury, and is particularly useful when an infarction pattern is seen. Otherwise the ECG is nonspecific, frequently showing ventricular hypertrophy and atrial enlargement.

A most useful ancillary test is the *echocardiogram*, often combined with *Doppler flow studies*. These noninvasive tests may aid etiologic diagnosis. For example, abnormalities of the cardiac valves can be identified and semiquantified by Doppler investigation. These tests also have contributed much to our current understanding of the importance of diastolic dysfunction. The echocardiogram can identify compensatory changes (dilatation, hypertrophy), assess the appropriateness of these compensatory changes (concentric versus eccentric hypertrophy), and assess regional and global systolic function. Determination of chamber size can help in management. The patient with a large left atrium is resistant to both electrical and pharmacological cardioversion of atrial fibrillation.

## TREATMENT

### General Measures

Correct management begins with accurate diagnosis. All too often, past medical records are inadequately reviewed, or a longstanding diagnosis goes unchallenged, when in fact other pathophysiological events (e.g., diastolic dysfunction) may be relatively more important. One should search aggressively for surgically correctable abnormalities. The absence of chest pain, particularly in a patient with risk factors for coronary atherosclerosis, does not exclude myocardial ischemia as the cause of heart failure.

Cardiac arrhythmias should be evaluated and treated. From the standpoint of cardiac pump function, a patient is better off with sinus rhythm than with atrial fibrillation. The atrial contribution to cardiac output is usually 20 percent, but may approach 40 percent in patients with diastolic dysfunction. When a permanent pacemaker is needed, heart failure can be avoided by using dual-chambered (physiological) pacing, which mimics the normal atrioventricular contraction pattern.

General treatment of heart failure includes the patient's achieving an ideal body weight and appropriate dietary salt intake. The workload of the heart should be reduced by appropriate changes in physical and emotional stress and by rigid control of elevated blood pressure.

### Diuretics

These agents alleviate congestive symptoms by decreasing elevated intracardiac pressures. In patients with diastolic dysfunction, over-diuresis may reduce cardiac output, in which case congestive symptoms are improved only at the expense of low-output symptoms. Patients refractory to oral diuretics may not be absorbing their medication. Hospitalization and intravenous diuretic administration may often break a vicious cycle of diuretic resistance and worsening congestion. A loop diuretic (such as furosemide) used with a proximal tubule agent (such as metolazone) makes a potent diuretic combination. Indeed, the danger of over-diuresis with accompanying electrolyte imbalance is real. Patients should ideally lose two to three pounds per day (when treated on an outpatient basis) and should be carefully monitored for electrolyte imbalance.

### Positive Inotropic Agents

Digitalis (most often digoxin) is effective when used orally or intravenously. It is most effective in patients with left ventricular dilatation, an $S_3$ gallop, and atrial fibrillation. Patients with diastolic dysfunction and preserved ejection fraction do not benefit from digitalis's inotropic effect. However, the drug may be useful in slowing the ventricular-rate response to atrial fibrillation, thereby allowing more time for ventricular filling. Amrinone (parenteral) and milrinone (oral) are phosphodiesterase inhibitors that enhance contractility by increasing cyclic AMP in myocardial cells. In chronic trials, milrinone appears no more effective than digitalis, and in one study milrinone was associated with an increased risk of sudden cardiac death. Aminophylline, a phosphodiesterase inhibitor, is often given to patients with florid pulmonary edema who have bronchospasm and arterial hypoxemia. Not only is it an effective bronchodilator, but it increases contractility and is a fair diuretic.

Dopamine and dobutamine are intravenous positive inotropic agents used in treatment of very advanced heart failure. Both drugs improve cardiac output. Dopamine produces a greater increase in mean arterial pressure but may also increase left ventricular filling pressures, particularly at higher doses. Dobutamine is preferred when low output is accompanied by elevated filling pressures, since it also decreases pulmonary capillary wedge pressures. Rarely, patients with refractory heart failure may be treated with prolonged infusions of dobutamine to acutely improve hemodynamics and enhance response to oral agents.

## Vasodilators

Vasodilators are now used earlier in the treatment of heart failure. As a class, they produce favorable hemodynamic effects, improve the quality of life, and increase life expectancy. Diuretics and positive inotropic agents have not been shown to increase life expectancy. When vasodilators are part of the treatment regimen, lower doses of diuretics and digitalis can be used.

Nitrates primarily dilate veins, thereby increasing venous capacitance. The subsequent reduction in preload alleviates congestive symptoms and may have an additional salutary effect in patients whose heart failure is due to myocardial ischemia. Intravenous nitroglycerin is frequently used in acute pulmonary edema.

Systemic arterial vasodilators (hydralazine, minoxidil) primarily dilate arterioles. The resulting reduction in impedance to left ventricular output improves cardiac output and low-output symptoms. Hydralazine is often combined with nitrates to relieve both low-output and congestive symptoms. The combination has been shown to improve life expectancy.

Nitroprusside, prazosin, and the angiotensin-coverting enzyme (ACE) inhibitors are balanced vasodilators that can alleviate congestive and low-output symptoms. A patient may develop a tolerance to chronic prazosin therapy. Termination of nitroprusside infusion can result in rebound vasoconstriction if high doses have been used. ACE inhibitors antagonize the renin-angiotensin-aldosterone system and thereby dilate veins and arterioles. The ACE inhibitors are the most effective and useful vasodilator therapy in heart failure and should be used relatively early in the course of the illness. However, they should be used cautiously in the presence of renal insufficiency or electrolyte imbalance (hyperkalemia, hyponatremia). When hyponatremia or hypovolemia is present, ACE inhibitors may produce hypotension. Recent data suggests that heart failure can be prevented by the early use of ACE inhibitors in patients with left ventricular dysfunction due to recent myocardial infarction. This cardioprotective effect is attributed to the prevention of dilatation and hypertrophy, as well as antagonism of neurohumoral-induced vasoconstriction.

## Other Therapy

Paradoxically, beta blockers, despite their negative inotropic effect, can relieve symptoms in selected patients with heart failure. The mechanism may be a change in beta receptor density or sensitivity. Dilated-cardiomyopathy patients with demonstrated tachycardia appear to benefit most. Perhaps the slowing of heart rate improves coronary blood flow. These drugs are also anti-ischemic agents, and may improve heart failure in the coronary disease patient by reducing myocardial oxygen demand. The use of beta blockers in heart failure is still investigational.

Calcium antagonists are potent systemic vasodilators and may be useful in patients with heart failure complicating hypertension or ischemic heart disease. However, they all have intrinsic negative inotropic effects and must be used very cautiously in patients with hypotension, low ejection fractions, or pulmonary congestion. In such patients the vasodilator effect fails to balance the negative inotropic effect and heart failure is worsened.

Cardiac transplantation is now a realistic alternative for appropriate patients. One-year survival rates exceed 90 percent. The cost of the procedure and the scarcity of available donors remain major obstacles to this otherwise definitive therapy.

## SUGGESTED READING

Cohn JN: Current therapy of the failing heart. *Circulation* 78:1099–1107, 1988.

Francis GS: Development of arrhythmias in the patient with congestive heart failure: Pathophysiology, prevalence and prognosis. *Am J Cardiol* 57:3–7B, 1986.

Katz AM: Changing strategies in the management of heart failure. *J Am Coll Cardiol* 13:513–523, 1989.

Kessler KM: Diastolic heart failure: Diagnosis and management. *Hospital Practice* 24(7):137–164, 1989.

Parmley WW: Pathophysiology and current therapy of congestive heart failure. *J Am Coll Cardiol* 13:771–785, 1989.

Spann JF, Hurst JW: The recognition and management of heart failure, in Hurst JW et al (eds): *The Heart,* 7th ed. New York, McGraw-Hill, Chap 27, pp 418–441, 1990.

## 2 | The Recognition and Management of Cardiogenic Shock

*David W. Ferguson, M.D.*

### DEFINITION

*Cardiogenic shock* is defined *clinically* as a primary cardiac disorder resulting in tissue perfusion that is inadequate for delivery of necessary substrates and removal of metabolic wastes. Tissue perfusion depends on the arterial pressure and vascular resistance of the particular organ bed. Arterial pressure is determined by cardiac output (stroke volume × heart rate) and total vascular resistance. Stroke volume depends on the preload, afterload, and contractile state of the heart. Often, in cardiogenic shock, an inadequate forward stroke volume is the primary physiological defect and forward cardiac output is inadequate to meet the metabolic demands of the body. Cardiogenic shock is defined *hemodynamically* as any primary cardiac condition resulting in *all* of the following: (1) systolic arterial pressure < 90 mmHg (absolute hypotension) or at least 60 mmHg below basal blood pressure (relative hypotension); (2) evidence of impaired major organ blood flow (decreased mentation, peripheral vasoconstriction, and oliguria [urine output < 30 ml/hr]); (3) absence of insufficient preload (which would be marked by pulmonary capillary wedge pressure < 15 mmHg) or other primary nonmyocardial processes as the etiology of the shock state (e.g., arrhythmias, acidosis, or pharmacological or physiological myocardial depressants); (4) presence of primary myocardial insult as defined by clinical and laboratory criteria.

### ETIOLOGY

Cardiogenic shock is usually due to an *acute* deterioration of cardiac function, but may also be the end result of chronic decline of the contractile performance of the heart. In common practice, cardiogenic shock implies a mechanical or myopathic disorder of cardiac function, rather than a primary electrical dysfunction. Cardiogenic shock most frequently results from acute myocardial infarction, with shock complicating 5 to 15 percent of infarction patients admitted to a general hospital. Shock resulting from inotropic impairment alone (i.e., absence of a mechanical lesion) is more common following anterior than inferior infarctions.

However, inferior infarction with significant right ventricular involvement may also result in cardiogenic shock. Acute mechanical lesions (e.g., mitral insufficiency or ventricular septal rupture) may result in cardiogenic shock; they complicate both anterior and inferior infarctions, with similar frequencies. Primary cardiac disorders other than myocardial infarction may result in cardiogenic shock. They include fulminant infectious myocarditis; critical valvular heart disease; cardiac tamponade; constrictive pericardial disorders; infective endocarditis; aortic valve disruption complicating aortic dissection; decompensation of chronic heart failure from any of diverse etiologies; spontaneous rupture of chordae tendineae in myxomatous mitral valves; and nonvalvular obstruction of left ventricular inflow (e.g., atrial myxoma) or outflow (e.g., hypertrophic obstructive cardiomyopathy). Cardiogenic shock may also occur as a perioperative complication of cardiopulmonary bypass.

## PATHOLOGY

In the absence of an acute mechanical defect, cardiogenic shock complicating acute myocardial infarction usually results from severe impairment of at least 35 percent of functioning left ventricular mass, either due to the acute infarction or as a total sum of acute and remote insults. Occasionally, cardiogenic shock may result primarily from massive right ventricular infarction. Mechanical lesions producing shock following acute infarction include ventricular rupture, mitral insufficiency, and ventricular septal rupture. Left ventricular free wall rupture accounts for approximately 10 percent of in-hospital deaths from acute infarction. Rupture occurs most frequently within the first 2 days following infarction, is often a complication of first infarctions, is more common with lateral infarctions, and occurs in patients with less severe narrowing of epicardial coronary arteries. Mitral insufficiency may be secondary to either ischemic papillary muscle dysfunction or dehiscence of a portion of the subvalvular apparatus. True rupture of a papillary muscle is a rare event, more commonly involves the posteromedial papillary muscle, and is often associated with a first myocardial infarction. Ventricular septal rupture complicates 1 to 3 percent of all infarctions, occurs with similar frequency in anterior and inferior infarctions, and accounts for approximately 5 percent of in-hospital deaths in infarct patients. Ventricular septal rupture complicating inferior infarction carries a poorer prognosis than that complicating anterior infarction. Associated involvement of right ventricular myocardium appears to be an important determinant of survival in patients with acute septal rupture.

Cardiogenic shock complicating acute infectious myocarditis results from extensive inflammatory involvement of large portions of both ventricles. In the setting of infective endocarditis, shock may arise from acute regurgitant lesions secondary to valve leaflet disruption. With acute aortic dissection, cardiogenic shock may result from rupture of the dissecting hematoma into the pericardial sac with resultant tamponade, or from free rupture into the thorax.

## CLINICAL MANIFESTATIONS

### History

Cardiogenic shock presents in one of three general patterns: (1) abrupt appearance within 4 to 6 h following onset of infarction, as a result of massive myocardial involvement or left ventricular free wall rupture; (2) slow gradual onset over several days in the presence of recurrent infarctions; or (3) abrupt onset remote from the index infarction (i.e., 2 to 10 days) with appearance of a new systolic murmur (mitral regurgitation or ventricular septal rupture) or electromechanical dissociation (ventricular rupture). These episodes may or may not be associated with chest pain, but are frequently associated with acute dyspnea and a sense of impending doom on the part of the patient.

### Physical Examination

The appearance of patients may range from acute anxiety to moribund obtundation. In addition to the hemodynamics listed above, frequent manifestations include tachypnea, tachycardia, narrow pulse pressure, diaphoresis, and peripheral vasoconstriction with cyanosis. Peripheral pulses may be absent. These signs may be altered in the presence of pharmacological blockade (e.g., beta blockers) or in the presence of high-degree atrioventricular block. Examination of the neck veins often reveals jugular venous distension, but this is an unreliable sign of left heart filling pressure. Auscultation of the chest frequently reveals diffuse rales. However, in a patient with acute infarction, the combination of a clear chest, profound hypotension, and neck vein distension suggests significant right ventricular infarction, massive pulmonary embolism, or cardiac tamponade. Cardiac auscultation frequently reveals atrial ($S_4$) and ventricular ($S_3$) gallops. The appearance of a new systolic murmur in the setting of acute infarction should raise the possibility of mitral insufficiency or ventricular septal rupture. In a patient with endocarditis, acute regurgitant murmurs may appear in the setting of valvular disruption. The clinician must remember, however, that a patient in shock must be able to generate some degree of effective forward cardiac output to produce a murmur.

Thus, significant valvular or myocardial pathology may be present without an audible murmur in a severe low-output state. Valuable bedside examination involves serial assessment of mental status, peripheral perfusion, and urine output.

## USUAL DIAGNOSTIC TESTS

The *chest roentgenogram* varies with the underlying pathophysiological process responsible for cardiogenic shock. In the setting of acute myocardial infarction, heart size is often normal and pulmonary edema is often present. The *electrocardiogram* is often markedly abnormal in the setting of cardiogenic shock complicating an acute myocardial infarction, with ST segment and T wave changes of transmural ischemia with or without associated Q waves. In the presence of a normal electrocardiogram, cardiogenic shock due to acute infarction is extremely rare and other diagnostic possibilities must be considered. Electrical alternans is suggestive of large pericardial effusion and possible cardiac tamponade. The most common electrocardiographic finding in cardiogenic shock from any etiology is sinus tachycardia.

## DIFFERENTIAL DIAGNOSIS

The differential diagnosis of cardiogenic shock includes a large number of disorders which account for the other three broad etiologic categories of shock: *hypovolemic shock*, *microcirculatory shock*, and *cellular membrane shock*.

## SPECIAL DIAGNOSTIC EVALUATION

During the initial assessment of the patient in cardiogenic shock, specialized diagnostic tests may be employed to increase the accuracy of diagnosis. The implementation of these tests should not interfere with standard resuscitative measures (see "Treatment," below). *Echocardiography* may be invaluable as a bedside tool for the determination of regional and global ventricular function, presence and significance of pericardial effusion, valvular pathology, and assessment of intracardiac shunts. *First pass radionuclide ventriculography* may be of benefit in assessment of right and left ventricular function. *Cardiac catheterization* is often an integral part of the initial assessment and resuscitation of the patient in cardiogenic shock. The performance of a complete right and left heart catheterization, serial oximetry analyses, left ventricular angiography, and selective coronary arteriography is often essential to define correctable lesions in the patient with cardiogenic shock complicating an acute myocardial infarction. In selected cases, the implementation of intraaortic balloon counterpulsation or other forms of percutaneous mechanical cardiac assistance is best performed in the catheterization suite. Recent studies suggest that emergent coronary angioplasty may be of benefit in cardiogenic shock complicating some acute myocardial infarctions.

## NATURAL HISTORY AND PROGNOSIS

The incidence of cardiogenic shock complicating acute infarction appears to be decreasing, perhaps in association with newer interventional therapies for acute myocardial infarction. However, the development of cardiogenic shock in the setting of acute infarction still carries a mortality of at least 60 to 70 percent in most medical centers. The use of emergency surgical approaches and mechanical circulatory assistance, and the rare implementation of urgent cardiac transplantation, may alter the outcome in rare cases of massive infarction. The mortality from cardiogenic shock due to etiologies other than acute infarction varies widely depending upon the reversibility of the underlying process.

## TREATMENT

Effective management of the patient with cardiogenic shock requires an initial high index of suspicion, rapid recognition of early warning signs, appropriate clinical history taking and physical examination, and, often, specialized diagnostic tests. The prognosis depends on the underlying pathophysiological process, the rapidity of clinical recognition of the shock state, the accuracy of diagnosis of the underlying defect, and the rapid initiation of primary and secondary therapies. Primary therapy is directed at the underlying defect (e.g., pericardiocentesis for tamponade), while secondary therapy is directed at reversing the deleterious processes associated with the shock state (e.g., acidosis, hypoxemia, electrolyte imbalances).

Rapid initiation of hemodynamic monitoring is essential. This includes continuous electrocardiographic monitoring and insertion of a thermodilution pulmonary artery balloon flotation catheter and an arterial catheter. These provide for minute-to-minute assessments of arterial and cardiac filling pressures and forward cardiac output. An indwelling Foley catheter with urimeter permits indirect assessment of renal perfusion. Rapid and repeated determinations of arterial blood gases, electrolytes, and hematologic parameters are essential. Oxygen should be administered by a high-flow delivery system (Venti mask) to the awake patient with hypoxemia (increased alveolar-arterial oxygen tension gradient). Assessment of the ability of the shock patient to protect his or her airway should be performed early; the obtunded patient or the patient in extreme respiratory distress should be intubated and mechanically ventilated.

All medications administered to the patient in cardiogenic shock must be given intravenously, due to unreliable absorption following subcutaneous or oral administration. Pain should be alleviated with the judicious administration of a reversible narcotic, such as morphine sulfate in 2- to 4-mg doses. Antiarrhythmic agents should be administered only for treatment of sustained, hemodynamically significant arrhythmias, because of the negative inotropic action of most such agents.

Documentation of adequate left ventricular preload, as assessed by pulmonary capillary wedge pressure (PCWP), must be obtained rapidly in all patients with presumed cardiogenic shock. As a guideline, volume replacement (normal saline solution or similar volume expander) should be administered to all patients if necessary to maintain PCWP $\geq$ 15 mmHg. Since cardiac preload (volume) is related to pressure by the compliance of the ventricle, frequent *in vivo* Starling curve assessments should be used to determine the optimal cardiac filling pressure (which supports adequate cardiac output, yet does not produce significant alveolar edema and impair oxygenation). Cardiac output should be determined by the thermodilution technique and indirectly verified by assessment of arterial–mixed venous oxygen content difference.

In the presence of cardiogenic shock due to inotropic failure of the ventricle without profound hypotension, stroke volume should be increased by intravenous administration of the synthetic (beta-1 and beta-2) adrenergic agonist dobutamine (2–10 µg/kg/min) to maintain cardiac index within acceptable ranges. An alternative agent would be the phosphodiesterase inhibitor amrinone, administered as a bolus of 0.75 mg/kg over 2 to 3 min followed by an infusion of 5–10 µg/kg/min. In the presence of profound hypotension and low forward output, the administration of dopamine (2–20 µg/kg/min) or norepinephrine (2–20 µg/min) may be required to support arterial blood pressure via alpha-adrenergic mechanisms in addition to beta-adrenergic–mediated increases in stroke volume.

Vasodilator therapy may be of significant benefit in the treatment of cardiogenic shock, although such agents must be employed with caution because of the potential for profound hypotension. Vasodilators are of particular benefit for the treatment of acute regurgitant lesions such as mitral insufficiency or ventricular septal rupture. Effective utilization of afterload-reducing agents requires the presence of adequate ventricular preload. Of the commercially available agents, the most appropriate vasodilator in this setting is intravenous sodium nitroprusside. This agent must be carefully titrated with respect to arterial and cardiac filling pressures and forward cardiac output. The initial starting dose for nitroprusside is 0.4 µg/kg/min; the infusion is titrated to achieve the hemodynamic goal.

*Mechanical circulatory assistance* is often required for the management of patients with cardiogenic shock. The most frequent form of this assistance is the intraaortic balloon counterpulsation pump. This technique provides for a beat-to-beat mechanical decrease in impedance to ventricular ejection with a resultant increase in forward ejection fraction, decrease in post-augmented ventricular preload, and decrease in ventricular regurgitant fraction. These effects are achieved with a concomitant increase in coronary artery peak diastolic perfusion pressure. Though often effective in initial stabilization of patients with certain forms of cardiogenic shock, the balloon pump is associated with a significant complication rate and should be used only as a temporizing measure, and only in selected patients with potentially correctable lesions. As a general guideline, the intraaortic balloon pump should be considered for early use in a patient with cardiogenic shock who fails to respond rapidly (i.e., within 4 to 6 h) to vigorous and hemodynamically-guided pharmacological therapy. Either before or soon after the patient is put on balloon support, a full diagnostic cardiac catheterization should be performed to define surgically correctable lesions. Most patients who will survive can be successfully weaned from balloon support within 4 to 5 days. Newer forms of mechanical cardiac assistance to be considered in carefully selected patients include left and right ventricular-assist devices, extracorporeal membrane oxygenators, bedside external cardiopulmonary bypass, and total mechanical heart devices.

Various acute medical and surgical interventional therapies for the treatment of patients with cardiogenic shock resulting from acute myocardial infarction (without mechanical lesions) have been described recently. These include thrombolytic therapy, coronary angioplasty, and coronary artery bypass surgery. Successful coronary reperfusion with thrombolytic therapy is associated with improved short- and long-term prognosis in patients with anterior infarction when administered in the early hours of infarction. Emergent coronary angioplasty has recently been described as effective in some patients with cardiogenic shock following infarction. The role of emergent coronary bypass surgery for evolving infarction, and especially for infarction shock, remains controversial.

In patients with cardiogenic shock due to acute infarction with a mechanical defect (e.g., papillary muscle or ventricular septal rupture), surgery can be very effective. The timing of such surgery remains controversial; recent data suggests that early intervention may be preferable. Whether such surgery should be accompanied by myocardial revascularization remains a matter of controversy.

Other forms of non-infarction cardiogenic shock that may respond well to interventional approaches include cardiac tamponade (pericardiocentesis or pericardiotomy), acute valvular insufficiency of infectious or myxomatous etiology (valve replacement), and severe valvular stenosis (valve replacement, or percutaneous valvuloplasty in selected cases). Mechanical circulatory support may be a useful temporizing adjunct in cardiogenic shock from potentially reversible causes, such as fulminant myocarditis.

## SUGGESTED READING

Barbour DJ, Roberts WC: Rupture of a left ventricular papillary muscle during acute myocardial infarction: Analysis of 22 necropsy patients. *J Am Coll Cardiol* 8:558–565, 1986.

Cummings RG, Reimer KA, Califf R, et al: Quantitative analysis of right and left ventricular infarction in the presence of postinfarction ventricular septal defect. *Circulation* 77:33–42, 1988.

Ferguson DW, Abboud FM: The recognition and management of shock, in Hurst JW et al (eds): *The Heart,* 7th ed. New York, McGraw-Hill, Chap 28, pp 442–461, 1990.

Hands ME, Lloyd BL, Robinson JS, et al: Prognostic significance of electrocardiographic site of infarction after correction for enzymatic size of infarction. *Circulation* 73:885–891, 1986.

Held AC, Cole PL, Lipton B, et al: Rupture of the interventricular septum complicating acute myocardial infarction: A multicenter analysis of clinical findings and outcome. *Am Heart J* 116:1330–1336, 1988.

Lee L, Bates ER, Pitt B, et al: Percutaneous transluminal coronary angioplasty improves survival in acute myocardial infarction complicated by cardiogenic shock. *Circulation* 78:1345–1351, 1988.

Mann JM, Roberts WC: Rupture of the left ventricular free wall during acute myocardial infarction: Analysis of 138 necropsy patients and comparison with 50 necropsy patients with acute myocardial infarction without rupture. *Am J Cardiol* 62:847–859, 1988.

Moore CA, Nygaard TW, Kaiser DL, et al: Postinfarction ventricular septal rupture: the importance of location of infarction and right ventricular function in determining survival. *Circulation* 74:45–55, 1986.

Pohjola-Sintonen S, Muller JE, Stone PH, et al: Ventricular septal and free wall rupture complicating acute myocardial infarction: Experience in the Multicenter Investigation of Limitation of Infarct Size. *Am Heart J* 117:809–818, 1989.

Reddy SG, Roberts WC: Frequency of rupture of the left ventricular free wall or ventricular septum among necropsy cases of fatal acute myocardial infarction since introduction of coronary care units. *Am J Cardiol* 63:906–911, 1989.

Schreiber TL, Miller DH, Zola B: Management of myocardial infarction shock: Current status. *Am Heart J* 117:435–443, 1989.

Stone PH, Raabe DS, Jaffe AS, et al: Prognostic significance of location and type of myocardial infarction: Independent adverse outcome associated with anterior location. *J Am Coll Cardiol* 11:453–463, 1988.

Thanavaro S, Kleiger RE, Province MA, et al: Effect of infarct location on the in-hospital prognosis of patients with first transmural myocardial infarction. *Circulation* 66:742–747, 1982.

## 3 | Clinical Assessment and Management of Arrhythmias and Conduction Disturbances

*Marilyn M. Cox, M.D.*
*Kenneth M. Kessler, M.D.*
*Robert J. Myerburg, M.D.*

Effective management of cardiac arrhythmias and conduction disturbances requires proper identification of the specific rhythm disturbances, analysis of the clinical settings in which they occur, and targeting of appropriate endpoints of therapy. Recognition and subsequent correction of any aggravating hemodynamic, electrolyte, metabolic, or respiratory abnormalities is essential to the treatment of any arrhythmia.

Arrhythmias may be primary or secondary. A *primary* arrhythmia is one occurring as a result of an electrophysiological disturbance caused by a disease process; it is independent of significant changes in hemodynamic function. In contrast, when a disease process causes a hemodynamic abnormality, which in turn initiates or contributes to an electrical disturbance, the arrhythmia is called *secondary*. Prevention or reversal of secondary arrhythmias may be accomplished through the use of hemodynamically active drugs, alone or in combination with antiarrhythmic medications.

The spectrum of arrhythmias ranges from bradyarrhythmias to tachyarrhythmias. Tachycardias may be divided into narrow—and wide—QRS complex tachycardias. Intracardiac electrograms permit identification of the site and pathway of a tachycardia, but are not usually available in an acute setting. Therefore, examination of the surface electrocardiogram (ECG), in addition to the use of physiological maneuvers, is the standard approach to the identification of arrhythmias at the bedside.

*Narrow-QRS tachycardias* are supraventricular in origin. Table 3-1 illustrates the Wellens stepwise approach to the diagnosis of a narrow-QRS tachycardia (QRS <0.12 s), which allows identification of the type of tachycardia based on atrial rate and on P wave location and configuration. *Wide-QRS tachycardias* may be ventricular or supraventricular in origin. In the presence of a left bundle branch block—like QRS configuration on surface ECG, the distinction between ventricular and supraventricular tachycardia with left bundle branch block or left bundle branch aberrancy can be especially difficult. Diagnosis of a wide—QRS complex tachy-

**17**

TABLE 3-1  Diagnosis of Narrow-QRS Tachycardia (QRS <0.12 s)

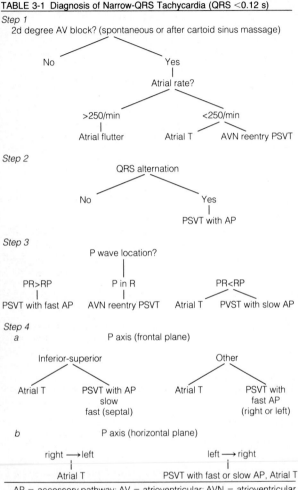

*Step 1*

2d degree AV block? (spontaneous or after cartoid sinus massage)

No — Yes

Atrial rate?

>250/min → Atrial flutter

<250/min → Atrial T — AVN reentry PSVT

*Step 2*

QRS alternation

No — Yes → PSVT with AP

*Step 3*

P wave location?

PR>RP → PSVT with fast AP

P in R → AVN reentry PSVT

PR<RP → Atrial T — PVST with slow AP

*Step 4*

*a*   P axis (frontal plane)

Inferior-superior → Atrial T — PSVT with AP slow fast (septal)

Other → Atrial T — PSVT with fast AP (right or left)

*b*   P axis (horizontal plane)

right → left : Atrial T

left → right : PSVT with fast or slow AP, Atrial T

AP = accessory pathway; AV = atrioventricular; AVN = atrioventricular nodal; PSVT = paroxysmal supraventricular tachycardia; T = tachycardia.
*Source:* Modified from Wellens HJJ: The electrocardiogram 80 years after Einthoven. *J Am Coll Cardiol* 7:484–491, 1986. Reproduced with permission from the author and the publisher.

cardia can be approached in a similar stepwise fashion (see Table 3-2).

Antiarrhythmic drugs are the mainstay of therapy for the majority of arrhythmias. Drugs may be categorized according to their electropharmacological and electrophysiological properties. The usual dosages and routes of antiarrhythmic drugs are discussed in Chap. 4. Other drugs currently under investigation for use as antiarrhythmic agents include adenosine, aprindine, bethanidine, avenzoline, ethmozin, imipramine, lorcainide, meoventine, nortriptyline, pirmenol, recainam, and sotolol.

Although the management of arrhythmias has been predominantly pharmacological, recently other forms of therapy have

TABLE 3-2 Steps in the Diagnosis of Wide-QRS Tachycardia (QRS > 0.12s)

| | |
|---|---|
| 1) AV dissociation? | Present → VT |
| 2) QRS width? | >0.14 s → VT<br>Rule out *a)* SVT with preexisting bundle branch block (BBB)<br>*b)* SVT with anterograde conduction over AP |
| 3) Left axis deviation (left of −30)? | Presence favors VT<br>Rule out *a)* SVT with preexisting BBB<br>*b)* SVT with anterograde conduction over Kent (septal or right-sided) or Mahaim bundle |
| 4) QRS configuration?<br>　　RBBB-shaped<br><br><br>　　LBBB-shaped | $V_1$: Mono- or biphasic QRS suggests VT<br>$V_6$: R/S <1 suggests VT<br>$V_1$: $R_{TACHY}<R_{SR}$ suggests SVT<br>　　$R_{TACHY}>R_{SR}$ suggests VT<br>$V_{1,2}$: $R_{TACHY}≥30$ ms suggests VT<br>$V_{1,2}$: Notching downslope S wave suggests VT<br>$V_{1,2}$: Beginning QRS to nadir S >70 ms suggests VT<br>$V_6$: qR suggests VT |

*Source:* Reproduced, with permission from the authors and the publisher, from Wellens HJJ, Brugada P: Diagnosis of ventricular tachycardia from the 12-lead electrocardiogram. *Cardiol Clin* 5:511–525, 1987.

become integral to the treatment of rhythm disturbances. These interventions include catheter ablation procedures and antiarrhythmic surgery for both supraventricular and ventricular arrhythmias, as well as implantation of electronic devices such as the automatic implantable cardioverter-defibrillator (AICD) and antitachycardia pacemakers.

## SUPRAVENTRICULAR ARRHYTHMIAS

### Premature Atrial Impulses

Atrial extrasystoles, or premature atrial contractions (PACs), are impulses that arise in an ectopic atrial focus and are premature in relation to the prevailing sinus rhythm. The significance of atrial extrasystoles depends on the clinical setting in which they occur. They may be seen in completely normal individuals; however, they may be associated with myocardial ischemia, rheumatic heart disease, myopericarditis, congestive heart failure, and a variety of systemic abnormalities including acid-base and electrolyte disturbances and pulmonary disease. Caffeine, tobacco, or alcohol use, as well as emotional stress, may initiate or exacerbate premature atrial contractions. Asymptomatic patients with no underlying heart disease require no treatment other than removal of the underlying or precipitating factors. Patients may complain of disturbing palpitations, and a low-dose beta-adrenergic blocking agent may provide relief. Both digitalis and verapamil have been tried, but their efficacy has not been proven.

Premature atrial impulses that initiate sustained arrhythmias, such as atrial fibrillation or atrial flutter, reentrant supraventricular arrhythmias, or, rarely, ventricular arrhythmias, should be treated. Conventional membrane-active antiarrhythmic agents, particularly the class IA antiarrhythmic drugs (procainamide, quinidine, or disopyramide), may be effective in suppressing the triggering PACs. The class IB and IC drugs may also be effective in selected individuals, but there are limited data on their use, and none are approved for this indication.

### Supraventricular Tachyarrhythmias

All tachyarrhythmias that originate above the bifurcation of the bundle of His or incorporate tissue proximal to it in a reentrant loop are classified as *supraventricular tachyarrhythmias*. By definition, in a supraventricular tachycardia the atrial rate must be 100 or more beats per minute. In rare instances, the atrial rate may be less than 100 beats per minute if the AV junctional rate exceeds 100 beats per minute and is accompanied by incomplete retrograde conduction. Atrial activity may be identified with the use of a long rhythm strip using multiple leads. Recording the rhythm strip at rapid paper speed (e.g., 50 mm/s) may be helpful. Other diagnostic aids include vagal manuevers to slow the ventricular response rate, or an esophageal lead to identify atrial activity. Intraatrial electrograms are occasionally required. Supraventricular tachyarrhythmias usually have narrow QRS complexes, but the presence of a wide QRS complex does not exclude supraventricular tachycardia in the presence of aberrant conduction, preexisting bundle branch block, or the Wolff-Parkinson-White syndrome (see below).

Supraventricular tachycardias (SVTs) may be classified as *paroxysmal* (lasting seconds to hours), *persistent* (lasting days to weeks), or *chronic* (lasting weeks to years). Consideration of not only the duration of the tachyarrhythmia but also its electrophysiological mechanism is essential to the appropriate management of supraventricular tachyarrhythmias.

### Sinus Tachycardia

*Sinus tachycardia* results from rapid discharge of the sinoatrial nodal pacemaker cells, and is defined as a sinus rate that exceeds 100 beats per minute. It is characterized by normal sinus P waves at a rapid rate, which usually does not exceed 130 to 140 beats per minute under resting conditions but can be as high as 180 to 200 beats per minute, particularly during exercise. Sinus tachycardia is a normal physiological response to exercise or emotional stress; persistence of this rhythm usually signals an underlying disorder (e.g., heart failure, hypovolemia, hypermetabolic states). Vagotonic manuevers, such as carotid sinus massage or Valsalva manuever, may help differentiate sinus tachycardia from other SVTs. Gradual slowing of the rapid rate, followed by gradual return to that rate, is typical for sinus tachycardia. In contrast, other SVTs may terminate abruptly with vagal manuevers. Sinus tachycardia usually requires no specific treatment; management should be directed toward the underlying disorder. When pharmacological slowing of sinus tachycardia is desired, beta-adrenergic blocking agents are often effective. However, it must be determined first that the tachycardia is not a necessary compensatory response.

### Paroxysmal Supraventricular Tachycardias

*Paroxysmal supraventricular tachycardia (PSVT)* may occur in the presence or absence of heart disease, and occurs in patients of all ages. Electrophysiologically, it is most often due to reentry, usually within the AV node or involving an accessory pathway; infrequently, sinus node reentry or intraatrial reentry is the mechanism.

**PSVT due to AV nodal reentry** *AV nodal reentry* is the most common cause of PSVT, and is characterized electrophysiologically by two functionally distinct pathways (slow and fast) within the AV node. During SVT, anterograde conduction occurs over one pathway (usually the slow pathway) and retrograde conduction over the other, resulting in almost simultaneous activation of the atria and ventricles. Electrocardiographically, retrograde P waves are buried within the QRS complex or appear immediately after it. In the unusual form, in which anterograde conduction occurs over the fast pathway, the retrograde P wave occurs well after the end of the QRS complex. In the absence of ischemia or significant valvular heart disease, PSVT due to AV nodal reentry is a benign rhythm and may be treated with rest, sedation, and vagotonic manuevers. If these physiological interventions are unsuccessful, intravenous calcium antagonists, digoxin, or beta-adrenergic blockers may be used. Verapamil, 5 mg IV, followed by one or two additional boluses 10 min apart if the initial bolus is unsuccessful, is the drug of choice; its use is contraindicated in patients with hypotension or high-grade AV block. Intravenous diltiazem has recently been shown to be effective also. Intravenous digoxin, 0.5 mg over 10 min, followed by an additional 0.25 mg every 4 h to a maximum dose of 1.5 mg in 24 h, may be used. Intravenous beta-adrenergic blockers—e.g., propranolol or esmolol—may be effective. Class IA antiarrhythmic agents may be effective occasionally if the other drugs fail. Hemodynamic instability dictates immediate cardioversion; low energy-shocks (10 to 50 W·s) are usually sufficient. Rapid atrial pacing is an alternative if other methods fail or if cardioversion should be avoided.

Although the QRS complexes are usually narrow in PSVT due to AV nodal reentry, occasionally aberrant intraventricular conduction with resultant wide QRS complexes (either right or left bundle branch block patterns) may occur. However, unless preexisting bundle branch block or aberrant conduction has *clearly* been documented, a wide–QRS complex tachycardia should be assumed to be ventricular tachycardia. The use of verapamil for the treatment of a wide-QRS tachycardia, on the *assumption* that it is a supraventricular tachycardia with aberration, may lead to severe hemodynamic compromise and even death if the arrhythmia is incorrectly diagnosed. Low-energy cardioversion or a class I antiarrhythmic agent is a logical alternative when the diagnosis of the arrhythmia is uncertain.

Decisions concerning long-term therapy for recurrent PSVT due to AV nodal reentry should be based on the frequency of episodes, the patient's symptoms, and the presence of underlying heart disease. Digoxin, beta-adrenergic blockers, or calcium antagonists may be useful. Chronic pharmacological therapy is useful in patients with frequent symptomatic or disabling episodes; otherwise, self-administered physiological manuevers or intermittent acute treatment (single oral or IV administration of an effective drug) may be preferred. Ablation of the electrical pathway, by catheter or surgery, and antitachycardia pacing devices are available alternatives to pharmacological therapy, but are currently reserved for patients in whom medical therapy is ineffective or poorly tolerated.

*PSVT due to Wolff-Parkinson-White (WPW) syndrome* This is the second most common form of reentrant SVT. When conduction during an SVT occurs anterograde through the AV node and retrograde via the accessory pathway, it is referred to as an *orthodromic* reciprocating tachycardia. This is the common form of PSVT in WPW syndrome. Vagal manuevers, verapamil, propranolol, and the class IA antiarrhythmic agents may be used to convert the arrhythmia acutely. However, digoxin is contraindicated since it may shorten the refractory period of the bypass tract and cause extremely rapid conduction across the bypass tract ($\geq 250$ beats per minute), leading to hemodynamic collapse or ventricular fibrillation. Likewise, if the patient has a history of atrial fibrillation or flutter, verapamil should be avoided as it may accelerate the ventricular rate. *Antidromic* SVT, referring to retrograde conduction through the normal pathway and anterograde conduction via the accessory pathway, is rare; its hallmark is retrograde atrial depolarization with a longer R-P interval than in orthodromic SVT. Therapy should be directed toward blocking accessory pathway conduction.

Intracardiac electrophysiological studies permit characterization of the accessory pathway and its associated tachyarrhythmias. Although electrophysiological testing may not be necessary for all patients, it is recommended for patients who have frequent or poorly tolerated tachyarrhythmias, a history of atrial fibrillation or atrial flutter (particularly with anterograde bypass tract conduction), and a family history of WPW syndrome and sudden death. Class IA antiarrhythmic agents are effective treatment, as are class IC and class III drugs. However, neither the class IC nor the class III drugs are approved for SVTs. Catheter ablation or surgical excision of the accessory pathway should be considered in any patient with a life-threatening arrhythmia who is not clearly responsive to antiarrhythmic medications.

Concealed WPW syndrome is an entity in which the accessory pathway is incapable of anterograde conduction. However, the ability to conduct retrogradely across the bypass tract permits orthodromic PSVT. There is little if any danger of atrial fibrillation degenerating to ventricular fibrillation in this case. Medical treatment is similar to that for other WPW syndrome patients, except that there is less cause for concern in the use of drugs that enhance bypass tract conduction.

*Other reentrant SVTs*  PSVT due to sinus node reentry or intraatrial reentry is distinguished electrocardiographically from PSVT due to AV node reentry of WPW syndrome by the presence of P waves preceding the QRS complexes, with normal or short PR intervals. There is no standard effective treatment for these PSVTs; membrane-active antiarrhythmic agents, beta-adrenergic blockers, and calcium antagonists have all been used. Intracardiac electrophysiological studies may be required for the optimization of therapy in some patients.

### Ectopic Atrial Tachycardias

These arrhythmias are characterized by an abnormal P-wave vector, a tendency to low P-wave amplitude, and rapid rates in the range of 160 to 240 beats per minute. When an ectopic atrial rhythm is associated with a high-grade block and a slow ventricular rate (so-called paroxysmal atrial tachycardia [PAT] with block), digitalis intoxication should be suspected.

Antiarrhythmic agents may offer effective treatment if no reversible cause can be found. Cardioversion is rarely helpful. However, since ectopic atrial tachycardias commonly have precipitating factors, removal, reversal, or control of the inciting factors (e.g., digitalis intoxication, decompensated chronic obstructive pulmonary disease, electrolyte imbalance, metabolic abnormalities, hypoxia, thyrotoxicosis) is the primary therapy.

**Multifocal atrial tachycardia**  This tachycardia is identified electrocardiographically by three or more ectopic P-wave morphologies and a chaotic, irregular rhythm. The rate is usually <150 beats per minute. When the average rate is <100 beats per minute it is not a tachycardia and is called chaotic or multifocal atrial *rhythm*, but the implications are similar. It occurs most commonly in the setting of chronic lung disease, but is also seen in patients with severe metabolic abnormalities or sepsis. Although calcium antagonists have been tried with some success, the most effective approach to therapy has been to correct the underlying hypoxia or other metabolic disturbance. There is no role for cardioversion.

### Atrial Flutter

*Atrial flutter* is characterized electrocardiographically by broad atrial deflections—"F" or flutter waves—which have a sawtooth configuration in leads II, III, and $aV_F$. The atrial rate in flutter ranges from 280 to 320 beats per minute. However, partial treatment with antiarrhythmic drugs (especially class IC drugs) may slow the flutter rate to as low as 220 beats per minute. The *paroxysmal* form of atrial flutter may occur in healthy individuals, or transiently in acute pulmonary embolism or thyrotoxicosis.

However, it is most commonly associated with some form of chronic heart disease.

Carotid sinus massage may slow the ventricular response, but tends to increase the flutter rate; occasionally it will convert the flutter to fibrillation, and very rarely to sinus rhythm. The treatment of choice in hemodynamically compromising atrial flutter is low-dose (10 to 50 W·s) electrical cardioversion. Otherwise treatment is directed first to slowing the flutter rate with either digoxin or verapamil, and then to adding a class IA antiarrhythmic agent to convert the rhythm to sinus rhythm. Class IC antiarrhythmic agents may also be effective in converting atrial flutter to sinus rhythm, but are not currently approved for this indication. If antiarrhythmic agents are unsuccessful, elective cardioversion is an alternative. A patient receiving digoxin who does not have signs of digoxin toxicity may safely undergo cardioversion if a class IA antiarrhythmic agent is given concomitantly. One recent study has shown that class I antiarrhythmic therapy for cardioversion is unnecessary in patients with digoxin levels under 1.9 ng/ml.[1]

The incidence of embolic events during paroxysmal atrial flutter or its reversion to sinus rhythm is little to none. Anticoagulation, therefore, is not necessary. If cardioversion is contraindicated, rapid atrial pacing may convert the atrial flutter to sinus rhythm or atrial fibrillation. Pacing is usually performed from the right atrium, with rapid bursts faster than the atrial flutter rate. A special pacemaker generator is required for overdrive pacing, and insertion of a right atrial catheter usually requires fluoroscopy. Alternatively, in the patient who has recently undergone open heart surgery, atrial pacing wires are usually in place and may be used. Chronic control of recurrences of paroxysmal and persistent atrial flutter includes class IA antiarrhythmics to prevent the arrhythmia, and digitalis to control the ventricular response rate during recurrences. In some centers surgical therapy is now being offered for patients with frequent symptomatic recurrences.

*Chronic atrial flutter* usually occurs in the setting of advanced heart disease, and commonly heralds atrial fibrillation. The goal of therapy for chronic atrial flutter is adequate control of the ventricular rate, rather than repeated attempts to revert the rhythm to sinus rhythm. Digoxin, beta-adrenergic blocking agents, and calcium antagonists are useful agents. In rare instances, catheter ablation or surgical sectioning of the AV node may be the only effective therapy.

### Atrial Fibrillation

*Atrial fibrillation* is characterized by disorganized atrial deflections and a variable AV conduction sequence resulting in a grossly irregular distribution of the QRS complexes.

*First episode of atrial fibrillation*   The first episode of atrial fibrillation requires a thorough clinical investigation to determine whether the arrhythmia is a primary electrical abnormality or secondary to a hemodynamic abnormality. Significant mitral or aortic valvular disease, hypertension, coronary artery disease, cardiomyopathy, atrial septal defect, and myopericarditis are all disease processes associated with the development of atrial fibrillation. Pulmonary emboli and thyrotoxicosis are well-known causes of atrial fibrillation. Coffee, tobacco or alcohol consumption, and extreme stress or fatigue also predispose to atrial fibrillation.

In the absence of organic heart disease or WPW syndrome, removal of precipitating factors and observation for recurrences is sufficient. However, in the presence of significant heart disease, therapy should be directed toward treatment of that particular cardiac abnormality; otherwise the risk of recurrence is high, even with pharmacological therapy and/or electrical cardioversion. Cardioversion is warranted for the first episode of atrial fibrillation if the patient requires the benefit obtained from the hemodynamic contribution of atrial contraction (e.g., aortic stenosis) or slowing of the ventricular rate to prolong the diastolic filling period (e.g., mitral stenosis).

*Paroxysmal atrial fibrillation*   In the absence of underlying heart disease a program of rest, sedation, and treatment with digitalis is the treatment of choice for short paroxysms. Chronic therapy is based on the need to control the ventricular rate during recurrences. This may be accomplished with digitalis, beta blockers, or calcium antagonists, as described for atrial flutter.

In the presence of heart disease, the development of hemodynamic compromise or congestive heart failure may require immediate reversion to sinus rhythm. When atrial fibrillation occurs in the presence of hemodynamically significant mitral or aortic stenosis, immediate cardioversion is mandatory to prevent or reverse the development of pulmonary edema. Direct-current countershock synchronized to the QRS complex, using energies ranging from 100 W·s for the initial shock to 200 W·s for the second and subsequent shocks, is the preferred method. If the patient is hemodynamically stable, the ventricular rate can be controlled with intravenous digoxin, beta blockers, or calcium antagonists. Currently, intravenous verapamil is preferred because of its rapid onset of action. Secondly, unlike digoxin, which loses its vagal effect as sympathetic tone predominates, verapamil maintains its depressant effect on the AV node. The class IA antiarrhythmic drugs, quinidine, procainamide, and disopyramide, are effective in chemically converting atrial fibrillation to sinus rhythm and maintaining sinus rhythm. Quinidine has been the most frequently used medication. Conventional dosing schedules

(200 to 600 mg orally every 6 to 8 h) are now used in contrast to the highly aggressive, potentially toxic quinidine protocols of the past. During attempted chemical cardioversion, careful monitoring of QT intervals for excessive prolongation (i.e., QTc 25 percent greater than QTc prior to initiation of treatment) should be performed, in addition to monitoring of serum drug levels. The class IC agents (flecainide and encainide) may convert atrial fibrillation to sinus rhythm when class IA agents have failed. They have also been useful for maintaining sinus rhythm. Currently, however, they are not approved for use in atrial fibrillation.

Amiodarone, a class III agent, is effective for preventing recurrences of atrial fibrillation. The major limitation of the use of amiodarone is its adverse side-effect profile; therefore, the threshold for its use should be high. In patients in whom atrial fibrillation is refractory to all medical therapy, both conventional and experimental, and in whom the arrhythmia is accompanied by severe disabling symptoms, catheter ablation adjacent to the His bundle to produce complete AV block is an alternative. However, because this often results in pacemaker dependency, this procedure should be used as a last resort for the control of ventricular rate during atrial fibrillation.

*Persistent atrial fibrillation* If recurrent episodes of persistent atrial fibrillation (lasting days to weeks) are well tolerated hemodynamically, most physicians avoid repeated electrical cardioversions. This pattern of atrial fibrillation eventually leads to chronic atrial fibrillation; therefore the best approach is control of ventricular rate during recurrences. Class IA antiarrhythmic agents may be used in an attempt to decrease the frequency of recurrence, but their efficacy is unpredictable. If symptoms during recurrences are disturbing enough, catheter ablation of the AV node should be considered.

*Chronic atrial fibrillation* Pharmacological or electrical cardioversion of chronic atrial fibrillation is indicated primarily if the patient will gain some hemodynamic benefit. Usually no more than one attempt at electrical cardioversion is warranted in the presence of adequate levels of a membrane-active antiarrhythmic agent, since the chance of long-term maintenance of sinus rhythm is very low if the patient reverts to chronic atrial fibrillation after cardioversion. Management of the patient is then directed to control of the ventricular response rate, as outlined above.

*Anticoagulation of patients with atrial fibrillation* The purpose of anticoagulation is to limit the morbidity and mortality from systemic and pulmonary embolization. The decision to initiate anticoagulation for atrial fibrillation depends on the relative risks of an embolic event and a major bleeding complication secondary to anticoagulant therapy. Table 3-3 lists indications and relative contraindications for anticoagulation in patients with atrial fibrillation. These same indications apply to elective cardioversion of persistent atrial fibrillation of recent onset and of chronic atrial fibrillation. Anticoagulation with warfarin is begun 2 to 3 weeks before elective cardioversion and maintained for 3 to 4 weeks after cardioversion, since there is higher risk of an embolic phenomenon in the early days after reversion to sinus rhythm. When anticoagulation is used, warfarin is given in doses sufficient to prolong the prothrombin time to 1.5 to 2.0 times control.

## AV JUNCTIONAL AND ACCELERATED VENTRICULAR RHYTHMS

*AV junctional rhythms* originate within or in the immediate vicinity of the AV node. This category includes those rhythms referred to as "AV nodal," "idiojunctional," and "idionodal." In AV junctional rhythm the impulse travels anterogradely and retrogradely

---

TABLE 3-3 Anticoagulation of Patients with Atrial Fibrillation

Indications
  Rheumatic mitral valve disease with recurrent persistent or chronic atrial fibrillation
  Dilated cardiomyopathy with recurrent persistent or chronic atrial fibrillation
  Elective cardioversion with mitral valve disease, prosthetic valves, dilated left atrium, or prior embolic events
  Coronary heart disease or hypertensive heart disease and prior embolic events related to atrial fibrillation
Controversial; limited data
  Coronary or hypertensive heart disease with normal left atrial size and no prior embolic events
  Chronic lone atrial fibrillation
  Atrial fibrillation in thyrotoxicosis (while awaiting long-term control; elective cardioversion)
Not indicated
  Paroxysmal or persistent lone atrial fibrillation
  Most clinical settings associated with short paroxysms
Relative contraindications
  Inability to control prothrombin times
  Dementia
  Malignancies
  Prior bleeding events
  Uncontrolled hypertension

*Source:* Reproduced, with permission of the authors and the publisher, from Myerburg RJ, Kessler KM: Clinical assessment and management of arrhythmias and conduction disturbances, in Hurst JW et al (eds): *The Heart,* 7th ed. New York, McGraw-Hill, Chap 32, pp 535–560, 1990.

at the same time from the AV junction, and is characterized by a normal QRS complex (unless coexistent bundle branch block or aberrancy is present) and a retrograde P wave. Depending on the site of origin and the rate of conduction in each direction, the P wave may occur shortly before the QRS complex, may follow the QRS, or may be lost within it. The rates of AV junctional escape rhythms are usually in the range of 40 to 60 beats per minute; therefore these rhythms can become manifest only when the sinus impulse fails to reach the AV node within physiological ranges of rate. These rhythms are secondary rhythms, occurring as a result of sinus depression, sinoatrial block, or AV block, and are normal physiological phenomena. Failure of these escape rhythms can result in significant bradycardia; this phenomenon is discussed under "Bradyarrhythmias," below.

The primary arrhythmias originating in the AV junction include premature junctional impulses, accelerated junctional rhythms, and AV junctional tachycardias. Various forms of reentrant tachyarrhythmias involve the AV node as part of the circuit. These have been discussed under "Paroxysmal Supraventricular Tachycardias," above.

Another type of secondary rhythm is an accelerated *ventricular* rhythm. This occurs because the sinus rate is slow enough to permit an ectopic ventricular rhythm to escape. The ectopic pacemaker is accelerated above its normal physiological rate of 20 to 40 beats per minute and overrides the sinus rate, which may be relatively depressed. The rate of an accelerated ventricular rhythm is usually between 50 and 100 beats per minute, and the QRS complexes are wide. The rhythm commonly begins with one or two fusion beats and then is regular; however, it may show progressive acceleration or deceleration until it terminates spontaneously.

## AV Junctional Premature Beats

*AV junctional premature beats,* or *AV nodal extrasystoles,* arise in an AV nodal focus and are premature in relation to the prevailing sinus rhythm. They are relatively uncommon and may be difficult to distinguish from atrial or ventricular extrasystoles. In the absence of heart disease, AV extrasystoles usually require no treatment; even in the presence of heart disease they usually require no active treatment. Correction of hemodynamic abnormalities, if any are present, may abolish the arrhythmias.

## Accelerated Junctional and Accelerated Ventricular Rhythms

If the AV junctional rate exceeds 60 beats per minute but is less than 100 beats per minute, it is called an *accelerated rhythm.*

These rhythms are seen commonly in patients with acute myocardial infarction (particularly inferior MI). They have also been associated with digitalis intoxication, electrolyte abnormalities, hypertensive heart disease, cardiomyopathy, and congenital and rheumatic heart disease. The mechanism of the accelerated AV junctional rhythm may be enhanced phase-4 depolarization in the AV junction or in the intraventricular conduction system, which accelerates the rate of the subordinate pacemakers at these sites. In ischemia, ventricular pacemaker acceleration is associated with sinus node depression. Accelerated ventricular rhythms are discussed with accelerated junctional rhythms because both phenomena are due to enhanced automaticity. However, AV junctional rhythms are supraventricular in origin, and accelerated ventricular rhythms originate in the His-Purkinje network of the ventricles. These rhythms usually require no treatment; in fact, the use of antiarrhythmic agents may suppress a subordinate pacemaker required for maintenance of an adequate heart rate. If a faster ventricular rate is required to maintain adequate hemodynamics, atropine 0.6 mg to 1.2 mg IV may be given to increase the sinus rate, or temporary pacing may be performed.

### AV Junctional Tachycardia

Occasionally, the rate of accelerated AV junctional rhythm abruptly increases to the tachycardia range (i.e., ≥100 beats per minute). This phenomenon probably represents an autonomic focus firing at the faster rate with 2:1 exit block, which abruptly changes to 1:1 conduction. Usually no treatment is needed except in the setting of ischemia, where faster heart rates are unacceptable.

Persistent AV junctional tachycardia (sometimes referred to as *nonparoxysmal* junctional tachycardia) occasionally occurs in patients with chronic heart disease. Conventional antiarrhythmic agents may be used when suppression of the arrhythmia is desired.

### VENTRICULAR ARRHYTHMIAS

The effective management of a ventricular arrhythmia depends on careful analysis of the patterns of the arrhythmia and the clinical setting in which it occurs. Electrocardiographically, ventricular arrhythmias may be analyzed quantitatively (frequency) or qualitatively (forms). To this end, we use a classification based on parallel hierarchies of frequency and forms (Table 3-4). For example, in regard to frequencies, most studies have shown that post–myocardial infarction patients with frequencies of ≥10 ectopic beats per hour (class III, or intermediate) are at increased

TABLE 3-4 Classification of Ventricular Arrhythmias

| Hierarchy of frequencies | | Hierarchy of forms | |
| --- | --- | --- | --- |
| Class 0 | Nil | Class A | Uniform morphology, unifocal |
| Class I | Rare (<1 ectopic impulse per h) | Class B | Multiform, multifocal |
| Class II | Infrequent (1–9 ectopic impulses per h) | Class C | Repetitive forms<br>Couplets<br>Salvos, repetitive responses (3–5 consecutive impulses) |
| Class III | Intermediate (10–29 ectopic impulses per h) | Class D | Nonsustained ventricular tachycardia (from 6 consecutive ectopic impulses to runs lasting up to 30 s) |
| Class IV | Frequent (≥30 ectopic impulses per h) | Class E | Sustained ventricular tachycardia (runs of ectopic activity ≥30 seconds) |

*Source:* Modified from Myerburg RJ, Kessler KM, Luceri RM, et al: Classification of ventricular arrhythmias based on parallel hierarchies of frequency and form. *Am J Cardiol* 54:1355–1358, 1984. Reproduced with permission from the authors and the publisher.

risk, although one study found that frequencies in the range of 1 to 9 impulses (class II, or infrequent) were significant.[2] Among the forms of ventricular arrhythmias, class C, or repetitive forms (couplets and salvos), indicate a higher risk than uniform and multiform premature ventricular contractions. Nonsustained ventricular tachycardia (VT) (class D) may constitute an even higher risk, but there is insufficient data to prove this. Sustained VT (≥30 s, class E) almost always indicates high risk, but there are exceptions (see below). VT has been traditionally defined as three or more consecutive ventricular impulses occurring at a rate of 120 beats per minute or greater. This definition, however, is inadequate for evaluation and treatment in the light of current knowledge.

In addition to considering the frequency and forms of ventricular arrhythmias, one must evaluate the severity of underlying structural heart disease and left ventricular ejection fraction, since these all contribute to the risk of developing potentially lethal arrhythmias. Risk increases as a function of the severity of organic heart disease and left ventricular dysfunction.

### Premature Ventricular Contractions

A ventricular extrasystole, or *premature ventricular contraction (PVC)*, is an impulse that arises in an ectopic ventricular focus and is premature in relation to the prevailing rhythm. PVCs are characterized by a tendency toward constant coupling intervals, wide QRS complexes, and secondary ST-segment and T-wave changes.

#### PVCs in the Absence of Significant Structural Heart Disease

Routine treatment of PVCs in this setting is not indicated; there is little or no increased risk of lethal arrhythmias in patients with no underlying cardiac disease. However, if a patient is bothered by symptoms of palpitations, particularly if frequent, the problem must be addressed to improve the quality of life. First, aggravating factors such as tobacco, caffeine, stress, or other stimulants should be removed. If the symptoms persist, therapy with a mild antianxiety medication or low-dose beta-adrenergic blocking agent may be helpful. Class I antiarrhythmic agents are rarely indicated, because of their potential side effects. In the absence of structural heart disease even more-advanced forms of PVCs, such as salvos, need not be treated, because there is no increased risk of sudden death.

A special subgroup of patients with mitral valve prolapse (MVP) appear to be at higher risk for serious ventricular arrhythmias. Some patients with nonspecific ST-T wave changes in leads II, III, and $aV_F$, sustained arrhythmia, and/or a redundant mitral valve by echocardiography, may require more aggressive treatment. Management of the MVP patient with sustained VT or ventricular fibrillation (VF) is similar to that carried out in other clinical settings.

#### Premature Ventricular Contractions in Acute Settings

PVCs are frequently seen in acute myocardial infarction (MI). Although the classic teaching is that PVCs are a "warning" for more severe arrhythmias and therefore require aggressive treatment, the predictive value of such warning arrhythmias is not substantiated. Clinical management of arrhythmias in acute myocardial infarction ranges from routine treatment of all patients to prevent PVCs, VT, or VF to a threshold for treatment of certain frequencies of PVCs. Intravenous lidocaine, in a 50- to 200-mg bolus followed by a continuous infusion of 2 to 4 mg/min, is the treatment of choice for PVCs associated with an acute MI. Second, intravenous procainamide, 100 mg every 5 min to a total dose of 10 to 20 mg per kg body weight, followed by a continuous infusion of 1 to 4 mg/min, may be used if lidocaine cannot be used or has been ineffective.

Other acute syndromes associated with the appearance of PVCs are those characterized by transient myocardial ischemia and coronary reperfusion, such as Prinzmetal's angina, thrombolysis in acute MI, and balloon deflation during percutaneous transluminal coronary angioplasty. Reperfusion arrhythmias are usually transient and self-limiting, but they do have the potential to progress to sustained VT or VF. Arrhythmias associated with acute ischemia may be treated initially with IV lidocaine or IV procainamide, although prevention of recurrences should include control of the ischemia. In the setting of reperfusion arrhythmias, IV lidocaine is used in the same dosages as for acute MI. Prophylactic administration may be used during thrombolysis or PTCA.

Frequent and advanced forms of PVCs are commonly seen in severe heart failure and acute pulmonary edema, as well as in acute and subacute myocarditis and myopericarditis. Antiarrhythmic therapy is given in these settings until the hemodynamic abnormality or acute disease process has resolved. In the case of myocarditis and myopericarditis, antiarrhythmic therapy should be continued for at least 2 months after resolution of clinical symptoms. At that time, the patient should be reevaluated by 24-h ECG monitoring while off all antiarrhythmic medications. If no advanced forms reappear, antiarrhythmic therapy is not restarted. If complex forms do reappear, drug therapy is reinstituted for 2 to 3 months, after which a drug-free 24-h ECG monitoring is repeated. Usually no antiarrhythmic therapy is required after 6 months.

*Premature Ventricular Contractions in Chronic Cardiac Diseases*

The presence of chronic heart disease heightens the clinical significance of PVCs. Sudden and total death rates are increased in patients having intermediate PVC frequency (class III—10 to 30 PVCs per h) or repetitive forms (class C forms) in the setting of either chronic ischemic heart disease or the cardiomyopathies. A reduced ejection fraction (<30 percent) further increases mortality risk. Conversely, patients with ejection fractions >40 percent and single PVCs have a significantly lower death rate. Although suppression of chronic PVCs in post-MI or cardiomyopathy patients is achievable, it is not known whether suppression affects sudden or total death rates.

At present, the approach to the management of frequent or advanced forms of PVCs after MI is controversial. A wide spectrum of clinical approaches exists: (1) no treatment, (2) beta blockers alone, (3) membrane-active antiarrhythmic drugs, and (4) electrophysiological testing in the subgroup with poor left ventricular function. Our approach is based on frequency and forms of ventricular arrhythmias and left ventricular ejection fraction. Patients with asymptomatic uniform or multiform single PVCs (class A or B) and an ejection fraction >40 percent after MI are treated with beta blockers if at least partial reduction or suppression of the PVCs can be achieved. Patients with salvos or nonsustained VT (class C or D forms) and ejection fractions <40 percent are treated with class I antiarrhythmics, although it is not known at this writing whether the risk of sudden death is thereby reduced.

Cardiomyopathies are the other major category of heart disease associated with PVCs. The risk of sudden cardiac death is high in both dilated and hypertrophic cardiomyopathies, and although the efficacy of antiarrhythmic medications in the suppression and prevention of ventricular arrhythmias is not certain, treatment is customary. Hospitalization of patients during initiation of therapy is recommended, because of the increased risk of proarrhythmia in patients with myopathic ventricles.

The selection of antiarrhythmic medications for suppression of chronic PVCs in high-risk patients involves several considerations: incidence of proarrhythmia, occurrence of intolerable side effects, and myocardial depression. Class IA agents all have significant risks of proarrhythmia, but the majority of these responses are not life-threatening. Among high-risk proarrhythmic effects, they may cause the polymorphic ventricular tachyarrhythmia known as *torsade de pointes,* particularly in the patient with a prolonged QT interval prior to treatment. Procainamide may be associated with a lupus-like reaction, gastrointestinal discomfort, or agranulocytosis. Quinidine most commonly causes diarrhea but is also associated with cinchonism, allergic reactions, and thrombocytopenic pupura. Disopyramide has side effects, such as urinary retention, dry mouth, and abdominal discomfort, that are attributable to its anticholinergic properties. More important, in the patient with a reduced ejection fraction disopyramide may induce congestive heart failure.

The oral class IB agents, tocainide and mexiletine, though they may be effective, have a high incidence of gastrointestinal and neurological side effects. Flecainide and encainide, class IC agents, currently are not indicated for the treatment of PVCs after MI, because of data from the CAST study.[3] The trial showed that post-MI patients with asymptomatic PVCs who were receiving active therapy with flecainide or encainide had significantly increased total mortality in comparison to patients receiving placebo. For this reason, flecainide and encainide are currently approved only for life-threatening arrhythmias.

Occasionally a combination of antiarrhythmic agents, such as a class IA and a class IB, may be effective when a single agent is not effective. Class III agents have been approved only for life-threatening arrhythmias, though amiodarone may be useful in patients with severe left ventricular dysfunction and long runs of nonsustained VT. The class II agents, beta blockers, suppress PVCs. The class IV agents, calcium antagonists, have no role in the treatment of chronic PVCs.

The appropriate endpoint of therapy for chronic PVCs appears to be suppression of advanced forms of PVCs (couplets, salvos, nonsustained VT) if these forms were present on baseline ambulatory monitoring. The goal of therapy includes suppression of 70 to 80 percent of total PVCs in a 24-h period, and complete suppression of salvos and nonsustained VT.

## Salvos and Nonsustained Ventricular Tachycardia

These classifications include salvos of 3 to 5 consecutive ventricular impulses (class C) and nonsustained VT of at least 6 consecutive impulses lasting up to a maximum of 30 s (class D). Patients with no underlying or with limited heart disease appear to be at low risk for potentially lethal arrhythmias. All other patients with these forms of ventricular arrhythmia, however, are at high risk for sustained VT or VF. Patients with cardiomyopathies or advanced coronary artery disease and low ejection fractions are among the highest-risk patients. Treatment for these patients is similar to that for those with other forms of PVC. The role of invasive electrophysiological testing in patients with nonsustained VT is controversial, and is being evaluated.

### Repetitive Monomorphic Ventricular Tachycardia

This form of VT is characterized by short paroxysms which last a few beats or a few seconds. It was first identified by Gallavardin in the early 1920s. The paroxysms may be separated by only one sinus beat, and are not aggravated by effort. Occasionally the paroxysms become continuous; then the arrhythmia becomes a sustained VT. This rhythm disturbance is more common in women, and usually is benign. Treatment usually is not needed unless there is concomitant structural heart disease.

## Sustained Ventricular Tachycardia

*Sustained VT* is defined as a rapid succession of ventricular impulses lasting more than 30 s or resulting in severe hemodynamic compromise requiring cardioversion. In the absence of hemodynamic compromise, intravenous antiarrhythmic therapy may be used. A 12-lead ECG should be recorded to characterize VT morphology, and a blood sample for measurement of plasma concentrations of known prescribed antiarrhythmic medications should be taken prior to institution of acute drug therapy. Although plasma drug levels are not usually available for initial acute management, knowledge of plasma drug concentrations may help later to determine whether the rhythm disturbance was secondary to inadequate treatment.

### Sustained Uniform-Morphology Ventricular Tachycardia

Management of this form of ventricular tachycardia depends on the clinical characteristics of the VT and the setting in which it occurs. When it appears within the first 24 h of an acute MI, aggressive treatment is mandatory because of the high risk of the VT degenerating into VF. If the patient is hemodynamically *unstable* then immediate DC cardioversion, followed by infusion of lidocaine for 24 to 48 h, is required. If the patient is hemodynamically *stable* then lidocaine, 75 to 100 mg IV, followed by a 1- to 4-mg/min infusion, is the first line of therapy. Cardioversion is necessary if the arrhythmia does not revert immediately or the patient develops hemodynamic compromise. If VT recurs despite lidocaine therapy, procainamide is the next drug of choice; 100-mg boluses of procainamide are infused at 5-min intervals to a total loading dose of 10 to 20 mg per kg body weight, followed by a constant infusion of 2 to 4 mg/min. If neither lidocaine nor procainamide is effective in suppressing the arrhythmias, bretylium tosylate, 5 mg per kg body weight, is infused over 15 min, repeated if necessary, and followed by a 0.5- to 2.0-mg/min infusion. The total dose should not exceed 25 mg/kg per 24 h. Bretylium is usually well tolerated, but it often causes an initial increased systemic arterial pressure followed by mild hypotension. Therefore, caution should be exercised when using it. Antiarrhythmic therapy may be discontinued 48 to 72 h later, since the risk of recurrence of VT is small at that point.

VT occuring during the convalescent phase of myocardial infarction, most common in patients with large anterior wall infarctions, has a far more serious long-term implication than the acute phase VT, because the mortality rate is high among these patients. They should undergo both cardiac catheterization and invasive electrophysiological studies to define the effective therapy. For both convalescent VT (up to 8 weeks after infarction) and VT appearing later (i.e., chronic phase), electrophysiological testing is used to demonstrate the characteristics of arrhythmias induced at baseline study, and to guide therapy. Left main coronary artery disease and unstable angina are relative contraindications to baseline testing. If electrophysiological testing is not available, antiarrhythmic therapy may be guided by ambulatory monitoring or exercise testing. This requires identification of intermediate (class III) to frequent (class IV) PVCs and/or complex PVCs (repetitive forms—classes C,D) at baseline monitoring, or VT induced during exercise testing. Reduction of PVC frequency by

80 percent or more, with abolition of complex forms, is an acceptable endpoint for therapy when ambulatory monitoring is used to define therapy.

Alternatives to antiarrhythmic therapy include surgery, catheter ablation, and electronic-device implantation. A patient with a discrete ventricular aneurysm and bypassable coronary artery lesion may undergo coronary bypass, aneurysmectomy, and/or surgical cryo-ablation, with prophylactic placement of AICD patches (for later use if needed) if a hemodynamically unstable VT was induced preoperatively. If the arrhythmia is still inducible after antiarrhythmic surgery, the patient may undergo repeat drug trials, since the substrate for arrhythmias may have changed. If this approach is unsuccessful, AICD implantation is indicated. AICDs are also indicated for patients who have life-threatening recurrent arrhythmias that cannot be managed surgically and are refractory to medical therapy.

Electrophysiologically guided therapy is applicable to patients with sustained VT and dilated cardiomyopathy, but mortality may not be altered by drug therapy. Patients who have had clinical VF or nonsustained VT do not appear to benefit from electrophysiological testing. AICD implantation is useful in these patients, although the degree of left ventricular dysfunction is probably more influential in determining long-term outcome.

### Less Common Causes of Sustained Ventricular Tachycardia

Sustained VT may be mediated by catecholamines or other neurophysiological influences. Beta blockers are useful for sustained VTs seen in association with high emotion and stress, as these are probably catecholamine-related.

Sustained VT or VF may be seen years after repair of complex congenital heart defects such as tetralogy of Fallot and transposition of the great vessels. Bidirectional VT is very infrequent, and usually is associated with digitalis toxicity.

### Torsade de Pointes

This polymorphic ventricular tachycardia occurs in the presence of repolarization abnormalities and a prolonged QT interval, although the same ECG patterns may occur in the presence of a normal QT interval. It occurs most commonly as a proarrhythmic response to a class IA antiarrhythmic agent, but may also be seen, infrequently, in association with class IC agents. Other causes of torsade de pointes include chronic bradycardia (complete AV block with a slow ventricular response rate), hypokalemia, chlorpromazine derivatives, and tricyclic antidepressants. This arrhythmia may also occur as part of a congenital prolonged QT syndrome, or in association with transient ischemia and reperfusion during myocardial infarction, thrombolytic therapy, or Prinzmetal's angina.

Treatment is first directed toward correction of the underlying cause or aggravating factors. Overdrive atrial or ventricular pacing is often necessary; cardioversion usually interrupts torsade de pointes only transiently. Isoproterenol effectively increases the heart rate and shortens the QT interval, but should be avoided in patients with active ischemia. Congenital QT prolongation with associated symptomatic ventricular arrhythmias may require beta-adrenergic blockade and/or partial sympathectomy.

### Ventricular Fibrillation

*Ventricular fibrillation* (VF) is a terminal rhythm and requires immediate defibrillation with 200 or more W·s. CPR should be performed until defibrillation is successful. Some antiarrhythmic drugs may increase the defibrillation threshold, and thresholds may be decreased by the use of bretylium, lidocaine, or epinephrine. Once the patient's rhythm has returned to normal, prophylactic antiarrhythmic agents (lidocaine or procainamide, or, in resistant recurrent cases, bretylium) should be administered and all metabolic and electrolyte disturbances corrected. VF occurs most commonly in acute ischemic settings.

VF is the underlying arrhythmia in the majority of patients with sudden cardiac arrest. If it is not associated with an acute MI, electrophysiological testing is warranted to guide therapy. Drug testing may be guided by ambulatory monitoring or exercise testing if electrophysiological testing is unavailable; however, this requires that the patient have high-risk forms on ambulatory monitoring or during exercise. Patients who are refractory to drug therapy and do not have cardiac disease amenable to surgery should undergo AICD implementation. Concomitant antiarrhythmic therapy may be necessary to avoid excessive shocks from the AICD due to recurrent arrhythmias.

### BRADYARRHYTHMIAS

Bradyarrhythmias may be secondary to abnormalities of cardiac impulse formation or to AV conduction abnormalities. Although they are often asymptomatic, symptoms of hypoperfusion may occur, necessitating immediate treatment. The first step in management is to increase the heart rate. Atropine sulfate, 0.5 to 1.0 mg (0.01 mg/kg) should be administered intravenously and repeated 2 to 3 times, if necessary. Sympathomimetic amines such as isoproterenol may be used, but with caution; they should be avoided in patients with ischemic symptoms. Temporary *external* pacing is a simple, noninvasive way to increase the heart rate, and in some instances has supplanted transvenous pacing. It offers a rapid alternative for patients in whom venous access is difficult or is relatively contraindicated (e.g., patients receiving thrombolytic agents). Moreover, it is ideal for patients who have transient bradycardic episodes. Its limitation is the number of patients in whom capture is inconsistent or fails. Temporary *transvenous* demand pacing provides a stable and reliable increase in ventricular rate when necessary. Dual-chamber pacing is indicated for patients who will benefit from synchronized atrial contraction (e.g., patients with inferior wall and right ventricular infarction).

In addition to increasing the heart rate, any medications known to cause bradycardia should be discontinued. Beta blockers, calcium antagonists, digitalis, clonidine, and methyldopa are common offenders; less frequently, quinidine, procainamide, and lidocaine cause bradyarrhythmias. Patients who have persistent symptomatic bradyarrhythmias with no identifiable reversible causes require permanent pacing.

## Failure of Impulse Formation

### Sinus Bradycardia

*Sinus bradycardia* is a rhythm in which each cardiac impulse arises normally from the sinoatrial node, but the rate is <60 beats per minute. The P-wave morphology is identical to that observed in normal sinus rhythm; occasionally the PR interval is prolonged. Sinus bradycardia occurs in patients with no underlying heart disease, in acute myocardial infarction, and in association with certain medications, autonomic imbalance, hypothermia, hypothyroidism, and hyperkalemia. The rhythm requires no treatment unless the patient is symptomatic. Removal of aggravating factors is the first step in therapy. If this is not successful, or if the patient requires negative chronotropic agents as part of medical management, permanent pacing may be necessary.

### Sick Sinus Syndrome

*Sick sinus syndrome* is a condition characterized by abnormal cardiac impulse formation, commonly accompanied by disordered intraatrial and AV conduction. The syndrome is associated with a wide spectrum of brady- and tachyarrhythmias. Some patients exhibit fixed or intermittent sinus bradyarrhythmias, while others have sinus bradyarrhythmias alternating with normal sinus rhythm and/or supraventricular tachyarrhythmias (the "tachy/brady syndrome"). Therapy should be reserved for patients with electrocardiographic documentation of bradyarrhythmias or tachyarrhythmias and symptoms corresponding to the periods of arrhythmias. Patients with sick sinus syndrome may be particularly susceptible to bradycardias induced by beta blockers, calcium antagonists, and antiarrhythmic drugs. Since these medications are frequently used to treat the tachyarrhythmias associated with sick sinus syndrome, concomitant permanent pacing may be required.

## AV Conduction Abnormalities

### First Degree AV Block

Isolated first degree AV block is characterized electrocardiographically by a PR interval that exceeds 200 ms. It may be seen in association with increased vagal tone, vagotonic drugs, digitalis, beta-adrenergic receptor blockade, hypokalemia, acute carditis, tricuspid stenosis, Chagas' disease, and some forms of congenital heart disease. A prolonged PR interval may occur in a normal individual, reflecting increased vagotonia. Patients with isolated first degree AV block are never symptomatic; neither temporary nor permanent pacing is indicated.

### Second Degree AV Block

Mobitz type I AV block, or the Wenckebach phenomenon, is characterized electrocardiographically by consecutively conducted impulses with PR intervals increasing progressively until an impulse is blocked and the P wave is not followed by a QRS complex. This is the most common form of second degree AV block and usually is not symptomatic. It usually does not progress to high-grade AV block; therefore, prophylactic pacing is not necessary, unless the patient is symptomatic and vagolytic therapy is ineffective. The presence of Mobitz type I AV block usually does not adversely affect a patient's prognosis.

In contrast, the less common Mobitz type II block implies more significant conduction system disease. It is characterized by consecutively conducted impulses with fixed PR intervals and a sudden blockage of impulse conduction. It is almost always associated with organic heart disease, including disease in the AV conducting system distal to the AV node, and may progress to complete AV block. For this reason permanent pacing is indicated, primarily to protect the patient from symptomatic events.

Paroxysmal AV block produces runs of consecutive atrial impulses that fail to conduct to the ventricles and may last for up to 10 to 20 s. Unless a reversible cause is clearly identified, permanent pacing is required.

### Complete AV Block

Complete heart block, or third degree AV block, is characterized by a complete interruption of conduction within the AV junctional tissues; supraventricular impulses are unable to propagate to, and activate, the ventricles. The ventricles are subsequently activated by a subsidiary idionodal or idioventricular pacemaker at a rate of 20 to 50 beats per minute. Two independent pacemakers then control the rhythm of the heart: one for the atria and one for the ventricles. The two rhythms are asynchronous, since each pacemaker discharges at its own rate.

Acute symptomatic complete heart block requires immediate treatment with either pharmacological agents (atropine or isoproterenol) or temporary external or intracardiac pacing. Isoproterenol should be avoided in the presence of ischemia. Complete heart block in the setting of an acute inferior MI is usually transient, but may take up to 2 weeks to resolve. In contrast, complete AV block in association with acute anterior wall MI may be permanent and require permanent pacing. Even if AV block in this setting is not permanent, it indicates high risk for future events, and some authors have proposed permanent pacemakers even after transient AV block in anterior infarction.

### Congenital AV Block

Complete heart block may occur as an isolated congenital anomaly. The QRS complex is usually normal or near normal, since the site of the block is almost always within the AV node or the bundle of His. The resting heart rate is usually in the range of 45 to 65 beats per minute, and patients are frequently asymptomatic; syncopal attacks are rare. Diagnostic evaluation should include exercise testing to ascertain whether the patient can mount an adequate heart rate in response to stress. If the patient is asymptomatic and heart rate increases appreciably with exercise, no further therapy may be needed. However, congenital complete AV block associated with structural congenital cardiac abnormalities implies higher risk.

### AV Dissociation

Electrocardiographically, the diagnosis of AV dissociation is made when the P waves of sinus rhythm (or other forms of atrial electrical activity) are dissociated from, and bear no fixed relation to, the QRS complexes of the ectopic idionodal or idioventricular rhythm. The presence of AV dissociation suggests an abnormality of normal intrinsic pacemaker activity. AV dissociation may occur as a result of either slowing of normal pacemaker activity or acceleration of a subordinate focus, or in the presence of complete AV block. The diagnosis of AV dissociation, however, is not synonymous with complete AV block.

If a patient with AV dissociation is symptomatic, the underlying rhythm disturbance responsible for the symptoms must be identified and treatment directed toward that rhythm disturbance. For example, a ventricular ectopic focus may become predominant during extreme sinus bradycardia. Suppression of these ventricular escape beats with antiarrhythmic therapy may worsen the underlying bradycardia and the patient's symptoms. Appropriate treatment in this instance would be directed toward the bradycardia; pacing would alleviate the bradycardia, abolish the patient's symptoms, and suppress the ventricular ectopy.

## Indications for Pacing

Cardiac pacing is indicated for the treatment of symptomatic bradyarrhythmias that are unresponsive to medical therapy. In the setting of an acute anterior wall MI, temporary pacing is indicated for AV block if it is associated with excessively slow heart rates and/or a reduction in cardiac output. The development of a new right bundle branch block, particularly in association with a left hemiblock, frequently heralds the development of complete heart block and traditionally requires prophylactic pacing. External pacing techniques, in some instances, have supplanted the need for insertion of temporary transvenous pacemakers. This is particularly applicable in the setting of acute inferior wall MI, where AV block usually is transient. New left bundle branch block, or a preexisting right or left bundle branch block, does not require pacing. Permanent pacing is often recommended for patients who have had transient complete heart block during an acute anterior wall MI, although it is unclear whether mortality is affected. Permanent pacing is rarely required after complete AV block in inferior wall infarction. In the absence of an acute or recent MI, permanent pacing is the therapy of choice for fixed or intermittent symptomatic bradyarrhythmias that have no identifiable reversible cardiac or noncardiac cause.

## REFERENCES

1. Mann DL, Maisel AS, Atwood JE, et al. Absence of cardioversion induced arrhythmias in patients with therapeutic digoxin levels. *J Am Coll Cardiol* 5:882–888, 1985.
2. Bigger JT, Fleiss JL, Kleiger R, et al: The relationship among ventricular arrhythmias, left ventricular dysfunction, and mortality in the 2 years after myocardial infarction. *Circulation* 69:250–258, 1984.
3. The Cardiac Arrhythmia Suppression Trial (CAST) Investigators: Preliminary report: effect of encainide and flecainide on mortality in a randomized trial of arrhythmia suppression after myocardial infarction. *N Engl J Med* 321:406–412, 1989.

## SUGGESTED READING

Chakko CS, Gheorghiade M: Ventricular arrhythmias in severe heart failure: Incidence, significance, and effectiveness of antiarrhythmic therapy. *Am Heart J* 109:497–504, 1985.

Cox JL: The status of surgery for cardiac arrhythmias. *Circulation* 71:413–417, 1985.

Marriott HJL, Myerburg RJ: Recognition of cardiac arrhythmias and conduction disturbances, in Hurst JW et al (eds): *The Heart*, 7th ed. New York, McGraw-Hill, Chap 31, pp 489–534, 1990.

Mirowski M, Reid PR, Winkle RA, et al: Mortality in patients with implanted automatic defibrillators. *Ann Intern Med* 98:585–588, 1983.

Myerburg RJ, Kessler KM: Clinical assessment and management of arrhythmias and conduction disturbances, in Hurst JW et al (eds): *The Heart*, 7th ed. New York, McGraw-Hill, Chap 32, pp 535–560, 1990.

Myerburg RJ, Kessler KM, Luceri RM, et al: Classification of ventricular arrhythmias based on parallel hierarchies of frequency and form. *Am J Cardiol* 54:1355–1358, 1984.

Olshansky B, Waldo AL: Atrial fibrillation: Update on mechanism, diagnosis, and management. *Mod Concepts Cardiovas Dis* 56:23–27, 1987.

Packer M: Sudden unexpected death in patients with congestive heart failure. A second frontier. *Circulation* 72:681–685, 1985.

Swerdlow CD, Winkle RA, Mason JW: Determinants of survival in patients with ventricular tachycardias. *N Engl J Med* 308:1436–1442, 1983.

Zipes DP: Cardiac electrophysiology: Promises and contributions. *J Am Coll Cardiol* 13:1329–52, 1989.

Zipes DP: Proarrhythmic events. *Am J Cardiol* 61:70A–76A, 1988.

Indications for Cardiac Pacemakers

*Harry G. Mond, M.D.*


Cardiac pacing is a rapidly advancing and ever-changing specialty. The value of pacing in the treatment of a variety of brady- and tachyarrhythmias cannot be challenged. During the early 1960s, the only indication for permanent cardiac pacing was incapacitating Stokes-Adams attacks, usually resulting from complete heart block (CHB). Recent advances in implantable pacing hardware, particularly with dual-chamber and rate-responsive pacemakers, have broadened the indications for pacing.

Today, the two major indications for permanent pacing are failure of cardiac impulse formation and failure of atrioventricular (AV) conduction. These usually result from degenerative atherosclerotic processes which damage pacemaker and conductive cells and surrounding tissues.

## DISORDERS OF THE AV NODE AND DISTAL CONDUCTING SYSTEM

A variety of ECG patterns can be described. Symptomatic patients usually have high-degree AV block.

### Complete Heart Block

Pacing is indicated irrespective of symptoms. Asymptomatic patients are rare; such patients usually attribute their "slowing down" to other age-related problems. Digitalis toxicity should be excluded. Results of pacing are impressive even in asymptomatic patients. Dual-chamber pacing (DDD) is indicated in patients with normal sinus activity. Atrial pacing as part of DDD pacing may help prevent supraventricular tachyarrhythmias. Ventricular rate-responsive pacing (VVIR) is indicated in patients with established atrial arrhythmias, such as atrial fibrillation.

### Second-Degree AV Block

Isolated Mobitz type I block (narrow QRS) is a stable arrhythmia and rarely requires permanent pacing.

Mobitz type II block (wide QRS) is unpredictable and progressive; syncope may result. The ventricular response may be very slow with a poor response to exertion. Pacing is usually indicated (DDD or VVIR).

## Bundle Branch Blocks

Bundle branch block may not be a predictor of complete heart block. Asymptomatic patients with isolated blocks, including bifascicular block, do not require permanent pacing.

Symptomatic patients (syncope) require electrophysiology (EP) studies to determine the infranodal conduction time.

Alternating right and left bundle branch blocks may require permanent pacing. The ultimate prognosis usually depends on the underlying heart disease.

## Congenital High-Degree AV Block

This condition in the young is often well tolerated, especially if the ventricular escape rhythm is satisfactory. Symptomatic patients require permanent pacing (DDD). Asymptomatic patients should have Holter monitoring, exercise testing, and EP studies. Pacing indications depend on the prognosis and on the stability of the ventricular pacemaker focus. Competing ventricular foci may lead to electrical instability and ventricular arrhythmias.

## High-Degree AV Block, Post Myocardial Infarction

*Indications for Temporary and Permanent Pacing*

- Inferior infarct—proximal block
- Temporary—for hemodynamic deterioration
- Permanent—rarely, for chronic block (usually in the elderly)

*Anterior Infarct—Distal Block with Extensive Septal Infarction*

- Temporary—for developing and progressive block
- Permanent—for persisting chronic high-degree AV block; possibly for transient blocks (controversial)

## His Bundle Ablation

Particularly for intractable supraventricular tachyarrhythmias. VVIR pacing; DDD pacing in cases of AV nodal pathways.

## DISORDERS OF IMPULSE FORMATION

The sick sinus syndrome entails episodic or persistent sinus bradycardia with periods of sinus arrest or sinoatrial block, with or without an escape AV junctional rhythm, and with varying degrees of AV block. Paroxysmal supraventricular tachyarrhythmias may also occur. The diagnosis is often made when spontaneous termination of tachyarrhythmia reveals a failure or slow recovery of sinus node function (this may cause syncope). Patients are usually elderly; pacing is indicated if patients are symptomatic. Symptoms may include syncope, tiredness, congestive cardiac failure, and angina. The ultimate prognosis often depends on the underlying cardiovascular disease.

There are three levels of severity:

- Sinus bradycardia (chronotropic incompetence)—often benign, though patients may be profoundly symptomatic. VVIR or rate responsive dual chamber pacing (DDDR) is indicated.
- Sinus arrest or sinoatrial block—patients may present with syncope. Standard ventricular inhibited (VVI) pacing is indicated if bradyarrhythmias are paroxysmal. DDDR or VVIR pacing is indicated if sinus bradycardia is present.
- Tachycardia/bradycardia syndrome—patients are usually symptomatic. DDD or DDDR pacing may prevent paroxysmal supraventricular tachyarrhythmias. Otherwise, VVI or VVIR pacing is indicated.

## OTHER SYMPTOMATIC BRADYARRHYTHMIAS

### Combined High-Degree AV Block and Sick Sinus Syndrome

This is called "pan conduction defect." The choice of pacing mode depends on the ECG. Usually, VVIR or DDDR is chosen.

### Atrial Fibrillation with Marked Pauses

VVI pacing is indicated in symptomatic patients. If this condition is associated with slow atrial fibrillation, VVIR pacing is indicated.

### Prolonged QT Interval and Torsade de Pointes

Atrial pacing (AAI) or rate responsive atrial pacing (AAIR) is indicated with beta blockade to prevent ventricular ectopic beats.

### Carotid Sinus Hypersensitivity and Vasovagal Syncope

Syncope may be life-threatening. DDD pacing is usually very successful. (VVI pacing does not help the profound vasodilatation. AAI pacing is not recommended, because of associated proximal AV block.)

### Atrial Inexcitability

In this condition there is no mechanical, electrical, or pacing activity in the atrium. VVIR pacing is indicated in symptomatic patients.

## Slow Junctional Rhythm

This is a part of the sick sinus syndrome. Symptomatic patients require VVIR or DDDR pacing.

## TACHYARRHYTHMIAS

Limited indications include relatively infrequent but severe tachycardia episodes, failure or refusal of drug therapy, and cases in which corrective heart surgery is inappropriate, has failed, or has been refused. Pacing is usually indicated for supraventricular, rarely for ventricular, tachycardia. The newer, complex, automatic systems are preferred. Patient-initiated radiofrequency devices are used rarely. For ventricular tachycardia, the automatic tachycardia-reverting system may be coupled to a cardioverter-defibrillator.

## EMPIRICAL INDICATION

On occasion a patient with intermittent life-threatening syncope thought to be cardiac in origin, but with no cause documented after extensive investigation, requires implantation of a permanent pacemaker. Retrograde conduction must be excluded before VVI pacing is considered. DDD pacing is indicated if vasovagal syncope is suspected.

## SUGGESTED READING

Hayes DL: Indications for permanent pacing, in Furman S, Hayes DL, Holmes DR (eds): *A Practice of Cardiac Pacing.* New York, Futura Publishing, p 1, 1986.

Hindman MC, Wagner GS, JoRo M, et al: The clinical significance of bundle branch block complicating acute myocardial infarction. 2 indications for temporary and permanent pacemaker insertion. *Circulation* 58:689–699, 1978.

Joint American College of Cardiology/American Heart Association Task Force on Assessment of Cardiovascular Procedures (Subcommittee on pacemaker implantation): Guidelines for permanent pacemaker implantation, May 1984. *J Am Coll Cardiol* 4:434–442, 1984.

Mond HG: *The Cardiac Pacemaker.* New York, Grune and Stratton, 1983.

Mond HG: The bradyarrhythmias: Current indications for permanent pacing (part 1). *PACE* 4:432–442, 1981.

Mond HG: The bradyarrhythmias: Current indications for permanent pacing (part 2). *PACE* 4:538–547, 1981.

Mond HG, Kertes PJ: *Rate Responsive Cardiac Pacing.* Sydney, Telectronics and Cordis Pacing Systems, 1988.

Mond HG, Sloman JG: The indications for and types of artificial cardiac pacemakers, in Hurst JW et al (eds): *The Heart,* 7th ed. New York, McGraw-Hill, Chap 33, pp 561–580, 1990.

Mond HG, Strathmore NF: The technique of using cardiac pacemakers: Implantation, testing and surveillance, in Hurst JW et al (eds): *The Heart,* 7th ed. New York, McGraw-Hill, Chap 126, pp 2100–2109, 1990.

Arnold M. Weissler, M.D.
Harisios Boudoulas, M.D.
Richard P. Lewis, M.D.
James V. Warren, M.D.

## CLASSIFICATION

Syncope can be classified into three broad categories: (1) syncope unassociated with cardiac disease (*noncardiac syncope*), (2) syncope associated with cardiac disease (*cardiac syncope*), and (3) *syncope of undetermined cause*. The frequency of syncope in each category and the estimated 1-year mortality rate, based on recent studies, is summarized in Table 5-1. Note the distinctly high mortality among patients with cardiac syncope, and the high frequency of syncope of undetermined cause.

## SYNCOPE UNASSOCIATED WITH CARDIAC DISEASE (NONCARDIAC SYNCOPE)

A subclassification of noncardiac syncope is summarized in Table 5-2. By far the most common cause is *vasodepressor syncope* (VDS), also termed *vasovagal syncope* or the *common faint*. VDS is frequent in early life. It often occurs as a response to emotional stress, real or perceived injury, sudden pain, the sight of blood, or an uncomfortable environment. Fatigue, hunger, fever, and blood loss are predisposing events. It occurs typically in the upright posture, and is preceded by pallor, perspiration, nausea, pupillary dilation, and blurred vision. Characteristic findings are systolic blood pressure below 50 mmHg and relative bradycardia. The arterial hypotension is caused by a sudden fall in arterial resistance accompanied by sympathetic nervous system withdrawal and an inadequate cardiac-output response. When VDS occurs in patients with heart disease it may carry an ominous prognosis—e.g., aortic stenosis or pulmonary hypertension.

*Orthostatic hypotension* is a syndrome characterized by a fall in arterial pressure and inadequate cerebral perfusion upon assumption of the upright posture. It may occur on the basis of (1) venous pooling and/or blood volume depletion, (2) pharmacologically induced vasodilation, or (3) a primary or secondary disorder of the autonomic nervous system. Often multiple inciting factors coexist. Uniquely prone to postural hypotension are the elderly

TABLE 5-1 Syncope: Frequency and Mortality Percentages by Category

|  | Frequency | 1-year mortality |
|---|---|---|
| Noncardiac | 45 | 0–12 |
| Cardiac | 19 | 19–30 |
| Undetermined | 36 | 6 |

*Source:* Adapted from Weissler AM, Boudoulas H, Lewis RP, et al: Syncope: pathophysiology, recognition, and treatment, in Hurst JW et al (eds): *The Heart,* 7th ed, New York, McGraw-Hill, Chap 34, 1990, with permission of the authors and publisher.

and patients with mitral valve prolapse, severe hypertension, and/ or prolonged bedrest. *Idiopathic orthostatic hypotension* and the *Shy-Drager syndrome* (multiple system atrophy) are causes of postural hypotension of unknown etiology.

Syncope in *cerebrovascular disease* is most commonly a complication of severe occlusive atherosclerosis of the major cerebral arteries wherein transient hypotension induces cerebral ischemia. Rarely syncope is a presenting symptom in patients with transient ischemic attacks (TIAs). Cerebral embolism, which is usually manifest by focal neurological findings, may cause syncope. Non-atherosclerotic occlusive disease (Takayasu's arteritis) and mechanical obstruction from skeletal deformities may cause cerebrovascular syncope. In the *subclavian steal syndrome,* caused by occlusive disease of the subclavian artery proximal to the vertebral artery, syncope occurs during upper-extremity exercise. Associated findings are diminished brachial arterial pulse and a supraclavicular bruit on the affected side.

TABLE 5-2 Syncope Unassociated with Cardiac Disease (Noncardiac Syncope)

Vasodepressor syncope (VDS)
Orthostatic syncope
Syncope in cerebrovascular disease
Carotid sinus syncope (CSS)
Reflex syncope
Situational syncope
   Cough syncope
   Valsalva syncope
   Micturition syncope
   Defecation syncope
   Diver's syncope
Neuropsychiatric and metabolic syncope

*Source:* Reprinted from Weissler AM, Boudoulas H, Lewis RP, et al: Syncope: pathophysiology, recognition, and treatment, in Hurst JW et al (eds): *The Heart,* 7th ed, New York, McGraw-Hill, Chap 34, 1990, with permission of the authors and publisher.

*Carotid sinus syncope* (CSS) is associated with a hypersensitive carotid sinus reflex and occurs in three forms: (1) cardioinhibitory with profound bradycardia, (2) vasodepressor with fall in arterial pressure, and (3) mixed type. A hyperactive carotid sinus in the absence of syncope is common in the elderly. The presence of a direct association between carotid sinus stimulation and syncope must be demonstrated to confirm the CSS diagnosis. CSS may be observed with neoplasms (e.g., carotid body tumor) and masses in the carotid sinus area. Impaired consciousness in CSS may be initiated by minor stimulation of the carotid sinus—e.g., turning the head, shaving, wearing a tight collar. Diagnostic testing for carotid sinus hypersensitivity should be performed with the patient supine and with brief (2 to 4s) massage on the first attempt. Digitalis, beta-blocking agents, and alphamethyldopa sensitize the response.

*Reflex syncope* results from vagal inhibition of the sinus pacemaker or AV node. It is often caused by painful stimulation of the pharyngeal, laryngeal, bronchial, esophageal, or visceral mucosa, or of the pleura or peritoneum. *Syncope in glossopharyngeal neuralgia* and *swallow syncope* have similar reflex mechanisms. The term *vagovagal syncope* is applied to this group.

*Situational syncopal disorders* are classified according to their precipitating events. Combined mechanical, reflex vagal, and vasodepressor responses are causative. Neuropsychiatric and metabolic causes of noncardiac syncope include *disorders of cerebral function* (convulsive disorders, syncopal migraine) and *generalized metabolic disturbances* (hypoxia, hypocapnia, hypoglycemia). *Hysteria* and *vertigo,* rarely associated with loss or impairment of consciousness, must be differentiated from other forms of syncope.

## SYNCOPE ASSOCIATED WITH CARDIAC DISEASE (CARDIAC SYNCOPE)

Cardiac syncope occurs when obstruction to cardiac output or disturbance in cardiac rhythm, or both, produce a marked diminution in cerebral perfusion. A differential diagnosis of disorders associated with cardiac syncope is summarized in Table 5-3.

### Syncope Related to Obstruction to Cardiac Output

Obstruction to cardiac output sufficient to cause syncope is classified, according to the predominant site of the hemodynamic impediment, as left- or right-sided. A vasodepressor response or transient arrhythmias may be accentuating mechanisms. Commonly, obstructive syncope is precipitated by exercise (*effort syncope*).

TABLE 5-3 Syncope Associated with Cardiac Disease (Cardiac Syncope)

Obstruction to cardiac output
   Predominant left-sided
      Aortic stenosis
      Hypertrophic cardiomyopathy
      Prosthetic valve malfunction
      Mitral stenosis
      Left atrial myxoma
   Predominant right-sided
      Eisenmenger syndrome
      Tetralogy of Fallot
      Pulmonary embolism
      Pulmonary valve stenosis
      Primary pulmonary hypertension
      Cardiac tamponade
Cardiac arrhythmia
   Conduction system disease (primary or secondary)
      Sick sinus syndrome
      AV block (Adams-Stokes syndrome)
         AV node disease
         His-Purkinje system disease
   Paroxysmal supraventricular tachycardias
      Wolff-Parkinson-White syndrome
   Paroxysmal ventricular tachycardia/fibrillation
   Long-QT syndromes
      Congenital
      Acquired
   Pharmacological and metabolic disorders
Pacemaker-induced syncope
   Malfunction
   Pacemaker-induced arrhythmias
   Pacemaker syndrome

*Source:* Reprinted from Weissler AM, Boudoulas H, Lewis RP, et al: Syncope: pathophysiology, recognition, and treatment, in Hurst JW et al (eds): *The Heart,* 7th ed, New York, McGraw-Hill, Chap 34, 1990, with permission of the authors and publisher.

## Syncope Related to Cardiac Arrhythmia

Syncope due to cardiac arrhythmia may complicate all forms of heart disease. Either extreme of heart rate can induce syncope. While arrhythmias can occur in isolation, they are frequently secondary to established heart disease. Arrhythmic syncope should be suspected when there is sudden onset, lack of relationship to posture, association with cardiac disease, and occurrence of immediately-preceding palpitations. The electrophysiological mechanisms causing arrhythmic syncope are summarized in Table 5-3.

Syncope in the *sick sinus syndrome* may be associated with episodes of either extreme bradycardia or supraventricular tachycardia. The association of bifascicular block and long PR interval with recurrent syncope suggests *Adams-Stokes syndrome*. *Supraventricular tachycardias,* including those associated with Wolff-Parkinson-White (WPW) syndrome, induce syncope on the basis of excessive heart rate or through a secondary hemodynamic effect in the cardiac patient. *Ventricular tachycardia,* probably the most common cause of arrhythmic syncope, occurs with all types of cardiac disease. Syncope in the *long-QT syndrome* is almost always due to ventricular arrhythmia, usually *torsade de pointes* tachycardia. Congenital long-QT syndromes include the autosomal recessive (*Jervell and Lange-Nielsen syndrome*), with deafness, and the autosomal dominant (*Romano-Ward syndrome*), without deafness. The *acquired long-QT syndrome* is caused by antiarrhythmic drugs, electrolyte disorders (hypokalemia, hypocalcemia, hypomagnesemia), antidepressants, phenothiazines, and liquid-protein diet. Drugs commonly implicated in arrhythmic syncope are antiarrhythmics, digitalis, beta-blocking agents, calcium channel blockers, theophylline, beta-agonist derivatives, caffeine, and alcohol. Pacemaker-induced syncope should be considered in all patients with syncope who have had cardiac pacemakers inserted.

## SYNCOPE OF UNDETERMINED CAUSE

This is a compromise diagnosis made only when thorough evaluation has failed to yield a specific etiologic definition. In most such cases the syncope is benign and nonrecurring. Nevertheless, the annual mortality among patients with this diagnosis exceeds that for a comparable normal population, suggesting undetected cardiac syncope in some of the patients. Before this diagnosis is made, the physician must perform an assiduous evaluation for subtle and less frequent forms of noncardiac and cardiac syncope.

## DIAGNOSTIC EVALUATION

The basic clinical and laboratory examination, along with the electrocardiogram and the chest x-ray, permit correct diagnosis in most patients and provide a firm differential diagnosis in the rest (see Fig. 5-1). The extent of evaluation for patients in whom no diagnosis is evident should be based on the perceived risk. A distinctly higher mortality and a uniquely greater risk for sudden death occur among elderly patients. Doppler echocardiographic studies provide invaluable noninvasive evaluation, particularly in the confirmation of the presence and extent of cardiac disease. While the initial diagnostic workup often establishes the diagnosis of obstructive cardiac syncope, additional invasive laboratory

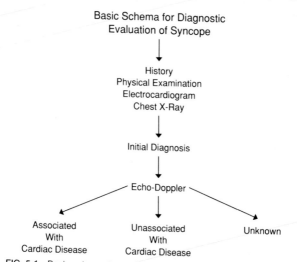

Basic Schema for Diagnostic
Evaluation of Syncope

↓

History
Physical Examination
Electrocardiogram
Chest X-Ray

↓

Initial Diagnosis

↓

Echo-Doppler

Associated
With
Cardiac Disease

Unassociated
With
Cardiac Disease

Unknown

FIG. 5-1  Basic schema for diagnostic evaluation of syncope. (Adapted from Weissler AM, Boudoulas H, Lewis RP, et al, with permission.

studies may be necessary to assess its severity, particularly when corrective cardiac surgery is contemplated. Table 5-4 summarizes various clinical tests for use in patients with suspected arrhythmic syncope. When no arrhythmia can be documented noninvasively and cardiac disease is present, invasive electrophysiological studies are usually indicated. These combined studies establish an arrhythmic cause in most patients.

## TREATMENT OF NONCARDIAC SYNCOPE

In *VDS* the patient must be placed recumbent until he or she has completely recovered; occasionally intravenous atropine or vasopressors are required. In *orthostatic hypotension,* primary emphasis must be placed on treatment of reversible causes, such as replenishment of blood volume, prevention of venous pooling, deletion of hypotensive drugs, and use of vasoconstrictors. Syncope in *cerebrovascular disease* demands treatment of the primary vascular disorder, including platelet antiaggregants (aspirin) for TIAs. The effectiveness of surgical endarterectomy remains controversial. CSS therapy includes anticholinergics, sympathomimetics, and avoidance of carotid sinus compression. Intractable CSS has been treated by surgical de-enervation and radiotherapy of the carotid sinus,

TABLE 5-4 Diagnostic Tests for Evaluation of Arrhythmic Syncope

| Test | Use |
|---|---|
| Electrocardiogram | Conduction disease, WPW syndrome, ischemic heart disease, ventricular hypertrophy, atrial and ventricular ectopy; occasionally defines arrhythmia |
| Signal-averaged electrocardiogram | Screen for ventricular tachycardia |
| Exercise testing | May document exertional arrhythmias |
| Ambulatory monitoring | Records rhythm disturbances during one or more 24-h cycles; relates arrhythmia to symptoms; aids in defining response to therapy |
| Transtelephonic | May document paroxysmal arrhythmias in low-risk subsets |
| Invasive electrophysiological study | Defines conduction system disease when noninvasive studies are inconclusive in high-risk patients. Elicits supraventricular and ventricular tachycardias, measures hemodynamic effects of arrhythmias and responses to pharmacological and pacing interventions |

*Source:* Reprinted from Weissler AM, Boudoulas H, Lewis RP, et al: Syncope: pathophysiology, recognition, and treatment, in Hurst JW et al (eds): *The Heart,* 7th ed, New York, McGraw-Hill, Chap 34, 1990, with permission of the authors and publisher.

intracranial section of the glossopharyngeal nerve, and permanent transvenous pacing. Ventricular pacing may accentuate hypotension; AV sequential pacing is preferred. *Reflex syncope* and *situational syncope* necessitate interventions directed at the initiating mechanisms. In *glossopharyngeal neuralgia syncope* anticonvulsants may be effective; intractable forms may require neurosurgical or pacemaker therapy. *Neuropsychiatric and metabolic syncope* demand specific attention to the primary cause.

## TREATMENT OF CARDIAC SYNCOPE

In syncope due to *obstructive heart disease,* surgical amelioration of the hemodynamic obstruction is often the treatment of choice. Syncope in hypertrophic cardiomyopathy may respond to pharmacotherapy; surgical management must be considered for intractable syncope. For severe pulmonary hypertension there are few effective therapeutic options; heart and lung transplantation has been attempted. Treatment of *arrhythmic syncope* should be directed at the underlying cardiovascular disease and mitigation of precipitating events. Use of arrhythmia-inciting agents (e.g., caffeine, alcohol) should be forbidden. The therapeutic effectiveness of antiarrhythmic agents needs documentation by ambulatory monitoring and, when applicable, exercise testing and electrophysiological studies. Combined use of pacemaker and antiarrhythmic therapy may be required when the latter induces severe bradycardia. The multicausal nature of syncope demands careful evaluation before the institution of permanent pacemaker therapy. In the *congenital long-QT syndrome,* beta-blocking drugs often control recurrent syncope; left sympathetic stellectomy may be attempted for intractable syncope. In *acquired long-QT syndromes,* discontinuation of offending drugs and restoration of metabolic balance usually prevents recurrence. A proarrhythmic cause must be considered when syncope occurs after antiarrhythmic therapy has begun. In *refractory tachycardias,* pacemaker therapy may prove useful in terminating and preventing episodes. Surgical section of bypass tracts in WPW syndrome with life-threatening supraventricular tachycardia, usually atrial fibrillation, has been uniquely effective. Intracardiac catheter ablation of bypass tracts in WPW is a new interventional approach. In selected patients with intractable ventricular arrhythmias, surgical procedures (aneurysmectomy, encircling ventriculotomy, and myocardial resection) have been effective. Coronary bypass may reduce ventricular arrhythmias in advanced coronary disease. The automatic implantable defibrillator is a promising new modality for syncope caused by malignant ventricular arrhythmias.

## SUGGESTED READING

Ben-Chetrit E, Flugelman M, Eliakim M: Syncope: A retrospective study of 101 hospitalized patients. *Isr J Med Sci* 21:950–953, 1985.

Day SC, Cook EF, Funkenstein H, et al: Evaluation and outcome of emergency room patients with transient loss of consciousness. *Am J Med* 73:15–23, 1982.

Eagle KA, Black HR, Cook EF, et al: Evaluation of prognostic classifications for patients with syncope. *Am J Med* 79:455–460, 1985.

Kapoor WN, Karpf M, Wieland S, et al: A prospective evaluation and follow-up of patients with syncope. *N Engl J Med* 309(4):197–204, 1983.

Kapoor W, Snustad D, Peterson J, et al: Syncope in the elderly. *Am J Med* 80:419–428, 1986.

Martin GJ, Adams SL, Martin HG, et al: Prospective evaluation of syncope. *Ann Emerg Med* 13(7):499–504, 1984.

Silverstein MD, Singer DE, Mulley AG, et al: Patients with syncope admitted to medical intensive care units. *JAMA* 248:1185–1189, 1982.

Weissler AM, Boudoulas H, Lewis RP, et al: Syncope: pathophysiology, recognition, and treatment, in Hurst JW et al (eds): *The Heart,* 7th ed. New York, McGraw-Hill, Chap 34, pp 581–603, 1990.

*Samuel J. DeMaio, M.D.*

## DEFINITION

Most authorities define sudden cardiac death as unexpected cardiac death preceded by no apparent symptoms or by symptoms less than 1 h in duration. Most cases are thought to result from cardiac arrhythmias. The incidence of sudden cardiac death in the United States approximates 400,000 cases annually, of which 80 percent are due to coronary atherosclerotic heart disease.

## ETIOLOGY

Most sudden cardiac deaths are thought to be precipitated by ventricular fibrillation (VF). However, electrocardiograms (ECGs) recorded at the onset of cardiac arrest often demonstrate that VF was preceded by a few beats of ventricular tachycardia (VT). In the ambulatory population, the distribution of Holter-recorded causes of sudden death has shown that 62 percent of cases were preceded by VT, 8 percent by primary VF, 16 percent by bradyarrhythmias, and 12 percent by torsade de pointes.

A relation between VF and acute myocardial ischemia has been shown in animal experiments in which a major coronary artery is acutely occluded. It has been suggested, in cases of patients' surviving sudden death without anatomic or electrophysiological substrate for reentrant ventricular arrhythmias, that plaque rupture, platelet aggregation, release of vasoactive substances, and thrombus fragmentation may lead to coronary microembolism and transient ischemia. However, from a clinical point of view, the importance of transient myocardial ischemia precipitating cardiac arrest is unclear.

## RECOGNITION OF HIGH-RISK PATIENTS

More than three-quarters of sudden deaths are due to coronary atherosclerotic heart disease, usually with obstruction of two or three coronary arteries. However, many other cardiac lesions may lead to unexpected cardiac death (see Table 6-1). In the absence of structural heart disease or evident conduction abnormalities, sudden death is unusual.

Three major risk factors have been associated with increased risk of sudden death in patients with coronary disease: (1)

TABLE 6-1 Noncoronary Causes of Sudden Death
_____

Cardiomyopathy
  Hypertrophic
  Dilated
  Restrictive
Valvular lesions
  Aortic stenosis
  Mitral valve prolapse (MVP) (uncommon)
Primary electrical disturbances
  Atrial ventricular block
  Ventricular preexcitation
  Prolonged QT syndromes
Congenital heart disease
  Drugs
  CNS injury
_____

ventricular electrical instability, (2) abnormal left ventricular function, and (3) repolarization abnormalities as determined by signal-averaged ECG.

Frequent ventricular premature depolarizations are predictors of sudden cardiac death in patients with known coronary atherosclerotic heart disease. However, in patients without demonstrable heart disease, ventricular ectopy has no proven prognostic significance.

There has long been recognized an association between left ventricular wall motion abnormalities, ventricular arrhythmias, and survival of sudden death—though it is debatable whether complex forms of ventricular ectopy are independent predictors of sudden death or reflect some predisposing, vulnerable myocardial substrate. Recently it has been shown that ventricular arrhythmias and left ventricular function are independent predictors of recurrent sudden cardiac death, and that left ventricular function is a significantly stronger predictor.

The ultimate factors that result in malignant ventricular arrhythmia and sudden cardiac death are not completely understood. The presence of an "electrophysiologic milieu," characterized by inhomogeneous propagation of conduction as identified by the signal-averaged ECG, has been shown recently to be at least as important as left ventricular function in the prediction of an arrhythmic event after myocardial infarction (MI).

## LESSONS LEARNED FROM SURVIVORS OF THE SUDDEN CARDIAC DEATH SYNDROME

A substantial number of patients with VF, when treated with early initiation of cardiopulmonary resuscitation (CPR) and prompt defibrillation, can be resuscitated and, ultimately, discharged after hospitalization.

It has been shown in the Seattle experience that the survival from out-of-hospital VF approaches 30 percent. Unfortunately, the outcome is dismal for patients whose first recorded rhythm is asystole or electromechanical dissociation. With the involvement of the general public in the initiation of CPR, the survival of patients has more than doubled (from 21 to 47 percent) when CPR was initiated prior to the arrival of emergency medical services (EMS) personnel.

## ACUTE MYOCARDIAL INFARCTION (MI) VERSUS SUDDEN CARDIAC DEATH

Although coronary atherosclerotic heart disease is responsible for most episodes of out-of-hospital ventricular fibrillation, only a minority of resuscitated patients appear to have developed ventricular fibrillation as a *consequence* of acute MI. New Q-wave MIs developed in approximately 20 percent of patients.

## RECURRENCE OF THE SUDDEN CARDIAC DEATH SYNDROME

During the first year following resuscitation, there has been a 20- to 30-percent mortality rate. The majority of deaths are due to recurrent cardiac arrest, usually with VF as the first recorded rhythm. The 1-year recurrence rate in patients with sudden cardiac death syndrome associated with Q-wave MI is 2 percent. In patients who did not develop Q-wave MIs, the 1-year recurrence rate is at least 10 times as high.

## PREDICTORS OF RECURRENT CARDIAC ARREST

Using data on survivors of out-of-hospital cardiac death syndrome, risk profiles have been developed and validated. Factors associated with increased risk of recurrent sudden death include: (1) remote MI, (2) congestive heart failure, (3) abnormal left ventricular function, (4) extensive coronary artery disease, (5) complex ventricular ectopy, (6) abnormal signal-averaged ECG, and (7) no associated Q-wave MI with the episode of VF.

## DIAGNOSTIC EVALUATION OF THE CARDIAC ARREST SURVIVOR

A patient whose cardiac arrest is the result of an acute Q-wave MI requires evaluation and therapy no different from that given to other patients with acute MI. Cardiac catheterization is recommended for most survivors of VF to determine the coronary anatomy, left ventricular function, and need for revascularization. It is important to identify any precipitating causes, such as drug toxicity and electrolyte imbalance.

Intracardiac electrophysiological study is useful in most patients surviving cardiac arrest. This is particularly true in those whose events are not associated with MI.

## THERAPY

Antiarrhythmic drug therapy, coronary artery bypass grafting, the automatic implantable cardioverter-defibrillator (AICD), aneurysmectomy, and endocardial resection, alone or in combination, are required by the vast majority of patients surviving sudden cardiac death syndrome.

### Antiarrhythmic Drug Therapy

Unlike patients with asymptomatic premature ventricular contractions (PVCs), patients with symptomatic sustained ventricular arrhythmias should be treated. Two methods of drug selection may be used: the noninvasive approach, using ECG monitoring and exercise tolerance testing, or the invasive approach, using program electrical stimulation. It has been shown that therapy based on the invasive approach prevents recurrence of ventricular tachycardia better than the noninvasive approach. Although the mechanism remains unknown, prophylactic beta-blocker therapy has been shown to reduce the risk of sudden cardiac death after a Q-wave MI.

### Automatic Implantable Cardioverter-Defibrillator (AICD)

The AICD is effective in preventing sudden cardiac death in patients whose ventricular arrhythmias cannot be controlled with medical therapy and who are not suitable candidates for surgical therapy. The AICD has reduced the incidence of sudden death to 2 to 3 percent per year. The device can continuously monitor both the rate and the morphology of the ventricular dysrhythmia. The device usually delivers shocks of 25 to 30 J until the tachyrhythmia is terminated, or until five shocks (per episode of ventricular dysrhythmia) have been delivered.

### Surgical Therapy

Multiple approaches to the treatment of ventricular arrhythmias have been proposed. They may be divided into the indirect and the direct (see Table 6-2). The indirect methods have been disappointing in their inability to control ventricular arrhythmias. The best results have been obtained with map-guided subendo-

TABLE 6-2 Surgery for Ventricular Tachycardia

| |
| --- |
| Indirect |
|    Sympathectomy–long QT |
|    Mitral valve replacement—MVP |
|    Coronary revascularization |
| Direct |
|    Map-guided subendocardial resection |
|    Non-map-guided surgery |
|       Left ventricular aneurysmectomy |
|       Encircling endocardial ventriculotomy |
|       Extended endocardial resection |

cardial resection, with or without cryoabulation. A candidate for map-guided subendocardial resection should be resistant to medical therapy. He or she should have concomitant ischemic or valvular heart disease requiring surgery, and a single ventricular tachycardia morphology that is well tolerated, allowing preoperative catheter and intraoperative mapping. The operative mortality remains high, at approximately 12 percent. Control of the arrhythmia with surgical therapy alone occurs in 40 to 50 percent of cases; with the addition of drug therapy, success of the operation is raised to 70 to 80 percent.

## SUGGESTED READING

Cobb LA: The mechanisms, predictors, and prevention of sudden death, in Hurst JW et al (eds): *The Heart,* 7th ed. New York, McGraw-Hill, Chap 35, pp 604–614, 1990.

Kelley PA, Cannon DS, Garan H, et al: The automatic implantable cardioverter-defibrillator: Efficacy, complications and survival in patients with malignant ventricular arrhythmia. *J Am Coll Cardiol* 11:1278–1286, 1988.

Kennedy HZ, Whitlock HA, Sprague MK, et al: Long term follow-up of asymptomatic healthy subjects with frequent and complex ventricular ectopy. *N Engl J Med* 312:193–197, 1985.

Mitchell LB, Duff JH, Manyari DE, et al: A randomized clinical trial of the noninvasive and invasive approaches to drug therapy of ventricular tachycardia. *N Engl J Med* 317:1681–1687, 1987.

| Congenital Heart Disease

*Elizabeth W. Nugent, M.D.*

## ATRIAL SEPTAL DEFECT

### Definition

An *atrial septal defect* is an opening in the interatrial septum due to a deficiency of septal tissue. This excludes a patent foramen ovale.

### Pathology

Most atrial septal defects are large enough to allow free communication between the atria. They are classified by anatomic location, as:

- *Ostium secundum defect,* the most common type, in the area of the fossa ovalis. Mitral valve prolapse may be associated.
- *Ostium primum defect,* a part of the complex known as *common atrioventricular canal defect,* in the area inferior to the fossa ovalis and frequently involving the atrioventricular valves and interventricular septum. (See also "Ventricular Septal Defect," below.)
- *Sinus venosus defect,* in the septum superior to the fossa ovalis near the orifice of the superior vena cava and frequently associated with partial anomalous pulmonary venous return.

All types of atrial septal defect have dilated right heart chambers and pulmonary arteries. Pulmonary hypertension may develop, but usually not before the patient's third decade. Pulmonary vascular disease can follow. (See "Eisenmenger's Syndrome," below.)

### Pathophysiology

There is no resistance to blood flow across the defect with a left-to-right shunt, due to lower resistance in the right heart and lungs than in the systemic circulation. Development of pulmonary hypertension and pulmonary vascular disease will lead to shunt reversal and cyanosis. Mitral regurgitation is common with ostium primum defects.

## Clinical Manifestations

### History

Most children are asymptomatic, except with primum defects complicated by mitral regurgitation. Mild fatigue and dyspnea may be noted in late adolescence. Most adults are symptomatic. Congestive heart failure and arrhythmias are common from the fourth decade. Atrial septal defects occur more commonly in females than in males.

### Physical Examination

Many patients are slender. There is a right ventricular lift along the lower left sternal border. The $S_1$ may be accentuated. The two components of the $S_2$ are widely split and do not vary (fixed splitting) with the respiratory cycle. There is a midsystolic crescendo-decrescendo murmur at the left upper sternal border due to increased right ventricular stroke volume. There is a diastolic flow rumble over the left lower sternal border denoting increased flow across the tricuspid valve during rapid ventricular filling. The holosystolic murmur of mitral regurgitation is common in patients with primum defects. With pulmonary hypertension and pulmonary vascular disease, the flow murmurs disappear, the pulmonary closure sound becomes accentuated, and cyanosis develops. Tricuspid and pulmonary regurgitation may result. (See "Eisenmenger's Syndrome," below.)

## Usual Diagnostic Tests

### Chest X-Ray

Mild to moderate cardiac enlargement and increased pulmonary arterial flow are characteristic. Absence of left atrial enlargement helps distinguish uncomplicated atrial septal defects from other left-to-right shunts. Left atrial and left ventricular enlargement occur in primum defects with significant mitral regurgitation. With pulmonary vascular disease, the pulmonary flow pattern appears diminished but the central pulmonary arteries remain enlarged.

### Electrocardiogram

An rsR' pattern in the anterior precordial leads is characteristic and indicates mild right ventricular conduction delay or hypertrophy. Most patients with secundum defects have a right, inferior QRS vector in the frontal plane. Most of those with primum defects have a superior QRS vector in the frontal plane. They may also have left atrial and left ventricular hypertrophy. Atrial fibrillation and flutter are the most common arrhythmias; they occur mainly in adults.

### Echocardiography

Echocardiography will demonstrate the chamber enlargement and flat or paradoxical septal motion. Most secundum and primum defects in children are visualized, whereas a smaller percentage of sinus venosus defects can be seen. Associated defects, such as mitral abnormalities in the primum defects, are visualized. Doppler flow study demonstrates the left-to-right shunt across the defect.

### Cardiac Catheterization

In young patients with the typical clinical findings (including the echocardiogram) of an uncomplicated secundum atrial septal defect, cardiac catheterization usually is not necessary. It is indicated in those with other types of defects, especially the primum defect, or with evidence of pulmonary hypertension.

There is a significant step-up in saturation at the right atrial level. The left atrium is usually easy to enter from the femoral approach. Similar pressures will be recorded in both atria, with a mean gradient between them of less than 3 mmHg. The degree of right ventricular and pulmonary arterial hypertension should be assessed, especially in older patients. Pulmonary vascular resistance should also be calculated. A systolic pressure gradient of up to 20 mmHg across the right ventricular outflow tract is due, if present, to increased flow, and does not represent true pulmonary stenosis. The site of pulmonary venous connections and the presence of associated defects can be demonstrated by selective biplane cineangiography.

## Natural History and Prognosis

Most children and adolescents are asymptomatic. In some cases, because of lack of symptoms and unimpressive findings, diagnosis is delayed for many years. Symptoms and complications occur with progressively increasing frequency and severity throughout the adult years. The most important problems are pulmonary hypertension and pulmonary vascular disease, atrial arrhythmias, and congestive heart failure. Pulmonary vascular disease may progress rapidly during pregnancy and with the use of contraceptive drugs. These complications lead to high morbidity and mortality with, and following, surgical correction. Congestive heart failure, pulmonary embolism, paradoxical emboli, brain abscess, and infection are causes of death in those who do not have surgical correction. Those with primum defects are subject to infective endocarditis.

**Treatment**

Surgery is recommended just prior to school age for those with typical findings and a significant shunt. If a catheterization is done, surgery is recommended if the pulmonary/systemic blood flow ratio is 1.5:1 or greater, provided there is no serious malfunction of the left side of the heart causing this. If pulmonary hypertension is present, surgery is also recommended for those with a flow ratio of 1.5:1 or greater if the systemic arterial saturation is at least 92 percent and the total pulmonary resistance is less than 15 units/m². With more severe pulmonary vascular disease, there is no benefit achieved by surgery.

Surgical closure is accomplished by direct suture repair or the use of a pericardial or Dacron patch. This choice is determined by the location, size, and shape of the atrial defect. Pulmonary venous connections should be inspected so that any anomalous veins may be redirected to the left atrium. In patients with primum defects, valvuloplasty of the mitral valve may also be necessary. The risk of surgery in childhood is quite low. Postoperative follow-up is necessary to determine adequacy of repair, document reversal or disappearance of previous abnormalities, and manage any associated arrhythmias.

## VENTRICULAR SEPTAL DEFECT

### Definition

A *ventricular septal defect* is an opening in the interventricular septum that permits communication between the two ventricles.

### Pathology

The size of ventricular septal defects varies greatly. They are classified by their anatomic location, as:

- Paramembranous defects, the most common type, in the superior septum immediately below the crista supraventricularis of the right ventricle.
- Conal or supracristal defects, in the right ventricular outflow tract and adjacent to the aortic valve, which tends to prolapse into these defects.
- Inlet or atrioventricular canal defects, in the posterior septum beneath the septal leaflet of the tricuspid valve.
- Muscular defects, commonly with multiple openings, in the trabecular and apical portions of the septum.

Cardiac chamber enlargement and hypertrophy depend on shunt volume and the degree of pulmonary hypertension.

**Pathophysiology**

Functional alterations depend on the defect's size and the status of the pulmonary vascular bed. A small defect (less than 0.5 cm²/m²) offers a large resistance to flow. The left-to-right shunt is small and there is no pulmonary hypertension. There is little additional work for the heart. A defect of moderate size (0.5 to 1.0 cm²/m²) still permits a gradient between left and right ventricular systolic pressures. Pulmonary pressure is generally less than 80 percent of the systemic systolic pressure. A large left-to-right shunt is present which imposes a significant volume overload on the left side of the heart. Pulmonary vascular disease can result, but is uncommon. (See "Eisenmenger's Syndrome," below.)

If the defect is large, approximately equal to or greater than the aortic valve orifice (at least 1.0 cm²/m²), it offers no resistance to blood flow. The systolic pressures in both ventricles and great arteries are the same. The relative proportion of flow to each circulation is governed by the relative resistances in the pulmonary and systemic vascular beds. These patients are at high risk for the development of pulmonary vascular disease.

At birth, the pulmonary vascular resistance is high and there is little left-to-right shunting across a ventricular septal defect. The resistance decreases over the first few days and weeks of life, and as it does so the magnitude of shunting increases. Congestive heart failure may then occur with the larger defects.

**Clinical Manifestations**

*History*

Infants with larger defects develop heart failure, usually by 3 months of age. Parents may note tachypnea, fatigue with feedings, poor weight gain, and excessive sweating. Infants and children with small ventricular defects are asymptomatic; their defects are ordinarily detected early by routine examination because of the loudness of the murmur. ·

*Physical Examination*

The diagnosis is supported by the typical loud, harsh holosystolic murmur at the lower left sternal border that is frequently accompanied by palpable thrill. In patients with significant left-to-right shunts (pulmonary/systemic flow ratio ≥ 2:1) there is a middiastolic rumble at the apex caused by excessive flow across the mitral valve. The right and left ventricular impulses are prominent. There also may be signs of congestive heart failure in these patients. Pulmonary rales and peripheral edema are signs of severe and long-standing heart failure in infants. The pulmonary component of the second heart sound $(P_2)$ is increased with pulmonary hypertension.

With advanced pulmonary vascular disease, these findings regress. The second sound is loud and single. Murmurs of pulmonary and tricuspid regurgitation may become audible. Cyanosis appears and gradually worsens. (See "Eisenmenger's Syndrome," below.)

Signs of a decreasing left-to-right shunt may also be obvious if the defect becomes smaller, as is common, or if infundibular pulmonary stenosis develops. The $S_2$ is helpful. Aortic regurgitation may also develop, especially when the defect is in the supracristal area.

## Usual Diagnostic Tests

### Chest X-Ray

Heart size—especially the size of the left atrium and left ventricle—and pulmonary vascularity reflect the magnitude of left-to-right shunting. Small defects cause no radiographic abnormalities. Larger defects cause cardiomegaly and pulmonary plethora.

### Electrocardiogram

With a small defect, the electrocardiogram may be normal or demonstrate slightly augmented left ventricular voltage. With larger defects, biventricular and left atrial hypertrophy are usual. Right atrial and right ventricular hypertrophy are seen with severe pulmonary vascular disease and when pulmonary stenosis develops.

### Echocardiography

Two-dimensional echocardiographic imaging permits visualization of most defects of significant size. A defect's position and diameter, as well as chamber sizes and ventricular function, can be determined. Doppler evaluation can estimate the gradient across the defect itself, or predict the right ventricular systolic pressure if tricuspid regurgitation is present. With the addition of color flow mapping, even tiny, muscular, or multiple defects can be identified.

### Cardiac Catheterization

There is a step-up in oxygen saturation at the right ventricular level. The degree of pulmonary hypertension can be measured, and pulmonary vascular resistance should be calculated. Selective biplane cineangiography in the left ventricle will outline the defect.

## Natural History and Prognosis

Fortunately, most ventricular septal defects are small and impose only the risk of infective endocarditis. Many become smaller or close spontaneously during childhood. Among patients with large defects, congestive heart failure is likely in infancy and causes death unless managed appropriately. Some such patients develop infundibular pulmonary stenosis that protects them from heart failure, but with time it will lead to a clinical picture indistinguishable from tetralogy of Fallot. (See below.) Those with larger defects who have significant pulmonary hypertension are at risk for developing progressive pulmonary vascular disease. Once there are irreversible vascular changes, the outlook is bleak. A few patients develop progressive aortic regurgitation, particularly if the defect is in the supracristal area of the septum.

### Treatment

It is important to identify those with moderate or large defects as early as possible, since they are at risk for developing congestive heart failure and pulmonary vascular disease. Congestive heart failure is treated with digoxin and diuretics as required. Cardiac catheterization is recommended for all infants with heart failure or evidence of important pulmonary hypertension.

Surgery is recommended in infancy if heart failure is difficult to manage medically or if the pulmonary arterial systolic pressure is greater than one-half the systemic level. Surgery is also recommended if there is any degree of pulmonary hypertension by age 2 years. In the remainder of cases it is advisable to correct the defect before the child enters school if there is still a large shunt (pulmonary/systemic flow ratio greater than 1.8:1) or if cardiac enlargement persists with a smaller shunt. If pulmonary vascular disease is already present at the time the diagnosis is made, surgery is still recommended if the pulmonary vascular resistance is less than 11 units/m$^2$ or if the pulmonary/systemic vascular resistance ratio is less than 0.7:1, provided the flow ratio is at least 1.5:1. Beyond this level the risk of surgery more than offsets any possible benefit.

Primary patch closure of the defect is the procedure of choice even in young infants. Paramembranous and inlet defects should be repaired through the right atrium and tricuspid valve. Supracristal defects usually require right ventriculotomy, whereas multiple apical defects may be best approached via apical or posterior left ventriculotomy. Avoidance of injury to the AV conduction tissue requires careful attention when repairing the paramembranous or inlet types.

## PATENT DUCTUS ARTERIOSUS

### Definition

*Patent ductus arteriosus* is patency of the fetal vessel that connects the aorta and pulmonary artery.

## Pathology

The ductus arteriosus connects the origin of the left pulmonary artery to the aortic arch just beyond the left subclavian artery. Normally it closes, and becomes a ligament, in the first few weeks of life.

## Pathophysiology

The diameter and length of the ductus determine the severity of the attendant hemodynamic abnormalities, which are similar to those described above for ventricular septal defects of varying sizes. The flow, however, occurs in diastole as well as in systole. The left-to-right shunt and the pulmonary arterial pressure increase with the magnitude of the communication.

## Clinical Manifestations

### History

Patent ductus arteriosus is more common in premature infants and those exposed to rubella during the first trimester of pregnancy with a nonimmune mother. It also is more common in situations associated with hypoxia. Symptoms are related to significant left-to-right shunting with poor growth or overt heart failure.

### Physical Examination

Peripheral pulses are bounding, especially with the larger shunts. Right and left ventricular impulses may be increased. The typical finding is a continuous or machinery murmur best heard at the left upper sternal border and below the left clavicle. This murmur peaks near the $S_2$. The length of the diastolic portion of the murmur may be abbreviated in newborns and in older patients with pulmonary hypertension. A middiastolic rumble at the apex is present with larger shunts. The pulmonary closure sound is increased when pulmonary hypertension is present. Findings of pulmonary vascular disease may predominate. In this case, the cyanosis usually involves only the left arm and hand and the lower segment of the body.

## Usual Diagnostic Tests

### Chest X-Ray

Findings are similar to those described for ventricular septal defects, except that the aorta may also be enlarged.

### Electrocardiogram

As for ventricular septal defect.

*Echocardiography*

Larger defects can frequently be imaged. Doppler echocardiography with color flow mapping is very valuable for delineating the shunt.

*Cardiac Catheterization*

Catheterization is not necessary in patients with a typical picture of uncomplicated patent ductus arteriosus and no pulmonary hypertension. At catheterization, there is a step-up in oxygen saturation at the pulmonary arterial level; the catheter usually crosses the ductus easily to enter the descending thoracic aorta from the pulmonary artery. Pulmonary arterial pressure and resistance should be ascertained. Aortography will outline the ductus. In specialized laboratories, the ductus may be closed by catheter introduction of an experimental occluding device.

## Natural History and Prognosis

Infective endarteritis can occur regardless of the size of the ductus. The risk increases with length of survival. Heart failure, pulmonary hypertension, and pulmonary vascular disease can occur in those with significant shunts. Infants with heart failure may die suddenly. Irreversible pulmonary vascular disease rarely is seen in the first year or two of life. Calcification of the ductal wall is common in adults.

## Treatment

Prophylaxis against infective endocarditis is appropriate in all cases. Indomethacin is often successful in causing closure of the ductus in premature infants. Diuretics and volume control are helpful in the treatment of heart failure. Patients unresponsive to medical treatment should have the ductus closed surgically. Surgery is recommended for all with continued patency beyond the first 6 months of life. This is usually done electively at 1 to 2 years of age. Severe pulmonary vascular disease is a contraindication to surgery.

The ductus is surgically obliterated by division or ligation, depending on the width, length, and wall thickness of the vessel. In adults with calcification, placement of a Dacron patch over the aortic orifice of the ductus may be advisable. Care is necessary to avoid injury to the adjacent left recurrent laryngeal nerve.

## COARCTATION OF THE AORTA

### Definition

*Coarctation of the aorta* is a discrete narrowing of the aortic arch (sometimes extending beyond the arch) due to a medial deformity in the wall.

**Pathology**

The deformity is usually in the distal segment of the aortic arch, either opposite the ductus or just proximal to it. There is an infolding of the wall in its anterior, superior, and posterior aspects that creates a narrowed and eccentric lumen. The principle cardiac abnormality is left ventricular hypertrophy. Prominent collateral vessels form in the older child and adult to carry blood to the distal aortic segment. A bicuspid aortic valve is present in approximately one-half of patients with coarctation.

**Pathophysiology**

Arterial pressures above the coarctation are elevated. There is a significant systolic and mean pressure gradient between the upper and lower extremities.

**Clinical Manifestations**

*History*

In infants, the symptoms are those of heart failure. There is often difficulty with feeding and poor weight gain. Older children usually are asymptomatic, but they may have mild fatigue or claudication in their legs when running.

*Physical Examination*

Signs of heart failure are common in infants. If a murmur is present, it is usually midsystolic and nondescript, unless best heard over the interscapular region. Prominent upper segment pulses and a left ventricular lift are present. Pulses in the lower extremities are much weaker (or absent) and delayed in timing. Blood pressure measurements in both arms and a leg will confirm the diagnosis. The frequency and degree of hypertension in the upper segment increase with age beyond infancy. An early systolic click at the apex suggests an associated bicuspid aortic valve.

**Usual Diagnostic Tests**

*Chest X-Ray*

Cardiomegaly and pulmonary venous congestion are common in infants. Left atrial and left ventricular enlargement are common in adults. Many children have a normal heart size. A figure-three configuration of the left aortic margin at the coarctation may be seen in overpenetrated films; and an "E" sign or reverse "3" is seen with a barium swallow. Rib notching due to the presence of collateral vessels is evident in older children and adults.

*Electrocardiogram*

Infants have right- or biventricular hypertrophy. Children may have a normal electrocardiogram, but left ventricular hypertrophy develops progressively with age.

*Echocardiography*

Often the coarctation can be imaged from the suprasternal approach. Left ventricular function should be assessed. Doppler flow pattern and gradient estimates offer diagnostic confirmation.

*Cardiac Catheterization*

Cardiac catheterization demonstrates left atrial and left ventricular hypertension and a significant systolic pressure difference across the coarctation. Associated defects are common in symptomatic infants. Aortography or magnetic resonance imaging will demonstrate the site and length of the coarctation.

## Natural History and Prognosis

Congestive heart failure is the most common problem associated with coarctation of the aorta in infancy. Persistent hypertension leads to complications in patients with uncorrected coarctation in the second and third decades. Premature death, in the form of dissecting aortic aneurysm, cerebral arterial rupture, heart failure, or myocardial infarction, is most common in those who are not operated on or whose surgery is delayed into the third decade. There is a significant risk of endocarditis or endarteritis.

Re-coarctation is common in patients who have undergone surgery in infancy. Residual or recurrent hypertension without re-coarctation is most common in those who are operated on after 6 years of age.

## Treatment

Vigorous treatment of heart failure is indicated. This includes temporary palliation with prostaglandin $E_1$ in the newborn, to maintain ductal patency. Surgery is recommended in all infants with significant complicating defects and in those who do not respond dramatically to decongestive measures. Elective surgery by 4 to 6 years of age is indicated in the remainder. Even older symptomatic patients, including adults, usually benefit from repair as soon as the diagnosis is recognized.

Repair by subclavian flap angioplasty is generally recommended in infancy. In older patients resection and direct end-to-end anastomosis is most commonly employed. Occasionally in children and commonly in adults, bypass of the coarctation using a tubular vascular prosthesis may be required because of the length of the obstruction or changes in the arterial wall.

Balloon angioplasty is an alternative to surgery and has been demonstrated to be particularly beneficial in patients with recurrent coarctation.

## VALVAR AORTIC STENOSIS (INCLUDING BICUSPID AORTIC VALVE)

### Definition

In *valvar aortic stenosis* there is subtotal obstruction to left ventricular outflow due to a congenital aortic valvar deformity.

### Pathology

Most commonly, the aortic valve is bicuspid. The degree of commissural fusion varies from case to case. Occasionally the valve is unicuspid and severely obstructive. Uncommonly the valve is tricuspid, again with variable commissural fusion. The valve leaflets are thickened and may be severely dysplastic. Calcification occurs in older adults. Left ventricular hypertrophy is present in patients with significant obstruction.

### Pathophysiology

The hemodynamics of congenital valvar aortic stenosis are similar to those of the acquired form. (See Chap. 8, "Aortic Valve Disease.") A bicuspid aortic valve may be unobstructive during the early years, but tends to become thickened and calcified in middle-to-late adult years.

### Clinical Manifestations

#### History

Most infants and children are asymptomatic. Symptoms of heart failure can occur in infants with critical aortic stenosis, and in older adults. Syncope, angina, and sudden death can also occur with severe disease, at any age. The remainder of patients come to medical attention because of the murmur.

#### Physical Examination

Most patients have a systolic thrill at the right upper sternal border and over the carotid arteries. Pulse amplitude may be diminished in severe disease. Paradoxical splitting of the $S_2$ is rare in children. A systolic click at the apex is characteristic and differentiates valvar stenosis from other forms of left ventricular outflow tract obstruction. A fourth heart sound in older children and adults signifies severe obstruction. There is a harsh crescendo-descrescendo murmur, which is loudest at the right upper sternal border. Louder and longer systolic murmurs generally indicate more important obstruction, except in the presence of heart failure, which may markedly diminish the murmur. Some children and adults also develop the murmur of aortic regurgitation.

## Usual Diagnostic Tests

### Chest X-Ray

Significant cardiac enlargement with or without pulmonary edema indicates severe disease. Poststenotic dilatation of the ascending aorta is characteristic. Calcification of the valve may be seen in adults.

### Electrocardiogram

Left ventricular hypertrophy seldom helps in judging severity. Diminished anterior forces, a deep $SV_1$ ($\geq 30$ mm), or absence of the Q wave in lead $V_6$ suggest severe stenosis. A normal T wave in lead $V_6$ is present in all patients with mild disease. The appearance of ST-segment depression in the left precordial leads with exercise testing is a reliable method for identifying those with at least a moderate gradient.

### Echocardiography

Echocardiographic imaging permits recognition of abnormal aortic valve motion and identification of the number of cusps, as well as differentiation from other types of aortic stenosis. Left ventricular function can be assessed. Doppler interrogation can accurately predict the systolic gradient as well.

### Cardiac Catheterization

Symptomatic patients and those with echocardiographic and Doppler evidence of severe obstruction do not require catheterization. Those with clinical evidence of only moderate obstruction should have this confirmed by cardiac catheterization to determine the proper method of management. In the absence of congestive heart failure (i.e., in the presence of a normal cardiac index) the peak left ventricular-aortic systolic pressure gradient or calculated valve area is used to assess severity. Moderate obstruction is commonly defined as a gradient between 50 and 75 mmHg or a valve area between 0.5 and 0.8 cm$^2$/m$^2$.

**Natural History and Prognosis**

Infants with severe obstruction develop heart failure early and require emergency surgical intervention. Mortality is significant with or without surgery and is often related to endocardial fibroelastosis, papillary muscle necrosis, or a small left ventricle.

In about one-third of patients with milder aortic stenosis, a gradual progression in severity is expected over the course of years during childhood. This is further complicated by calcification and associated atherosclerosis in older adults. Progression also occurs after successful surgical palliation. Sudden death can occur in those with at least a moderate gradient. Infective endocarditis poses a serious threat due to systemic embolization and serious aortic regurgitation.

**Treatment**

Medical treatment of the symptomatic infant should be instituted, but surgery should also be performed without delay. Careful evaluation and follow-up of all patients with aortic stenosis is mandatory. Surgery is recommended for any patient with a gradient of 75 mmHg or more or a valve area of less than 0.5 cm²/m². Surgery is also recommended for those with symptoms or ischemic electrocardiographic findings, but with a lower gradient of 40 to 75 mmHg. Balloon valvuloplasty is an alternative to surgery, but is still considered experimental by some.

Exercise restrictions are usually recommended for all patients except those with mild disease.

Surgical relief of valvar aortic stenosis is accomplished by a carefully placed incision in the middle of each fused, but well-supported, true commissure. A conservative approach is essential to prevent an intolerable degree of aortic regurgitation. Calcification and restenosis eventually force aortic valve replacement in most patients who have undergone valvotomy in infancy or early childhood.

# VALVAR PULMONARY STENOSIS

**Definition**

In *valvar pulmonary stenosis* there is subtotal obstruction of right ventricular outflow due to a congenital deformity of the pulmonary valve.

**Pathology**

The most common type is dome-shaped stenosis, with the valvar tissue appearing as a cone- or dome-shaped structure perforated at its distal end. There may be findings similar to those described above for the bicuspid aortic valve. Less commonly there is severe dysplasia of the valvar leaflets. There is poststenotic dilatation of the pulmonary trunk, and the ventricular septum is intact. The degree of right ventricular hypertrophy is a function of the severity of the obstruction. Muscular infundibular stenosis may occur secondarily.

## Pathophysiology

There is a systolic pressure gradient of varying severity between the right ventricle and the pulmonary artery. If there is right ventricular failure, the gradient is low because of the low flow. In infants, severe obstruction often causes the foramen ovale to remain patent; cyanosis results.

## Clinical Manifestations

### History

Most infants and children are asymptomatic, though mild fatigue may bother some. Only infants and adults with severe pulmonary stenosis tend to develop right ventricular failure.

### Physical Examination

A systolic thrill at the left upper sternal border and in the suprasternal notch is characteristic. The right ventricular impulse becomes increasingly forceful with more severe obstruction. An early systolic ejection click accentuated with expiration is audible at the left upper sternal border. As severity increases, the $P_2$ becomes progressively softer and more delayed until it finally becomes inaudible. There is a harsh systolic crescendo-decrescendo murmur best heard at the left upper sternal border. With mild or moderate stenosis, the murmur peaks in midsystole and ends at, or before, the aortic component of the $S_2$. In severe stenosis, the murmur peaks late in systole and extends beyond the aortic closure sound. Right-sided heart failure with tachypnea, hepatomegaly, and tricuspid regurgitation occurs in infants with very critical obstruction and in adults with long-standing severe stenosis. Cyanosis may be present if there is an atrial communication.

## Usual Diagnostic Tests

### Chest X-Ray

The only common abnormality is poststenotic dilatation of the main and proximal left pulmonary arteries. Significant cardiac enlargement signals critical disease; pulmonary flow may be diminished in a patient with a right-to-left shunt at atrial level.

*Electrocardiogram*

Right ventricular forces in the anterior precordial leads correlate reasonably well with the severity of stenosis. Right axis deviation and right atrial hypertrophy occur with significant obstruction.

*Echocardiography*

Abnormal pulmonary valve motion and thickness may be seen. Doppler evaluation can accurately predict the systolic gradient.

*Cardiac Catheterization*

There is elevated right ventricular systolic pressure with a distinct systolic pressure difference across the valve. If right ventricular output is normal, the gradient defines the severity. An atrial shunt can be detected. Right ventricular biplane cineangiography demonstrates the valvar anatomy as well as any associated infundibular hypertrophy.

**Natural History and Prognosis**

In most patients with mild to moderate pulmonary stenosis the clinical course is favorable, with no significant tendency for the gradient to increase with time. Some patients do have significant increases in infancy or early childhood. Growth of the young child or development of infundibular stenosis is usually thought to be the cause. The prognosis for those with critical obstruction in infancy, or severe obstruction of many years' duration, is poor. Right ventricular dysfunction ensues. Heart failure and arrhythmias lead to premature death in adults. Infective endocarditis is a risk.

**Treatment**

In the infant with critical stenosis, measures to treat heart failure should be instituted. This should be followed promptly by surgical intervention. Cyanosis, or a right ventricular pressure at or above systemic levels, is also an indication for prompt surgery. In asymptomatic older infants or beyond, elective surgery is usually recommended when the right ventricular systolic pressure is near 70 mmHg or the gradient is near 50 mmHg. Balloon valvuloplasty is often done as an alternative to surgery; in skilled hands it is quite successful, except in patients with a dysplastic valve or severe infundibular stenosis. Prophylaxis against infective endocarditis is recommended regardless of whether surgery is performed.

Surgical technique is tailored to fit the anatomy. Fused commissures are excised, very dysplastic leaflets are removed, subvalvar muscle bundles are excised, and patch augmentation of a small annulus can be done. Since pulmonary regurgitation is well tolerated, all obstructing tissue should be removed.

## TETRALOGY OF FALLOT

### Definition

*Tetralogy of Fallot* is characterized by a large ventricular septal defect, overriding aorta, right ventricular hypertrophy, and pulmonary stenosis.

### Pathology

The aorta is enlarged, straddles the ventricular septal defect, and arises to a varying degree from both ventricles. Fibrous continuity of the aortic and mitral valves is maintained. The crista supraventricularis is displaced, and there is significant narrowing. This is the dominant site of obstruction to pulmonary flow characteristic of tetralogy. The pulmonary valve is often malformed and the pulmonary arteries are often small. A right aortic arch is common.

### Pathophysiology

Because the ventricular septal defect is large, the systolic pressure is equal in both ventricles and the aorta. The degree of right ventricular obstruction determines the direction and volume of shunting. In most cases this is severe enough to overcome systemic resistance, causing a right-to-left shunt and cyanosis.

### Clinical Manifestations

#### History

The majority of cases are recognized in the first few months of life because of cyanosis. In some patients, the pulmonary stenosis slowly becomes more severe and may not cause cyanosis until later childhood or, rarely, even in adulthood. Dyspnea with exertion is common. Attacks of suddenly increasing cyanosis and hyperpnea, called *hypoxic spells,* occur in infants and young children.

#### Physical Examination

The degree of cyanosis varies. Clubbing is seen in those with cyanosis of more than 3 months' duration. Signs of congestive heart failure do not occur during childhood unless there is severe superimposed illness. A right ventricular lift is present. A crescendo-decrescendo murmur is audible at the left midsternal border. It is usually harsh, but may be quite soft, or become inaudible, with very severe stenosis or hypoxic spells. The $S_2$ is single.

### Usual Diagnostic Tests

#### Chest X-Ray

Right ventricular enlargement, a concave pulmonary segment, and diminished pulmonary flow are characteristic. The coeur en sabot (boot-shaped contour of the heart) is classic during childhood. A right aortic arch may be seen.

### Electrocardiogram

The mean QRS vector in the frontal plane is right and inferior. There is right ventricular hypertrophy.

### Echocardiography

All of the structural components of tetralogy of Fallot can be demonstrated, including the level(s) of right ventricular outflow tract obstruction. Color flow Doppler will confirm the direction of shunting across the ventricular septal defect.

### Other Laboratory Studies

The *hemoglobin* and *hematocrit* should be frequently evaluated so that the development of severe polycythemia or relative anemia may be avoided. Because bleeding may be associated with poly-cythemia, *platelet and coagulation studies* may be advisable if surgery is planned. Elevated uric acid levels and gout can occur if the cyanosis is severe and long-standing.

### Cardiac Catheterization

The diagnosis is confirmed by establishment of the presence of a nonrestrictive ventricular septal defect with right-to-left shunting and by delineation of the severity and location of the right ventricular outflow tract obstruction. Coronary artery anomalies that might influence surgical approach should be excluded.

## Natural History and Prognosis

The severity of right ventricular outflow obstruction is progressive. Prognosis is poor because of complications of the cyanosis and polycythemia, such as stroke and brain abscess. Sudden death can occur; survival beyond age 30 years is unusual. Infective endocar-ditis is common.

## Treatment

Hypoxic spells are treated with the knee-chest position, oxygen, and morphine. If the spells are severe, sodium bicarbonate and a beta-adrenergic blocking drug may be required. In newborns, administration of prostaglandin $E_1$ improves cyanosis temporarily by opening the ductus.

Complications such as endocarditis, dehydration, and anemia should be prevented or appropriately treated.

Prompt surgical intervention is indicated at any age for patients with progressive symptoms, or with polycythemia with the he-matocrit approaching 65 percent. For the remainder of patients, elective surgical corrections should not be delayed beyond early childhood.

Infants may be palliated with chronic administration of beta blockers or systemic-to-pulmonary arterial shunt procedures. The latter are preferable, especially when the pulmonary arteries are very small or there are other anatomic abnormalities, such as a major coronary artery across the right ventricular outflow tract. Early correction is preferable in most other infants, since it can now be done with an acceptable low mortality if the anatomy is favorable.

Surgical correction requires patch closure of the ventricular septal defect and resection of obstructive infundibular muscle. Pulmonary valvotomy and patch augmentation of the infundibulum, valvar annulus, and central pulmonary arteries are also frequently needed.

## EBSTEIN'S ANOMALY OF THE TRICUSPID VALVE

### Definition and Pathology

In *Ebstein's anomaly,* varying portions of the posterior and septal leaflets of the tricuspid valve are displaced downward and attached to the ventricular wall below the annulus. The proximal part of the right ventricle is thin-walled and continuous with the right atrium. The papillary muscles and chordae are usually malformed, with multiple direct attachments of valvar tissue to the mural endocardium. An interatrial communication—a stretched patent foramen ovale—is present in most cases.

### Pathophysiology

There is obstruction to right ventricular filling because of the decrease in the size of the functional right ventricle. Tricuspid regurgitation is also usual. A right-to-left shunt occurs through the stretched patent foramen ovale.

### Clinical Manifestations

#### History

Approximately one-half of reported cases present with cyanosis and right-sided heart failure in infancy. The remainder present at all ages, with symptoms of dyspnea on exertion and palpitations most common.

#### Physical Examination

The newborn may have severe cyanosis initially, due to high pulmonary vascular resistance. Cyanosis and clubbing in older patients tend to be mild. Only the rare patient with an intact atrial septum is not cyanotic. The liver is enlarged and the jugular venous pulse is elevated. The precordium is quiet even in the presence of striking cardiomegaly. The holosystolic murmur of tricuspid regurgitation is commonly heard, and may be accompanied by a "scratchy" diastolic murmur of tricuspid stenosis. The $S_1$ is split and loud. The $S_2$ is widely and persistently split. $S_3$ and $S_4$ sounds are audible in older patients.

## Usual Diagnostic Tests

### Chest X-Ray

Heart size varies; ordinarily it is very large due to a very dilated right atrium. Pulmonary blood flow is diminished in proportion to the degree of cyanosis.

### Electrocardiogram

Severe right atrial hypertrophy, a prolonged PR interval, and right ventricular conduction delay or right bundle branch block are common. In approximately 10 percent of cases the pattern of preexcitation, or Wolff-Parkinson-White syndrome, is present.

### Echocardiography

Delayed tricuspid closure is seen. The exact anatomy of the valve and its attachments, as well as associated defects, are clearly demonstrable.

### Cardiac Catheterization

Caution should be exercised, since the risk of rhythm disturbances is greater than usual. Right atrial pressure is elevated. The characteristic right ventricular pressure recording is not obtained until the catheter reaches the apex or outflow tract. An electrode catheter can demonstrate the area of atrial pressure with a ventricular electrogram. The pulmonary artery may be difficult to enter. Biplane cineangiography will demonstrate the anomaly and associated defects.

## Natural History and Prognosis

The natural history varies greatly with the severity of the anomaly. Infants and those with associated defects are at highest risk of early death; survival to old age has been reported with mild disease.

Symptoms tend to progress in most patients. Severe symptoms, cardiomegaly, and cyanosis correlate with mortality. Death usually is the result of heart failure, complications of cyanosis, arrhythmias, or low cardiac output if there is an intact atrial septum.

**Treatment**

Medical management includes treatment of heart failure, arrhythmias, and complications of cyanosis as well as prevention of endocarditis.

Surgery is generally recommended only for those with very severe disease. Reconstruction or replacement of the tricuspid valve is necessary, along with closure of the atrial communication. In some cases the atrialized portion of the right ventricle is plicated. Interruption of accessory conduction pathways can also be accomplished if needed.


## EISENMENGER'S SYNDROME

*Pulmonary arterial hypertension* usually is the result of transmission of systemic arterial pressure to the pulmonary artery via a large communication. Less commonly, it is due to obstruction in the left side of the heart. *Pulmonary vascular obstructive disease* is the process of structural changes in the smaller muscular arteries and arterioles of the lungs that gradually diminishes their ability to transport blood. Patients with defects that cause both increased pulmonary flow and pressure are most likely to develop their feared complication.

*Eisenmenger's syndrome* consists of a large communication between the left and right sides of the heart, pulmonary arterial hypertension at the systemic level, and pulmonary vascular obstructive disease of a degree that elevates pulmonary vascular resistance to a level that reverses the shunt and causes cyanosis. (See also Chap. 14, "Pulmonary Hypertension.")


## Clinical Manifestations

*History*

The age at which cyanosis and its symptoms appear varies greatly with the complex underlying cardiac defects causing an early presentation. Exertional fatigue and dyspnea are common. Syncope from inadequate cardiac output or arterial oxygen saturation, arrhythmias, hemoptysis, and chest pain occur when the disease progresses to a very severe level.

*Physical Examination*

A right ventricular lift, loud pulmonary closure sound, and cyanosis with clubbing are typical findings. The murmurs of pulmonary and tricuspid regurgitation may be audible.

## Usual Diagnostic Tests

### Chest X-Ray

The right ventricle is hypertrophied, but the overall heart size may not be large. The central pulmonary arteries are enlarged, with rapid tapering or "pruning" to small vessels distally.

### Electrocardiogram

Right axis deviation and right atrial and right ventricular hypertrophy are present.

### Echocardiography

The underlying cardiac defect can be outlined along with supporting evidence of the presence of pulmonary arterial hypertension.

### Cardiac Catheterization

The presence of pulmonary hypertension and elevated pulmonary vascular resistance is established and the underlying defects outlined. Pulmonary resistance should be evaluated after inhalation of 100 percent oxygen and again after intravenous tolazoline to rule out a reversible component of the disease.

## Natural History and Prognosis

The disease is a progressive one with a poor prognosis of survival beyond young to mid-adult years. Sudden death, heart failure, and stroke all contribute to this. Pregnancy is associated with a very high mortality.

## Treatment

Medical therapy usually is not effective in combating the complications of severe pulmonary vascular disease, but it should be tried. Pregnancy and the use of oral contraceptives should be avoided. Prevention of infective endocarditis is important.

Corrective surgery is contraindicated when the pulmonary vascular resistance is 11 units/m$^2$ or more, or the pulmonary/systemic resistance ratio is 0.7:1 or greater with a pulmonary/systemic flow ratio less than 1.5:1. Heart and lung transplantation is the only surgical means of treatment for these patients.

## LONG–TERM POSTOPERATIVE FOLLOW–UP

With the dramatic advances that have occurred in the surgical treatment for congenital heart defects, more patients are reaching adulthood.

It must be recognized that there are residua, sequelae, and complications that result from this type of surgery. A residual part of the defect may deliberately have been avoided in surgery. Sequelae are unavoidable consequences of the surgery; complications are unexpected, but related, events that occur after surgery. Of surgery for all congenital heart defects, only surgical correction of patent ductus arteriosus is likely to have no long-term problems.

Patients usually have residual murmurs. Careful evaluation of the hemodynamic abnormalities that they represent is very important. Doppler and two-dimensional echocardiography are particularly helpful. Continued cyanosis signals complex uncorrectable defects or pulmonary vascular disease. Dysrhythmias are particularly important late problems, especially among patients who have had complex surgery. Serious ventricular dysfunction may also occur late after surgery for complex defects. Ambulatory electrocardiographic monitoring and stress exercise testing are very helpful in guiding management.

Sick sinus syndrome with bradytachyarrhythmias can occur after repair of atrial septal defect. The most serious late problems after repair of ventricular septal defect or tetralogy of Fallot are development of complete heart block and serious ventricular arrhythmias. Significant residual shunts should have been repaired in childhood.

Valvar aortic stenosis continues to progress over the years, and may also be associated with progressive aortic regurgitation even in the face of successful surgery in childhood. Coarctation repair can be complicated by recurrence or by systemic hypertension.

In general, all patients who have had surgery for congenital heart defects with the exception of a patent ductus should be followed longitudinally throughout life for the development of problems.

## SUGGESTED READING

Adams FH, Emmanouilides GC, Riemenschneider TA (eds): *Moss' Heart Disease in Infants, Children, and Adolescents,* 4th ed. Baltimore, Williams and Wilkins, 1989.

Freedom RM, Culham JAG, Moes CAF: *Angiocardiography of Congenital Heart Disease.* New York, Macmillan, 1984.

Kidd BSL, Rowe RD (eds): *The Child with Congenital Heart Disease After Surgery.* Mount Kisco, NY, Futura Publishing Co Inc, 1976.

Kirklin JW, Barratt-Boyes BG: *Cardiac Surgery.* New York, John Wiley and Sons, Part IV, pp 463–1344, 1986.

Nugent EW, Plauth WH Jr, Edwards JE, et al: The pathology, abnormal physiology, clinical recognition, and medical and surgical treatment of congenital heart disease, in Hurst JW et al (eds): *The Heart,* 7th ed. New York, McGraw-Hill, Chap 37, pp 655–794, 1990.

Park MK: *Pediatric Cardiology for Practitioners,* 2d ed. Chicago, Year Book Medical Publishers, Inc, 1988.

Perloff JK: *The Clinical Recognition of Congenital Heart Disease,* 3d ed. Philadelphia, WB Saunders Co, 1987.

Roberts WC (ed): *Adult Congenital Heart Disease.* Philadelphia, FA Davis Co, 1987.

Seward JB, Tajik AJ, Edwards WD, et al: *Two-Dimensional Echocardiographic Atlas.* New York, Springer-Verlag, 1987.

| Aortic Valve Disease

*Douglas C. Morris, M. D.*

## AORTIC STENOSIS

### Definition, Etiology, and Pathology

*Aortic stenosis* is obstruction to the flow of blood from the left ventricle. It may be valvular, supravalvular, or subvalvular in location.

*Valvular aortic stenosis* is caused primarily by leaflet degeneration. These degenerative changes occur most often on a congenitally bicuspid valve; in the elderly they may occur on a tricuspid valve. Other causes of aortic stenosis are congenital and rheumatic. The age at which significant aortic stenosis becomes clinically manifest is an important clue to the etiology. Significant valvular aortic stenosis developing in a person under the age of 30 is almost always congenital. In the decades extending from age 30 to 70, the most prevalent cause of isolated aortic stenosis is a congenitally bicuspid valve with secondary degenerative calcification. It is during these same decades that rheumatic valvulitis gains significance as a cause of aortic stenosis, particularly in multivalvular disease. Patients developing significant stenosis after age 70 frequently show degenerative calcification of a tricuspid aortic valve.

*Supravalvular and subvalvular aortic stenosis* are usually congenital. The exception may be hypertrophic cardiomyopathy, which has a bimodal distribution with that portion that presents later in life possibly being an acquired variety. (See Chap. 17.)

The bicuspid valve usually is not inherently stenotic. Stenosis is the most frequent complication, however. Immobilization of the cusps by the deposition of calcium appears to be the most important factor in converting the bicuspid valve into a stenotic lesion. The process of collagenous degeneration, lipid deposition, and calcification occurring in the biscuspid valve is similar to that noted much later in life in some tricuspid valves. This similarity in pathological findings suggests that stenosis in the bicuspid valve is a degenerative change accelerated by the abnormal mechanical stress imposed on the valvular tissue by its bicuspid configuration.

The aortic valve is rendered stenotic by rheumatic valvulitis either through extensive fusion of commissures or by fusion of a single commissure with secondary calcium deposition. Commissural fusion stems from healing of the active rheumatic endocarditis. The fusion converts the aortic valve into a bicuspid configuration subject to the same abnormal stresses and degenerative changes as the congenital bicuspid valve.

## Abnormal Physiology

Stenosis of the aortic valve creates resistance to ejection, and a systolic pressure gradient develops across the valve. The outflow obstruction imposes a pressure overload on the left ventricle, which compensates by an increase in ventricular wall thickness and mass. This concentric hypertrophy normalizes systolic wall stress and preserves ventricular function. Even though systolic function may be preserved, abnormal diastolic compliance accompanies the development of concentric hypertrophy. A sustained pressure overload on the left ventricle will eventually result in impaired contractility and chamber dilatation.

## Clinical Manifestations

### History

The characteristic clinical manifestations of aortic stenosis are angina pectoris, syncope, heart failure, and sudden death. Unlike the setting of mitral stenosis, however, symptoms cannot be relied upon as the harbingers of significant disease in aortic stenosis. Symptoms tend to occur late in the course of this condition.

*Angina pectoris* is usually the initial clinical manifestation and is the most common, occurring in 50 to 70 percent of symptomatic patients. It does not necessarily reflect the presence of coronary atherosclerosis.

The *syncope* characteristic of aortic stenosis either immediately follows exertion or interrupts it. This manifestation occurs much less commonly than angina, with a reported frequency of 15 to 30 percent of symptomatic patients. Most of these patients experience angina just before the syncope.

The significance of *dyspnea* in a patient with aortic stenosis seems to depend on the age of the patient. In younger, more active patients, exertional dyspnea, which may be an early symptom, usually is not associated with nocturnal dyspnea or cardiac enlargement. In older, less active patients, exertional dyspnea, despite possible early appearances to the contrary, usually *is* associated with nocturnal dyspnea, and has a more sinister significance.

*Sudden death* may occur in 15 to 20 percent of symptomatic patients with aortic stenosis. Although most patients who die suddenly with aortic stenosis have been symptomatic, about 15 percent have had no previous symptoms.

*Physical Examination*

Typical physical findings of significant aortic stenosis include a delayed upstroke of the carotid pulse, a spindle-shaped systolic murmur, and evidence of left ventricular hypertrophy.

While the pulse pressure typically is narrow in aortic stenosis because of depression of the systolic pressure, elderly patients with loss of arteriolar elasticity may occasionally present with pulse pressures of 60 mmHg or more and systolic pressures reaching or exceeding 180 mmHg.

The characteristic murmur of aortic stenosis is a basal harsh crescendo-decrescendo systolic murmur. The murmur is commonly loudest in the second right intercostal space, with radiation into the carotids and to the apex. In children and young adults the murmur is preceded by an ejection sound. This high-pitched sound is usually loudest at the apex. A delay in aortic closure is the most common alteration of the $S_2$ sound in aortic stenosis. This delay results in a single or paradoxically split $S_2$ sound. One-third to one-half of patients with essentially "pure" aortic valvular stenosis have an early diastolic murmur at the base. Generally, this high-pitched decrescendo murmur reflects mild, insignificant valvular reflux.

In the elderly, the murmur of aortic stenosis frequently masquerades as a pure-frequency, musical, cooing murmur that is loudest at the apex.

*Electrocardiogram*

Sinus rhythm is the rule in aortic valvular stenosis, regardless of severity. Except in elderly patients, atrial fibrillation suggests coexisting mitral valve disease. The typical ECG of aortic stenosis shows increased QRS voltage accompanied by depression of ST segments and T-wave inversion in the leads with the most prominent R waves. Conduction defects are common and range from first-degree heart block to left bundle branch block.

*Chest X-Ray*

The concentric left ventricular hypertrophy of aortic stenosis may produce a prominent curvature of the apex of the cardiac silhouette on chest x-ray, but produces only moderate enlargement, if any, of the silhouette. Poststenotic dilatation of the ascending aorta is a common feature on chest x-ray. Although calcification of the aortic valve cannot be confidently identified on plain films, it should be present on fluoroscopy in any patient over age 40 years with severe aortic stenosis.

### Echocardiography

Echocardiography can delineate aortic-root and left ventricular outflow tract structure, and leaflet mobility, in valvular and nonvalvular forms of aortic stenosis. The thickening, calcification, and decreased mobility characteristic of all types of acquired valvular aortic stenosis will be manifest on the echocardiogram. Doppler echocardiography can be used to estimate the pressure difference across the aortic valve and to calculate the aortic valve area.

### Cardiac Catheterization

Cardiac catheterization is indicated upon the development of symptoms or the development of left ventricular hypertrophy with secondary ST-T wave changes on ECG. The catheterization should be directed toward determining the gradient across the aortic valve, measuring cardiac output, assessing left ventricular function, and excluding other explanations (e.g., coronary atherosclerosis) for the symptoms in question.

## Treatment

### Medical Therapy

There is no good medical therapy for symptomatic severe aortic stenosis. The mechanical obstruction to left ventricular outflow will not be altered by medical therapy. Symptoms warrant mechanical improvement of flow across the stenotic valve. Balloon valvuloplasty is a palliative procedure which should be limited to high-risk elderly patients with advanced symptoms.

Asymptomatic patients with aortic stenosis require prophylactic antibiotics to prevent bacterial endocarditis.

### Surgical Therapy

Patients with symptomatic severe aortic stenosis should undergo prompt aortic valve replacement. Asymptomatic patients with significant aortic valvular stenosis and the presence of left ventricular hypertrophy and strain on the ECG should also be advised to have aortic valve replacement.

Two general types of valve replacement are available: mechanical prostheses and tissue prostheses. The mechanical prostheses have the advantage of greater durability, but the disadvantage of a propensity for thromboembolism. The tissue prostheses lessen the risk of thromboembolism but tend toward degeneration. This degenerative process appears to occur more rapidly in younger patients.

## AORTIC REGURGITATION

### Definition, Etiology, and Pathology

*Aortic regurgitation* is the diastolic flow of blood from the aorta into the left ventricle due to incompetence of the aortic valve.

The disease mechanisms that impair the competence of the aortic valve have changed with time. In the past, rheumatic fever and syphilis were major causes of aortic regurgitation. As these diseases have become rarer, *myxomatous transformation of the leaflets* has become a more common cause. The Marfan syndrome including aortic root dilatation may accompany these myxomatous changes. *Connective-tissue disorders,* including ankylosing spondylitis, Reiter's syndrome, osteogenesis imperfecta, and rheumatoid arthritis, can be associated with aortic regurgitation. *Congenital abnormalities,* including bicuspid aortic valve and a supracristal type of ventricular septal defect, may contribute to the development of aortic regurgitation. *Chronic systemic arterial hypertension* can result in mild incompetence of the aortic valve. Sudden severe aortic regurgitation may be produced by *aortic dissection* or *bacterial endocarditis.* Incompetence of the aortic valve can result from *alteration of the leaflets,* including contracture scarring, perforation, redundance, loss of intrinsic rigidity, and tissue destruction, or from *dilatation or laceration of the aortic wall.*

### Abnormal Physiology

In aortic regurgitation, volume overload of the left ventricle is the basic hemodynamic abnormality. The magnitude of this volume overload depends on the volume of the regurgitant blood flow, which is determined, in turn, by the area of the regurgitant orifice, the diastolic pressure gradient between the aorta and left ventricle, and the duration of diastole. The compensatory response of the left ventricle is dilatation and development of eccentric hypertrophy. The increased end-diastolic volume is accompanied by an increased stroke volume. The left ventricular dilatation may occur with no increase in left ventricular end-diastolic pressure, because of increased myocardial compliance. In time, however, the hemodynamic burden imposed by volume overloading will result in depressed myocardial contractility and decreased compliance.

In acute aortic regurgitation the volume overload will be suddenly imposed on a left ventricle unable to dilate acutely and to adapt to increased diastolic filling. These sudden hemodynamic changes lead to pulmonary venous hypertension and acute pulmonary edema.

## Clinical Manifestations

### History

Patients with chronic aortic regurgitation remain asymptomatic for many years. The onset of disability is usually insidious. The earliest symptoms may be an awareness of the increased force of cardiac contraction and, later in the course, exertional dyspnea and easy fatigability. Angina pectoris may occur in aortic regurgitation, but it is much less common than in aortic stenosis. The chest pain in aortic regurgitation is more likely to occur at rest, and is likely to last longer and be frequently associated with vasomotor phenomenon and dyspnea.

### Physical Examination

The physical findings in severe chronic aortic regurgitation are related to a wide pulse pressure, a large ventricular diastolic volume, and the regurgitant blood flow. The absence of a wide pulse pressure (pulse pressure greater than 50 percent of peak systolic pressure or of a diastolic blood pressure greater than 70) in a patient without congestive heart failure makes severe aortic regurgitation unlikely. The dilatation of the left ventricle with severe aortic regurgitation displaces the apical impulse inferiorly and laterally. The regurgitant flow is characterized by a high-pitched diastolic blow along the left sternal border. An $S_3$ gallop and a diastolic rumble may be audible at the apex, secondary to the regurgitant flow.

The wide pulse pressure and left ventricular dilatation are not features of acute aortic regurgitation.

### Electrocardiogram

Increased QRS amplitude is a common early finding. Occasionally in the early stages this change is accompanied by tall T waves in the left precordial leads. The advanced stages of aortic regurgitation are typified by ST depression and negative T waves in association with the increased QRS voltage.

### Chest X-Ray

The characteristic chest x-ray finding in chronic severe aortic regurgitation is dilatation of the left ventricle with posterior and inferior elongation of the cardiac apex. Moderate-to-marked dilatation of the ascending aorta is not a feature of aortic regurgitation, except in the cases of the Marfan syndrome and aortic dissection.

### Cardiac Catheterization

Cardiac catheterization is indicated in aortic regurgitation if valve replacement is contemplated. Cardiac catheterization can give a visual estimate of the regurgitant flow, and by quantitative angiocardiography can quantitate the regurgitant flow. Cardiac catheterization also provides an assessment of left ventricular size, contractility, and compliance, and allows identification of abnormalities in the aorta, mitral valve, and coronary arteries.

### Natural History and Prognosis

Significant aortic regurgitation is well tolerated for many years before the development of heart failure. Eighty-five to ninety-five percent of patients with mild-to-moderate regurgitation will survive for 10 years. Three-fourths of patients with significant aortic regurgitation survive 5 years, and 50 percent live for 10 years after diagnosis. Once symptoms have developed, however, the patient deteriorates rather rapidly. Survival after the development of congestive heart failure is often less than 2 years.

## Treatment

### Medical

All patients with aortic regurgitation should receive prophylaxis against bacterial endocarditis. If heart failure develops in this condition, therapy should include digitalis, diuretics, and vasodilators. (Ideally, though, aortic valve replacement should have been proposed and completed before heart failure developed.)

### Surgical

Aortic valve replacement should be performed before heart failure or refractory left ventricular dilatation can develop. Serial evaluation of end-systolic dimensions seems the best guide in this decision making. Echocardiography provides an easy way to make this assessment. Surgery should be considered when the end-systolic dimension on M-mode echocardiography exceeds 55 mm.

The development of heart failure in acute aortic regurgitation from *infective endocarditis* requires valve replacement under intensive antibiotic coverage.

## SUGGESTED READING

Bonow RO, Rosing DR, McIntosh CL, et al: The natural history of asymptomatic patients with aortic regurgitation and normal LV function. *Circulation* 68:509–517, 1983.

Goldschlager N, Pfeifer J, Cohn K, et al: The natural history of aortic regurgitation: A clinical and hemodynamic study. *Am J Med* 54:577–588, 1973.

Hegglin R, Scheu H, Rothlin M: Aortic insufficiency. *Circulation* 38(suppl 5):V77–V92, 1968.

Perloff JK: Clinical recognition of aortic stenosis: The physical signs and differential diagnosis of the various forms of obstruction to left ventricular outflow. *Prog Cardiovasc Dis* 10:323–352, 1968.

Pomerance A: Pathogenesis of aortic stenosis and its relation to age. *Br Heart J* 34:569–574, 1972.

Rackley CE, Edwards JE, Wallace RB, et al: Aortic valve disease, in Hurst JW et al (eds): *The Heart,* 7th ed. New York, McGraw-Hill, Chap 40, pp 799–819, 1990.

Rahimtoola SH: Perspective on valvular heart diseases: an update. *J Am Coll Cardiol* 14:1–23, 1989.

Roberts WC, Perloff JK, Costantino T: Severe valvular stenosis in patients over 65 years of age. *Am J Cardiol* 27:497–506, 1971.

Ross J Jr, Braunwald E: Aortic stenosis. *Circulation* 38(suppl5):V61–V76, 1968.

Rotman M, Morris JJ, Behar V, et al: Aortic valvular disease: comparison of types and their medical surgical management. *Am J Med* 51:241–257, 1971.

Wigle ED, Labross CJ: Sudden, severe aortic insufficiency. *Circulation* 32:708–720, 1965.

## 9 | Mitral Valve Disease

*Douglas C. Morris, M. D.*

## MITRAL STENOSIS

### Definition, Etiology, and Pathology

*Mitral stenosis* is an obstruction to blood flow from the left atrium into the left ventricle caused by the mitral apparatus.

Mitral stenosis almost always is a result of rheumatic valvulitis, though there can be other causes of obstruction to diastolic flow into the left ventricle, such as atrial thrombi or myxoma. A rare cause of mitral stenosis in adults is a calcified mitral anulus; in children, dysplasia of the valve or "parachute" deformity of the valve may cause mitral stenosis. Rheumatic valvulitis results in scarring and contracture of the leaflets and chordae tendineae. There are often adhesions and fusion of the commissures. This process results in a funnel-shaped structure of the leaflets.

### Pathophysiology

Obstruction to flow across the mitral valve increases left atrial pressure and volume; these increases are reflected back into the pulmonary venous system. Chronic elevation of left atrial and pulmonary venous pressures produces hyperplasia and hypertrophy of pulmonary arteries, which, in turn, causes pulmonary arterial hypertension. Thus chronic mitral stenosis imposes a pressure overload on the left atrium and, ultimately, on the right ventricle.

### Clinical Manifestations

#### History

No more than one-half of patients with mitral stenosis have histories of rheumatic fever. The principal symptom of mitral stenosis is dyspnea due to pulmonary venous hypertension. Other frequent complaints include fatigue due to reduced cardiac output and palpitations due to atrial fibrillation. Symptoms of right ventricular failure (hepatomegaly, edema, and ascites) may predominate in those patients with severe pulmonary hypertension. Hemoptysis, hoarseness, and systemic embolus are dramatic, but infrequent, manifestations of mitral stenosis.

*Physical Examination*

The typical auscultatory features of mitral stenosis are an accentuated $S_1$ sound, an opening snap, and a diastolic rumble at the cardiac apex. In the early stages of mitral stenosis the diastolic rumble may not be audible unless the patient exercises and auscultation is then performed with the patient in the left lateral decubitus position. The opening snap, considered to be the most important physical sign of mitral stenosis, is a high-pitched sound loudest at the cardiac apex.

If pulmonary hypertension accompanies the mitral stenosis then a loud pulmonic sound, right ventricular heave, systolic murmur of tricuspid regurgitation, and/or distended neck veins may be present.

*Electrocardiogram*

The characteristic electrocardiographic findings in mitral stenosis include a broad, notched P wave most prominent in lead II and a P wave with terminal negative deflection of .04 s or more in $V_1$. Atrial fibrillation, though common, certainly is not the rule. A rightward deviation of the QRS vector suggests pulmonary hypertension.

*Chest X-Ray*

The radiographic hallmark of mitral stenosis is left atrial enlargement without left ventricular enlargement. Other frequent abnormalities on chest x-ray include an increase in upper-lobe vascular markings, prominence of the pulmonary arteries, and right ventricular enlargement. Kerley B lines are frequently seen; fluoroscopy often reveals mitral valve calcification.

*Echocardiography*

Echocardiography is the most reliable means of diagnosing mitral stenosis. The characteristic M-mode echocardiographic features are a decreased EF slope of the anterior leaflet, anterior diastolic motion of the posterior leaflet, and thickened dense echoes indicative of calcification. Two-dimensional echocardiography will demonstrate the valve orifice and allow calculation of its area. Doppler echocardiography will provide estimates of the gradient across the valve and pulmonary artery pressures.

*Cardiac Catheterization*

Cardiac catheterization confirms the echocardiographic assessment of the presence and severity of mitral stenosis. In addition, catheterization allows assessment of the degree of mitral regurgitation, the size and function of the left ventricle, and the degree of pulmonary hypertension. In general, however, the only information that cardiac catheterization provides that is not available on echocardiography is an assessment of the coronary arteries.

## Natural History and Prognosis

In the United States, most cases of acute rheumatic fever occur in the early teenage years. Usually another ten years elapse before a murmur is audible. Symptoms will then begin in another ten years, and will progress to the point that surgery is required in the fourth or fifth decade of life. About 50 percent of patients develop symptoms gradually; the rest experience a sudden deterioration in their clinical condition. The development of atrial fibrillation, fever, emotional stress, or pregnancy can produce this deterioration. Atrial fibrillation develops in about 40 percent of patients with mitral stenosis. The additional threat to patients with mitral stenosis who develop atrial fibrillation is systemic embolization.

## Treatment

Prophylaxis against recurrence of rheumatic fever should be continued until the age of 35. Endocarditis prophylaxis, of course, is a lifelong requirement.

If atrial fibrillation develops, digitalis and/or *either* diltiazem or verapamil should be used to control the ventricular rate. Quinidine or procainimide can be used to restore sinus rhythm. If these drugs are not successful, electrical cardioversion may be used. With chronic atrial fibrillation, oral anticoagulation should be given for 4 weeks prior to elective cardioversion.

Systemic embolization necessitates permanent anticoagulation. A single systemic embolus, however, is not an absolute indication for mitral valve surgery; emboli can occur in milder forms of mitral stenosis. Symptoms of pulmonary venous congestion unresponsive to medical therapy should prompt an evaluation for surgical intervention.

Balloon mitral valvuloplasty is still being refined, but has already proved useful in patients who are not candidates for surgery.

## Surgery

Surgery is offered to patients with symptoms that, despite medical therapy, prevent them from leading normal lives. The decision to intervene surgically may be made earlier in the course of the illness if mitral commissurotomy is likely—i.e., if there is little or no mitral calcification on echocardiography and there is absent or mild mitral insufficiency.

Mechanical prostheses are inserted in most patients; porcine prostheses are reserved for the elderly. The exception to this rule are potentially childbearing females: In order to avoid the use of anticoagulants during pregnancy, porcine valves should be suggested for these patients, despite the likely early degeneration of these prostheses.

## MITRAL REGURGITATION

### Definition, Etiology, and Pathology

*Mitral regurgitation* is the ejection of blood into the left atrium during left ventricular systole due to abnormalities in the mitral apparatus.

While rheumatic valvulitis remains an important cause of mitral regurgitation, it is no longer the most common cause. Mitral valve prolapse is probably the most common cause of mitral regurgitation nowadays; among patients requiring mitral valve replacement for pure mitral regurgitation, myxomatous transformation of the leaflets is the most common finding. Most of these patients (demonstrating myxomatous transformation on surgical specimens) have associated rupture of chordae tendineae. Other common causes of mitral regurgitation are papillary muscle ischemia or infarction, and dilatation of the left ventricle. Less common etiologies of mitral regurgitation include mitral annular calcification, infective endocarditis, idiopathic hypertrophic subaortic stenosis, trauma, heritable connective tissue disorders (Marfan syndrome, Ehlers-Danlos syndrome, osteogenesis imperfecta), and congenital deformities (partial atrioventricular canal, isolated cleft of the mitral valve).

The competence of the mitral valve depends on the normal anatomy and function of every part of the mitral apparatus. Those parts include the leaflets, the chordae tendineae, the anulus, the papillary muscles, and the left ventricular myocardium surrounding the papillary muscles. Every known cause of mitral regurgitation is associated with an abnormality in at least one of these.

### Pathophysiology

In chronic mitral regurgitation the portion of left ventricular stroke volume ejected into the left atrium determines the degree of left atrial and left ventricular enlargement. The left ventricle responds to the chronic volume overload by dilatation. This dilatation is accompanied by an increase in wall thickness which helps to maintain mechanical function. The diastolic volume of the left ventricle in mitral regurgitation includes the systolic output of the right ventricle and the volume regurgitated into the left atrium during the previous systole. The elastic recoil of the atrium and the increased compliance of the left ventricle allow rapid diastolic filling of the left ventricle without significant increases in left ventricular, left atrial, and pulmonary capillary diastolic pressures.

In acute mitral regurgitation the hemodynamic burden is different: the sudden regurgitation imposed on normal chambers does not allow compensatory dilatation of the left atrium and left ventricle. Consequently, marked elevations of left atrial and pulmonary capillary pressure are produced. This pressure overload on the pulmonary vascular tree produces acute pulmonary edema.

## Clinical Manifestations

### Symptoms

Chronic mitral regurgitation is well tolerated for years, without symptoms. When symptoms eventually develop, the earliest problems are fatigue and dyspnea, which progress to orthopnea, paroxysmal nocturnal dyspnea, and peripheral edema. Often the history provides clues to the etiology of the mitral regurgitation. A history of myocardial infarction or angina suggests papillary muscle involvement. Sudden appearance or sudden worsening of symptoms in a middle-aged male suggests chordal rupture. A patient with an enlarged heart and chronic symptoms of heart failure prior to the detection of mitral regurgitation probably has a dilated cardiomyopathy. A remote history of rheumatic fever implies rheumatic heart disease, and a recent history of fever raises the possibility of infective endocarditis.

### Physical Examination

The clinical manifestations of mitral regurgitation vary according to the hemodynamic spectrum of this condition. Usually if the left atrium remains small, as with acute mitral regurgitations, the patient is in sinus rhythm. Conversely, the markedly enlarged left atrium associated with chronic severe mitral regurgitation predisposes the patient to atrial fibrillation. In these chronic situations, the systolic murmur usually begins immediately after the $S_1$ sound and extends to, or through, the aortic closing sound. This high-pitched holosystolic murmur is heard at the cardiac apex and radiates to the axilla. If the left atrium is noncompliant (as in the acute setting), regurgitation may cease before the end of systole, causing the murmur to terminate before the $S_2$ sound. With a flail anterior leaflet the murmur may radiate to the spine, and with a flail posterior leaflet it may radiate to the second intercostal space near the sternum. The bidirectional ejection of blood (left atrium and aorta) frequently leads to early closing of the aortic valve and increased splitting of the $S_2$ sound.

The increased diastolic left ventricular volumes associated with chronic mitral regurgitation result in displacement of the cardiac impulse and hyperdynamic motion over a diffuse area, usually accompanied by a ventricular gallop.

### Electrocardiogram

Chronic mitral regurgitation produces left atrial and left ventricular enlargement, typically manifested by increased amplitude of the P wave and QRS complex. If atrial fibrillation is present, the left atrial enlargement usually causes a coarse fibrillatory pattern. When papillary muscle ischemia or infarction is the mechanism of the regurgitation, evidence of previous inferior or posterior myocardial infarction is often present.

### Chest X-Ray

In chronic severe mitral regurgitation, the chest x-ray reveals left atrial and left ventricular enlargement. With rheumatic disease, calcification of the leaflets may be visible; with degenerative disease a calcified anulus often is evident.

Acute severe mitral regurgitation is usually manifested by a normal cardiac size and pulmonary edema.

### Echocardiography

The echocardiogram is frequently helpful in establishing a diagnosis of the mitral regurgitation (e.g., flail leaflets, severe prolapse, mitral annular calcification, thickened poorly mobile leaflets, systolic anterior motion of anterior leaflet). Also, the sizes of the left atrium and left ventricle, as well as left ventricular function, are evident. Doppler echocardiography can give an estimate of the severity of the regurgitation.

Transesophogeal echocardiography is very helpful during the surgical repair of the mitral valve, as it allows for immediate assessment of the adequacy of the repair.

### Cardiac Catheterization

Cardiac catheterization confirms the diagnosis of mitral regurgitation, may provide a clue to the etiology (though not so well as echocardiography), assesses ventricular function, identifies other valve dysfunction, and defines the coronary anatomy.

A large *v* wave in the pulmonary capillary wedge pressure tracings suggests mitral regurgitation, but its absence does not exclude mitral regurgitation. A balloon flotation catheter, inserted at the bedside to determine oxygen saturations in the right heart chambers and determine the presence or absence of a v wave in the pulmonary capillary pressures, is helpful in establishing the diagnosis of a new systolic murmur after an acute myocardial infarction.

## Treatment

### Medical

Patients with mitral regurgitation of rheumatic etiology require prophylaxis against rheumatic fever until age 35. Prophylaxis against endocarditis is required for all etiologies of mitral regurgitation. If atrial fibrillation develops, digitalis and/or *either* verapamil or diltiazem should be used to slow the ventricular rate. Electrical cardioversion should be considered. Anticoagulation is generally advisable for patients who remain in atrial fibrillation. Early treatment of symptoms includes digitalis, diuretics, and afterload reducers. The optimal time for valve repair or replacement remains poorly defined. Ideally, surgery should be done before clinical evidence of impaired left ventricular contractility is evident. Since unloading of the left ventricle may be augmented by emptying into the low-pressure left atrium, deterioration of left ventricular function may remain clinically obscure.

### Surgery

Symptomatic patients with significant left ventricular enlargement due to mitral regurgitation should be advised to have mitral valve surgery. Surgery also seems advisable for asymptomatic patients with progressive left ventricular enlargement that reaches the point of marked left ventricular dilatation. The mitral valve surgery may be reconstructive, rather than replacement, surgery.

In symptomatic acute mitral regurgitation, medical therapy—primarily diuretics and afterload reduction with nitroprusside—serves as palliative therapy until surgery can be performed. Aortic balloon counterpulsation will help to stabilize some severely compromised patients.

## MITRAL VALVE PROLAPSE

### Definition, Etiology, and Pathophysiology

*Mitral valve prolapse* is a clinicopathological entity characterized by billowing or prolapse of one or both leaflets into the left atrium during systole. The etiology of the condition is unknown; it seems to arise from an alteration in leaflet and chordal structure.

### Clinical Manifestations

#### History

Most patients with this condition are asymptomatic, with detection occurring only on routine physical examination or echocardiography. Most estimates suggest that the prevalence of this condition is about 6 percent of the general population.

Frequently-reported symptoms include palpitations, chest pain, dyspnea, fatigue, lassitude, anxiety, hyperventilation, syncope, and orthostatic hypotension. The chest pain associated with mitral valve prolapse is not like the typical chest pain of angina; often it is prolonged and nonexertional, and of a stabbing quality.

### Physical Examination

Patients with mitral valve prolapse frequently have a distinct habitus. Typical features are narrower anterior-to-posterior chest diameters, straight back, pectus excavatum, long extremities, and hyperreflexic joints.

The mitral prolapse is manifested by a systolic click and/or a late systolic murmur. The click is loudest at the lower left sternal border or apex, the murmur loudest at the apex. Maneuvers that reduce left ventricular volume (standing, taking amyl nitrite) make the valve prolapse earlier and make the murmur and click occur earlier in systole. Maneuvers that increase the left ventricular volume (lying, squatting) make the click and murmur appear later in systole.

### Electrocardiogram

The ECG may be normal or may show nonspecific ST-T wave changes, particularly inversion of the T waves in leads III and $aV_F$. Paroxysmal supraventricular tachyarrhythmias, ventricular ectopy, or preexcitation may be present.

### Chest X-Ray

The chest x-ray may be normal, or may show a straight back or pectus excavatum. Cardiac enlargement, if present, suggests severe mitral regurgitation.

### Echocardiography

Echocardiography usually demonstrates the posterior systolic prolapse of the mitral leaflets. Two-dimensional echocardiography is superior to M-mode echocardiography in the diagnosis of mitral valve prolapse. False-positive and false-negative studies may occur, however, with either technique. Usually the false-negative studies with two-dimensional echocardiography result from inadequate visualization. False-positive studies may result from such conditions as inferior angulation of the transducer, pericardial effusion, presence of ventricular ectopy, and volume depletion. Besides confirming the diagnosis of mitral valve prolapse, echocardiography is helpful in detecting associated tricuspid and aortic valve prolapse and diagnosing chordal rupture. Doppler ultrasound is useful in assessing the presence and severity of mitral regurgitation and of regurgitation in other valves.

### Cardiac Catheterization

Left venticulography frequently demonstrates the prolapse of the mitral leaflets. In addition, the mitral prolapse may be accompanied by unusual ventriculographic silhouettes during systole. An estimate of the degree of mitral regurgitation can be made; and in patients with chest pain, the coronary anatomy can be defined.

## Natural History

The prognosis for most patients with mitral valve prolapse is good. While that majority will follow a benign clinical course, some patients will develop complications. The major complications are cardiac arrhythmias, transient ischemic attacks (TIAs), bacterial endocarditis, ruptured chordae tendineae, severe mitral regurgitation, and sudden death. Unfortunately, patients at risk for these complications cannot be accurately identified by current means.

## Treatment

### Medical

The patient should be reassured that mitral valve prolapse is usually benign. Patients with simple ventricular ectopy and non-ischemic chest pain should likewise be treated with reassurance, and beta blockers used only if palpitations or pain continue to provoke anxiety. Prophylaxis against endocarditis is recommended for prolapse associated with the murmur of mitral regurgitation. Patients with TIAs should receive daily aspirin. If systemic embolism occurs on this regimen, chronic anticoagulation with warfarin should be instituted.

### Surgical

Surgery is indicated to reconstruct or replace the mitral valve in the occasional patient who has severe regurgitation and *either* symptoms of heart failure or evidence of progressive deterioration of left ventricular function.

## SUGGESTED READING

Aranda JN, Befeler B, El-Sherif N, et al: Mitral valve prolapse: Recent concepts and observations. *Am J Med* 60:997–1004, 1976.

Barlow JB, Pocock WA: The problem of nonejection systolic clicks and associated mitral systolic murmurs: Emphasis on the billowing mitral leaflet syndrome. *Am Heart J* 90:636–655, 1975.

Oliveira DBG, Dawkins KD, Kay PH, et al: Chordal rupture: Aetiology and natural history. *Br Heart J* 50:312–317, 1983.

O'Rourke RA, Crawford MH: Mitral valve regurgitation. *Curr Probl Cardiol* 9:1–52, 1984.

Perloff JK, Child JS, Edwards JE: New guidelines for the clinical diagnosis of mitral valve prolapse. *Am J Cardiol* 57:1124–1130, 1986.

Perloff JK, Roberts WC: The mitral apparatus: Functional anatomy of mitral regurgitation. *Circulation* 46:227–239, 1972.

Rackley CE, Edwards JE, Karp RB: Mitral valve disease, in Hurst JW et al (eds): *The Heart,* 7th ed. New York, McGraw-Hill, Chap 41, pp 820–851, 1990.

Rahimtoola SH: Perspective on valvular heart disease: an update. *J Am Coll Cardiol* 14:1–23, 1989.

Salomon NW, Stinson EB, Griepp RB, et al: Surgical treatment of degenerative mitral regurgitation. *Am J Cardiol* 38:463–468, 1976.

Selzer A, Katayama F: Mitral regurgitation: Clinical patterns, pathophysiology and natural history. *Medicine* 51:337–366, 1972.

Wood P: An appreciation of mitral stenosis. *Br Med J* 1:1051–1063 and 1113–1124, 1954.

Pulmonary Valve Disease;
Tricuspid Valve Disease

*Douglas C. Morris, M.D.*

## PULMONARY VALVE DISEASE

### Definition, Etiology, and Pathology

*Pulmonary valve stenosis* is the obstruction of right ventricular outflow by pulmonary valvular deformity. With rare exception, it is congenital.

*Pulmonic regurgitation* is the diastolic flow of blood from the pulmonary trunk into the right ventricle due to incompetence of the pulmonary valve. Pulmonary hypertension from any cause, such as mitral stenosis, chronic lung disease, or pulmonary emboli, can produce pulmonary-valve incompetence.

Inflammatory lesions that involve the pulmonary valve include rheumatic fever, bacterial endocarditis, and, on rare occasions, tuberculosis. Rheumatic involvement of the pulmonary valve is unusual. It occurs in patients with severe myocardial involvement and involvement of the aortic and mitral valves and, usually, the tricuspid valve. Organisms that infect the pulmonary valve are usually highly virulent, staphylococcus being the most common. Carcinoid syndrome with cardiac involvement can create a pearly-white fibrous scarring, with retraction of the pulmonary leaflets, that resuts in both stenosis and regurgitation.

### Pathophysiology

Pulmonary regurgitation is the most frequently acquired lesion of the pulmonary valve. Pulmonary regurgitation imposes a volume overload on the right ventricle. If pulmonary hypertension has preceded regurgitation, the overload is superimposed on hypertrophied myocardium.

### Clinical Manifestations

*Symptoms*

Clinical manifestations depend on the severity of the deformity and the etiology of the disease process. Severe hemodynamic changes resulting from injury to the pulmonary valve are unusual. Patients with severe stenosis may have syncope or symptoms of right-sided heart failure. Pulmonary regurgitation is usually well tolerated, but may contribute to cardiac decompensation when associated with other valvular lesions.

### Physical Examination

The murmur of pulmonary valve stenosis is a spindle-shaped systolic murmur which may persist past the aortic $A_2$ sound. The murmur is usually loudest in the second left intercoastal space at the sternal border. The murmur of pulmonary regurgitation may be confused with aortic regurgitation or a middiastolic flow rumble. Its onset is generally delayed after the $S_2$ sound, and its duration is variable. If pulmonary hypertension is present, the $P_2$ sound is accentuated. The absence of peripheral findings of aortic regurgitation can be useful in suggesting that a diastolic high-pitched murmur arises from the pulmonary valve.

### Electrocardiogram

There are no characteristic electrocardiographic changes associated with pulmonary valvular lesions. Preexisting pulmonary hypertension produces evidence of right ventricular hypertrophy.

### Chest X-Ray

Pulmonary hypertension is characterized by pulmonary artery prominence and an increase in right ventricular dimensions.

### Echocardiography

Doppler echocardiographic techniques allow estimation of the severity both of the regurgitation and of the stenosis of the valve. They also provide a reliable estimate of pulmonary artery pressure.

### Cardiac Catheterization

Right-sided heart pressures define the severity of pulmonary hypertension and the severity and site of obstruction in pulmonic stenosis. Pulmonary regurgitation is not accurately demonstrated on angiography.

### Treatment

Endocarditis prophylaxis is indicated in the presence of pulmonary valve lesions. If the pulmonary valve regurgitation is secondary to pulmonary hypertension, therapy should be directed toward lowering pulmonary vascular resistance. Pulmonary regurgitation, of whatever cause, is generally well tolerated if pulmonary vascular resistance is normal.

When pulmonary valve replacement is required, a bioprosthetic valve is preferred because of the tendency for mechanical valve thrombosis in this position.

## TRICUSPID VALVE DISEASE

### Definition, Etiology, and Pathology

*Tricuspid regurgitation* is the flow of blood into the right atrium during right ventricular contraction. *Tricuspid stenosis* is the obstruction of diastolic flow across the tricuspid valve.

The most common cause of tricuspid stenosis is rheumatic valvulitis, but instances of stenosis secondary to congenital heart disease, carcinoid syndrome, fibroelastosis, endomyocardial fibrosis, and systemic lupus erythematosus have been reported. Clinically significant *organic* tricuspid regurgitation is uncommon. Most cases of isolated tricuspid regurgitation arise in IV drug abusers and are due to infectious endocarditis. Other causes of organic tricuspid regurgitation include Ebstein's anomaly, atrioventricular cushion defects, carcinoid heart disease, and trauma. A more frequent occurrence than organic tricuspid regurgitation is *functional* tricuspid regurgitation. Presumably, functional regurgitation develops because the weak anatomic support structure cannot adequately anchor the tricuspid leaflets as the right ventricle dilates in response to primary or secondary pulmonary hypertension.

Rheumatic valvulitis is characterized by fibrosis with contracture of the leaflets and commissural fusion. Unlike the case in the mitral valve, the chordae are not severely deformed. In malignant carcinoid tumor, the tricuspid and pulmonary valves may be affected. Fibrous plaques can develop on the surfaces of these valves as well as on the endocardial surfaces of the right atrium and ventricle. The hemodynamic effects result from the rigidity and contracture of the fibrous tissue deposited on the valves.

### Pathophysiology

The major hemodynamic alterations of tricuspid stenosis are a decrease in cardiac output and an increase in right atrial pressures. Inability of the right atrium to propel blood across the stenotic tricuspid valve accounts for the reduction in cardiac output. The greater reduction in output associated with tricuspid stenosis, in comparison with mitral stenosis, is probably related to the relatively small force of contraction of the right atrium in comparison with that of the right ventricle. Right atrial pressure is a critical factor in the production of peripheral edema; most patients begin to develop peripheral edema when the right atrial pressure reaches 10 mmHg.

In tricuspid regurgitation the normal decrease in right atrial pressure during ventricular contraction is replaced by an abrupt increase in pressure due to regurgitation of a portion of the right-ventricle stroke volume. This alteration of the right atrial pressure curve produces an increase in the mean right atrial pressure which is reflected throughout the venous system.

## Clinical Manifestations

### Symptoms

The most common symptoms of tricuspid stenosis are effort intolerance and easy fatigability. The most common presenting case would be a 20- to 50-year-old woman with coexisting, and usually dominant, mitral stenosis.

Since tricuspid regurgitation usually accompanies left ventricular failure or mitral stenosis, symptoms associated with the condition are dyspnea, orthopnea, and peripheral edema. The tricuspid regurgitation often ameliorates the pulmonary symptoms associated with the left-sided heart failure. Tricuspid regurgitation due to infective endocarditis typically is found in an IV drug abuser with fever.

### Electrocardiogram

Tall, peaked P waves in the absence of evidence of right ventricular hypertrophy are the most diagnostic electrocardiographic pattern for tricuspid stenosis. Atrial fibrillation is the customary rhythm in tricuspid regurgitation. A significant proportion of these patients show right bundle branch block.

### Chest X-Ray

The most characteristic roentgenographic pattern of tricuspid stenosis is conspicuous dilatation of the right atrium without significant enlargement of the pulmonary arteries. Tricuspid regurgitation may produce some degree of right atrial enlargement, but there is usually accompanying right ventricular enlargement.

### Echocardiography

A pattern of motion very similar to the mitral-valve manifestations of mitral stenosis is characteristic of the stenotic tricuspid valve on echocardiography. Doppler echocardiography can give an estimate of the diastolic gradient across the valve.

In a patient with tricuspid regurgitation echocardiography may reveal systolic prolapse, ruptured chordae, or shaggy, irregular echoes of vegetation. Contrast echocardiography with peripheral venous injections can detect the back-and-forth movement across the tricuspid valve. Doppler echocardiography can give estimates of the severity of regurgitation and the systolic pressure in the right ventricle.

*Cardiac Catheterization*

If tricuspid stenosis is clinically suspected, simultaneous pressures must be recorded in the right atrium and right ventricle. Since a mean gradient of 3 mmHg or more suggests significant tricuspid stenosis, the presence of tricuspid stenosis might go undetected on "pullback" pressure recording from the right ventricle to the right atrium.

A prominent CV, or regurgitant, wave in the right atrium suggests tricuspid regurgitation. Angiographic documentation of tricuspid regurgitation is imprecise because the catheter overrides the tricuspid valve.

## Treatment

*Medical*

Usually the management of a patient with tricuspid stenosis is determined by the more severely stenotic mitral valve. Prior to surgical intervention, the patient's management is not altered by the additional presence of tricuspid stenosis.

For tricuspid regurgitation, treatment of right ventricular failure requires management of the left ventricular failure or early surgical intervention for correction of mitral stenosis.

The decision to proceed with surgery is usually based on the severity of the aortic and mitral valve disease. The usual questions pertaining to the tricuspid valve are whether a procedure for it should be added to the planned mitral or aortic valve surgery and, if so, whether that procedure should be annuloplasty or valve replacement.

## SUGGESTED READING

Edwards JE: The spectrum and clinical significance of tricuspid regurgitation. *Practical Cardiol* 6:86–95, 1980.

Glancy DL, Marcus FL, Cuadra M, et al: Isolated organic tricuspid valvular regurgitation. *Am J Med* 46:989–996, 1969.

Holmes JC, Fowler ND, Kaplan S: Pulmonary valvular insufficiency. *Am J Med* 44:851–862, 1968.

Kitchin A, Turner R: Diagnosis and treatment of tricuspid stenosis. *Br Heart J* 26:354–379, 1964.

Morgan JR, Forker AD: Isolated tricuspid insufficiency. *Circulation* 43:559–564, 1971.

Perloff JK, Harvey WP: Clinical recognition of tricuspid stenosis. *Circulation* 22:346–364, 1960.

Rackley CE, Edwards JE. Wallace RB, et al: Pulmonary valve disease, in Hurst JW et al (eds): *The Heart,* 7th ed. New York, McGraw-Hill, Chap 42, pp 852–854, 1990.

Rackley CE, Wallace RB, Edwards JE, et al: Tricuspid valve disease, in Hurst JW et al (eds): *The Heart,* 7th ed. New York, McGraw-Hill, Chap 43, pp 855–862, 1990.

*11* | Angina Pectoris, Angina Equivalents, and Prolonged Myocardial Ischemia Without Evidence of Myocardial Infarction

*Hisham A. Ba'albaki, M.D.*
*J. Willis Hurst, M.D.*

## DEFINITION

*Angina pectoris* is not a disease. It is a clinical manifestation of acute myocardial ischemia, which, in turn, is a consequence of coronary artery disease, certain types of valve disease, cardiomyopathy, etc. (see "Etiology of Myocardial Ischemia," below). Heberden described angina pectoris as a "sense of strangling and anxiety" and "a painful and most disagreeable sensation in the breast." Angina pectoris usually lasts from 1 to 10 min and, while it can occur at rest, is usually precipitated by emotional and/or physical stress. The discomfort is usually located in the retrosternal area but may radiate to, or be confined to, the jaw, throat, right or left arm, wrist, or back. The physician must always distinguish between stable and unstable angina pectoris (see corresponding sections below).

Angina pectoris is not a sensitive marker of myocardial ischemia, since "painless" or "silent" ischemic episodes are three to five times more frequent than painful ones. Many patients with silent myocardial ischemia may never complain of angina pectoris.

There are four types of angina pectoris: stable angina, unstable angina, variant (Prinzmetal's) angina, and angina equivalents. Prolonged myocardial ischemia, with or without angina, but with no evidence of myocardial infarction (MI), is also a well-recognized clinical entity. The recognition and treatment of each of these types of myocardial ischemia will be discussed in this chapter.

## ETIOLOGY OF MYOCARDIAL ISCHEMIA

The causes of myocardial ischemia include the following:

- Coronary atherosclerotic narrowing (the common cause).
- Nonatherosclerotic coronary disease: coronary spasm, coronary thromboembolism, congenital anomalies, and coronary vasculitis.

- Valvular heart disease: aortic stenosis and/or insufficiency, mitral stenosis with pulmonary hypertension, mitral valve prolapse, and pulmonic stenosis.
- Pulmonary hypertension.
- Hypertrophic or dilated cardiomyopathies.

## STABLE ANGINA PECTORIS

Angina pectoris is said to be *stable* when there has been no change in the frequency, duration, precipitating factors, or ease of relief of angina attacks during the last 60 days. In making this diagnosis one must ascertain that the patient's activity level has not decreased during that period. Grading of effort angina, using the guidelines of the Canadian Cardiovascular Society (Table 11-1), allows the physician to determine the functional capacity of the patient. Unstable angina (see below) is more serious and has a poorer prognosis than stable angina pectoris, but the intensity of episodes of stable angina is a poor indicator of seriousness compared to other markers to be discussed below. The physician should identify the major modifiable and nonmodifiable risk factors for coronary disease.

### Pathophysiology

In patients with stable angina pectoris, myocardial ischemia occurs when an increase in myocardial oxygen demand occurs in the

TABLE 11-1 The Canadian Cardiovascular Society's Classification of Angina Pectoris*

1. Ordinary physical activity does not cause . . . angina, such as walking and climbing stairs. Angina with strenuous or rapid or prolonged exertion at work or recreation.
2. Slight limitations of ordinary activity. Walking or climbing stairs rapidly, walking uphill, walking or stair climbing after meals, or in cold, or in wind, or under emotional stress, or only during the few hours after awakening. Walking more than two blocks on the level and climbing more than one flight of ordinary stairs at a normal pace and in normal conditions.
3. Marked limitation of ordinary physical activity. Walking one to two blocks on the level and climbing one flight of stairs in normal conditions and at normal pace.
4. Inability to carry on any physical activity without discomfort—anginal syndrome may be present at rest.

* This classification of angina pectoris has replaced the New York Heart Association classification, which was abandoned in 1973.[1]
*Source:* Campeau L: Letter to the Editor. *Circulation* 54:522, 1976. Reproduced with permission from the American Heart Association, Inc., and author.

presence of fixed myocardial oxygen supply. This is why stable angina pectoris commonly occurs when the patient walks rapidly or climbs a slight incline. Factors that affect myocardial oxygen demand include heart rate, myocardial contractility, and myocardial wall stress. The latter is determined by left ventricular pressure, volume, and wall thickness. Factors that affect myocardial oxygen supply include oxygen content of the blood, and coronary blood flow. The latter is determined by coronary perfusion pressure and coronary arterial narrowing (fixed, dynamic).

## Usual Diagnostic Tests

The *resting ECG* is normal in approximately one-half of patients with angina pectoris. The presence of abnormal Q waves in the ECG usually indicates prior MI, but a pseudoinfarction pattern should be considered (e.g., cardiomyopathy, infiltrative disease, pre-excitation syndromes).

*Twenty-four hour Holter monitoring* is helpful in evaluating the *total ischemic burden*—i.e., episodes of *painful* and *painless* myocardial ischemia. While the presence of ST-segment changes on Holter monitoring has been associated with unfavorable outcome in patients with stable angina, the exact role of Holter monitoring in the management of these patients has not been defined. The presence and severity of ventricular arrhythmias can also be determined using this technology.

*Exercise stress testing,* with or without myocardial perfusion imaging, using treadmill protocols, is frequently used in patients with stable angina. As a *diagnostic tool,* exercise testing is helpful in individuals in whom the pretest probability of coronary atherosclerosis is intermediate (i.e., predictive value of history less than 80 to 90 percent but greater than 10 to 20 percent). *Stress testing is not needed, and should not be used as a diagnostic procedure, when the pretest probability of stable angina pectoris is 90 percent.* The addition of thallium ($^{201}$Tl) perfusion imaging and radionuclide ventriculography to stress ECG testing improves its accuracy, especially in individuals in whom the likelihood of a false-positive stress ECG is high (young females, users of certain drugs, patients with preexcitation or with abnormal baseline ECGs). A false-positive $^{201}$Tl scan may occur in patients with left bundle branch block or females whose breasts are large. Stress testing is also helpful in determining the *prognosis* of patients with stable angina and in assessing the therapeutic efficacy of anti-ischemic medication or revascularization procedures (angioplasty, bypass grafting). For patients who are not able to exercise on the treadmill, bicycle ergometers may be used.

Dipyridamole $^{201}$Tl scintigraphy has been introduced as an alternative to exercise testing. It is used when the patient cannot exercise on the treadmill or bicycle. Recently *exercise echocardiography* has been investigated, but more research is needed before it can be used as a diagnostic tool.

In general, *coronary arteriography* is indicated for patients with stable angina who are clinically determined to be at high risk for future cardiac events (ischemia at low cardiac workload, reduced ejection fraction, high-grade ventricular ectopy); whose angina pectoris is unacceptable to the patient and is poorly controlled by medications; or in whom coronary spasm is suspected. In deciding whether to perform diagnostic coronary arteriography in a particular patient, other factors such as the patient's age, risks of the procedure, and the patient's overall health must be considered. The reader is referred to guidelines for coronary arteriography recently published by the American College of Cardiology/American Heart Association Task Force on Assessment of Diagnostic and Therapeutic Cardiovascular Procedures (subcommittee on coronary arteriography).

## Treatment

The choice of therapy (medical or revascularization) depends on each patient's perceived functional status, response to anti-ischemic medications, and risk of future cardiac events. The latter depends primarily on the results of exercise testing and on coronary anatomy and left ventricular function as determined by coronary arteriography and ventriculography.[2] In general, the following recommendations can be made:

- Patients with significant left main coronary artery obstruction (or left main equivalent) should undergo surgical revascularization.
- Patients with single-vessel disease and class 1 or 2 stable angina should be treated medically when the obstructing lesions are located in the circumflex or right coronary arteries. Patients with class 3 or 4 stable angina pectoris, or patients with class 1 or 2 angina pectoris in whom there is obstruction of the proximal portion of the left anterior descending coronary artery, should be considered for coronary angioplasty (or bypass surgery, if the lesion is not suitable for angioplasty).
- Patients with class 1 or 2 angina due to significant multivessel (two or three vessels) disease not involving the proximal left anterior descending, and in whom exercise performance on the treadmill is good and left ventricular function is preserved, should be treated medically. However, crossover to revascularization therapy should be anticipated in up to one-third of these patients within a 5-year period.
- Patients with Class 1, 2, 3, or 4 angina pectoris due to significant multivessel disease in whom the proximal left anterior descending

coronary artery is involved and left ventricular function is depressed, should have coronary bypass surgery. Whether angioplasty can substitute for bypass grafting cannot be stated until the results of several randomized trials become available.

- Patients with stable angina and very poor left ventricular ejection fraction (less than 25 percent) should be considered for surgical revascularization if the coronary anatomy is suitable and surgical experience with such patients in the particular institution is favorable.
- Whenever surgical revascularization is performed, the use of one or both of the internal mammary arteries should be attempted.
- Patients in whom revascularization is indicated but cannot be performed because of severe diffuse disease of the coronary arteries should be treated medically.
- Medical management should be adequate to prevent and relieve episodes of angina pectoris. This treatment should include adequate doses of nitrates, beta blockers, or calcium antagonists. Combination antianginal therapy has gained widespread use. While combination therapy may be helpful in patients whose symptoms persist despite maximal therapy with one agent, combination therapy may be accompanied by unfavorable hemodynamic and electrophysiological interactions.
- Aspirin (80 to 325 mg daily) may be helpful. Aspirin should also be given following bypass grafting.
- The use of antithyroid medications or radioactive iodine to suppress the thyroid gland may be required in patients in whom antianginal therapy is inadequate to control class 4 angina pectoris and in whom revascularization is not feasible.
- It has not yet been determined how aggressively one should treat episodes of silent myocardial ischemia in patients who have angina pectoris.
- With all patients, attempts should be made to modify major risk factors (hyperlipidemia, cigarette smoking, hypertension). Disorders that increase myocardial oxygen demand, such as anemia and hyperthyroidism, should be looked for and corrected when present.

## UNSTABLE ANGINA PECTORIS

This syndrome comprises angina of recent onset; angina occurring with increasing frequency; anginal attacks occurring with progressively less effort; and angina pectoris occurring at rest. The time frame in which these events take place is crucial to understanding the syndrome—the events have taken place *during the last 60 days*. Unstable angina often progresses to acute MI (especially within 2 to 4 weeks from diagnosis). Significant left main coronary artery stenosis is found in approximately 10 to 15 percent of patients with unstable angina. However, a similar percentage have normal-appearing coronary arteries on angiography. An aggressive management approach is needed, especially when these patients present in the *acute phase* of unstable angina.

## Pathophysiology

The roles of plaque rupture, platelet activation and aggregation thrombus formation, and coronary spasm in the pathogenesis of unstable angina have been emphasized by recent angiographic, angioscopic, and hematopathological studies. Another mechanism is coronary vasoconstriction related to endothelial dysfunction (deficiency of endothelium-derived relaxing factor) leading to platelet activation, thrombosis, and coronary artery spasm. Thus, in unstable angina, myocardial ischemia results from a primary decrease in oxygen delivery rather than an increase in myocardial oxygen demand.

## Usual Diagnostic Tests

The *resting ECG* may reveal electrocardiographic changes suggestive of myocardial ischemia, especially in the acute phase of the illness. Rapidly reversible ST-segment elevation is less common than transient ST-segment depression.

The majority of patients with unstable angina can be "stabilized" by intensive medical therapy. However, because of the relatively high incidence of significant left main coronary stenosis and high frequency of future cardiac events, *exercise stress testing should be avoided* and *coronary arteriography should be performed soon after admission to the hospital.*

### Coronary Arteriography

It is generally recommended that all patients with unstable angina undergo coronary arteriography, not only to aid diagnosis but also to assess the need and feasibility of coronary revascularization, which is frequently required in these patients.

## Treatment

- Patients with unstable angina pectoris should be hospitalized and placed under close supervision and cardiac monitoring.
- Oxygen administration and sedation are helpful.
- Therapy with IV nitroglycerin should be initiated, especially in patients in the acute phase of the illness. Therapy with calcium antagonists and beta blockers is also frequently needed.

- A recent double-blind, randomized, placebo-controlled trial[3] involving 479 patients with unstable angina demonstrated that the use of heparin or aspirin (325 mg twice a day) during the acute phase of the illness is associated with a reduced incidence of MI (trend favoring heparin over aspirin) and refractory angina (heparin only). The combination of heparin and aspirin was inferior to heparin alone and was associated with slightly increased incidence of major bleeding.
- The role of thrombolytic therapy in the treatment of unstable angina is still controversial and requires further study.
- Most patients with unstable angina should undergo revascularization without delay. The factors determining whether bypass surgery or angioplasty is used are discussed under "Stable Angina Pectoris," above. Patients with an obvious coronary thrombus identified by coronary arteriography who have been medically stabilized should probably receive IV heparin for a few days before coronary angioplasty is attempted.
- All patients, including those treated medically, should be discharged on daily aspirin because of its beneficial effects in reducing the incidence of nonfatal infarction and mortality as demonstrated by a Veterans Administration cooperative study and a Canadian multicenter trial.
- The importance of risk factor detection and modification cannot be overemphasized.

### Postinfarction Angina

*Postinfarction angina pectoris* is a serious form of angina pectoris and is discussed under "Unstable Angina Pectoris" because it often carries similar prognostic implications. Patients should be approached and managed in a similar fashion to those with unstable angina. Postinfarction angina can occur within hours following acute MI or may occur days or several weeks after infarction. While postinfarction angina may occur in up to one-third of patients, the majority of episodes of ischemic ST-segment changes on Holter monitoring are silent. The presence of these electrocardiographic changes in high-risk postinfarction patients (ejection fraction less than 40 percent and/or Lown ventricular arrhythmias of class III or greater) is associated with an increase in 1-year mortality.

#### Evaluation and Treatment of Postinfarction Angina

As a rule, patients with postinfarction angina should have coronary arteriography and, if feasible, revascularization. This is true for immediate and delayed angina after infarction.

## VARIANT (PRINZMETAL'S) ANGINA PECTORIS

The episodes of myocardial ischemia that characterize variant angina last several minutes, occur at rest, are frequently worse in the morning, and are associated with transient ST-segment elevation detected on a 12-lead ECG made during chest pain or Holter monitoring. Transient abnormal Q waves may be seen during an episode of angina. Angina usually appears after the onset of ST-segment changes. Up to two-thirds of episodes of ST-segment elevation are painless. AV heart block, ventricular arrhythmias, and transient ventricular dysfunction may occur during these episodes.

### Pathophysiology

It is believed that coronary vasospasm is responsible for episodes of myocardial ischemia in this syndrome. Local endothelial changes may be responsible for the hyperactivity of coronary artery segments. The majority of patients also have atherosclerotic coronary artery disease. When significant atherosclerotic narrowing is present, exercise-induced angina may also be present.

### Usual Diagnostic Tests

Every effort must be made to record an ECG during an episode of chest discomfort; ST-segment elevation during the episode is characteristic of variant angina.

All patients with suspected or proven variant angina should be considered for coronary arteriography. When coronary arteriography does not show significant coronary stenoses, it is useful for the arteriographer to attempt to provoke vasospasm. IV ergonovine is commonly used for this purpose. Patients undergoing this test should not receive therapy with nitrates or calcium antagonists for at least 12 to 24 h prior to the test. *The ergonovine test should not be performed outside the cardiac catheterization laboratory.* The use of shorter-acting acetylcholine (intracoronary) is currently being investigated as another spasm-provoking maneuver.

### Treatment

In the absence of significant atherosclerotic coronary artery disease, nitrates and calcium antagonists are the mainstay of medical therapy.[4] The efficacy of therapy can be monitored via changes in the frequency of anginal episodes and the occurrence of electrocardiographic changes on Holter monitoring. Verapamil should be used with caution if ischemic episodes are accompanied by bradyarrhythmias. Beta blockers may, theoretically, exacerbate variant angina if unopposed alpha-receptor-mediated vasoconstriction occurs. Exposure to cold environments should be avoided. Tobacco smoking must be discontinued.

The prognosis of medically treated patients with variant angina in whom there is no coronary atherosclerosis is generally good. Patients who present with an acceleration of their anginal pain pattern or in whom there is significant obstructive atherosclerotic coronary artery disease are at increased risk of both nonfatal infarction and death, especially in the first 3 to 6 months after the diagnosis of variant angina is made. Spontaneous remission of vasospastic ischemic episodes may occur.

Coronary bypass surgery should be considered if significant coronary artery stenosis is present. Patients undergoing bypass grafting are at low risk of cardiac events after hospital discharge.

Coronary angioplasty may be used in selected patients when significant obstruction is present in one coronary artery. These patients may, however, be particularly susceptible to angioplasty-induced coronary spasm.

## ANGINA EQUIVALENTS

Acute transient myocardial ischemia can cause angina pectoris or produce signs of left ventricular dysfunction or arrhythmias. Many ischemic episodes, irrespective of underlying pathophysiology, are *silent*. Lack of angina pectoris despite myocardial ischemia can be explained by the frequency of events that occur during myocardial ischemia—the *ischemic cascade* (Nesto et al). In general, left ventricular diastolic dysfunction (decreased compliance, elevated end-diastolic pressure) and systolic dysfunction (reduced myocardial contractility and ejection fraction) precede the development of ischemic electrocardiographic changes. Angina pectoris, if it develops at all, may be the final step in the cascade.

*Dyspnea* and *exhaustion* are symptoms that reflect the pathophysiological consequences of early myocardial ischemia and are therefore referred to as *angina equivalents*. They may occur *with or without* angina pectoris. *Dyspnea* results from elevation of pulmonary venous pressure and can be viewed as transient ischemia-induced partial electromechanical dissociation—i.e., *ischemic paralysis*. In its most dramatic presentation, acute pulmonary edema may occur. Dyspnea usually is exercise-induced, but may occur at rest. Other causes of dyspnea should be considered and excluded. Episodic or chronic *fatigue* and *exhaustion* reflect reduced cardiac output secondary to ischemia-induced depression of myocardial contractility. In individuals who are at risk of having coronary artery disease, the presence of these symptoms—dyspnea and exhaustion—should alert the physician to the possibility of myocardial ischemia, and this, in turn, should provoke further diagnostic evaluation. While ischemia may result in symptoms of brady- and tachyarrhythmias (palpitation, syncope, and sudden death), these are not usually called angina equivalents.

### Diagnostic Evaluation and Management of Angina Equivalents

The same principles of diagnosis and management that apply to patients with angina pectoris apply to patients with angina equivalents. Stress testing must be done with great caution; it should not be done at all when the symptoms have occurred within the preceding 60 days. As a rule, coronary arteriography is the procedure of choice to determine the status of the coronary arteries and ventricular contractility.

## PROLONGED MYOCARDIAL ISCHEMIA WITHOUT EVIDENCE OF MYOCARDIAL INFARCTION

Transient myocardial ischemia usually lasts less than 15 min. Prolonged myocardial ischemia may result in myocardial necrosis and acute MI. However, *prolonged myocardial ischemia without evidence of MI* also occurs. There may be no electrocardiographic abnormalities present, and the level of creatine kinase (CK) in the blood may remain normal. Chest pain may or may not be present. Two types of this subset of myocardial ischemia have been recognized: *prolonged chest discomfort* and *hibernating myocardium*.

### Pathophysiology

*Prolonged chest discomfort* due to myocardial ischemia but with no evidence of MI is, in reality, rather common. Patients with this syndrome often have severe obstructive coronary atherosclerosis in which superimposed coronary thrombosis is thought to play a significant role. There is a high incidence of cardiac events, especially in the weeks following its onset.

Patients with *hibernating myocardium* have severe coronary artery narrowing associated with severe myocardial wall motion abnormality (severe hypokinesis, akinesis, rarely dyskinesis).[5] Myocardial tissue is, at least in part, still viable according to the evidence provided by myocardial $^{201}$Tl perfusion scintigraphy, metabolic imaging, and improvement in response to positive inotropic agents and coronary revascularization. Myocardial function is depressed (to reduce oxygen demand), as a protective mechanism against the development of myocardial necrosis, as long as ischemia is present. Hibernating myocardium is a chronic form of prolonged myocardial ischemia. Thus it is unlikely that coronary thrombosis is important in the pathophysiology of this syndrome.

### Treatment of Prolonged Myocardial Ischemia Without Evidence of Myocardial Infarction

Patients with *prolonged chest discomfort due to myocardial ischemia without evidence of myocardial infarction* should be admitted to the intensive care unit, and IV nitroglycerin and IV heparin should be administered. Therapy with calcium antagonists and beta blockers is also helpful. The role of thrombolytic therapy requires further investigation before it can be recommended routinely. Coronary arteriography should be performed without delay. Exercise testing is contraindicated. Definitive treatment with angioplasty, bypass grafting, or medical therapy is based on results of coronary catheterization (coronary anatomy, ventricular function). In general, the majority of these patients require some form of coronary revascularization.

The presence of *hibernating myocardium* should be suspected in patients with angina pectoris (or objective evidence of ischemia) with severe wall motion abnormality in whom there is no history of MI and the ECG does not show abnormal Q waves. Cardiac catheterization is often required. Improvement in regional and overall ventricular function may be expected after myocardial perfusion is restored by an appropriate revascularization procedure.

### REFERENCES

1. Campeau L: Letter to the editor. *Circulation* 54:522, 1976.
2. Silverman JK, Grossman W: Current concepts of angina pectoris: Natural history and strategies for evaluation and management. *N Engl J Med* 310:1712–1717, 1984.
3. Theroux P, Ouimet H, McCans J, et al: Aspirin, heparin, or both to treat acute unstable angina. *N Engl J Med* 319:1105–1111, 1988.
4. Feldman RL: A review of medical therapy for coronary artery spasm. *Circulation* 75(Part 2):96–102V, 1987.
5. Rahimtoola SH: A perspective on the three large multicenter randomized clinical trials of coronary bypass surgery for chronic stable angina. *Circulation* 72(Suppl V):V123–135, 1985.

### SUGGESTED READING

ACC/AHA Task Force on Assessment of Cardiovascular Procedures: Guidelines for clinical use of cardiac radionuclide imaging. *J Am Coll Cardiol* 8:1471–1483, 1986.

ACC/AHA Task Force on Assessment of Diagnostic and Therapeutic Cardiovascular Procedures (Subcommittee on Coronary Arteriography): Guidelines for coronary arteriography. *J Am Coll Cardiol* 10:935–950, 1987.

ACC/AHA Task Force on Assessment of Diagnostic and Therapeutic Cardiovascular Procedures (Subcommittee on Exercise Testing): Guidelines for exercise testing. *J Am Coll Cardiol* 8:725–738, 1986.

ACC/AHA Task Force on Assessment of Diagnostic and Therapeutic Cardiovascular Procedures (Subcommittee on Percutaneous Transluminal Coronary Angioplasty): Guidelines for percutaneous transluminal coronary angioplasty. *J Am Coll Cardiol* 12:529–545, 1988.

Cairns JA, Gent M, Singer J, et al: Aspirin, sulfinpyrazone, or both in unstable angina. *N Engl J Med* 313:1369–1375, 1985.

Crawford MH: The role of triple therapy in patients with chronic stable angina pectoris. *Circulation* 75(Part 2):122–127V, 1987.

Gottlieb SO, Weisfeldt ML, Ouyang P, et al: Silent ischemia as a marker for early unfavorable outcomes in patients with unstable angina. *N Engl J Med* 314:1214–1219, 1986.

Heberden W: Some account of a disorder of the breast. *Med Trans Roy Coll Physicians* 2:59–67, 1772.

Hurst JW: The recognition and treatment of four types of angina pectoris and angina equivalents, in Hurst JW (ed): *The Heart,* 7th ed. New York, McGraw-Hill, Chap 53A, pp 1046–1052, 1990.

Hurst JW: The recognition and treatment of prolonged myocardial ischemia with no evidence of infarction, in Hurst JW (ed): *The Heart,* 7th ed. New York, McGraw-Hill, Chap 53B, pp 1052–1054, 1990.

Lewis HD, Davis JW, Archibald DG, et al: Protective effects of aspirin against acute myocardial infarction and death in men with unstable angina: Results of a Veterans Administration Cooperative Study. *N Engl J Med* 313:1369–1375, 1985.

Loop FD, Lytle BW, Gosgrove DM, et al: Influence of the internal-mammary-artery graft on 10-year survival and other cardiac events. *N Engl J Med* 314:1–6, 1986.

Nesto RW, Kowalchuk GJ: The ischemic cascade: Temporal sequence of hemodynamic, electrocardiographic and symptomatic expressions of ischemia. *Am J Cardiol* 59:23–30C, 1987.

Takaro, T, Hultgren HN, Tipton MJ, et al: The VA cooperative randomized study of surgery for coronary arterial occlusive disease: II. Subgroups with significant left main lesions. *Circulation* 54(Suppl 3):107–117, 1977.

Tillisch J, Brunken R, Marshall R, Schwaiger M, Mandelkern M, Phelps M, Schelbert H: Reversibility of cardiac wall motion abnormalities predicted by positron tomography. *N Engl J Med* 314:884–888, 1986.

Varnauskas E and The European Coronary Surgery Study Group: Twelve-year follow-up of survival in the randomized European Coronary Surgery Study. *N Engl J Med* 319:332–337, 1988.

Waters DD, Bouchard A, Theroux P: Spontaneous remission is a frequent outcome of variant angina. *J Am Coll Cardiol* 2:195–199, 1983.

## 12 | Acute Myocardial Infarction

*Angel Leon, M.D.    Douglas Morris, M.D.*

## EVOLVING MYOCARDIAL INFARCTION

### Definition

An *evolving myocardial infarction* is a process in which a segment of the myocardium is progressing from ischemia to actual necrosis because of occlusion of a coronary artery. This concept implies that the progression may be arrested prior to completion.

### Pathophysiology

Pathological and angiographic data implicate coronary thrombosis as the cause of coronary occlusion in over 80 percent of acute transmural myocardial infarctions. Three factors are necessary for the development of a coronary thrombosis: (1) abnormalities in the intima or coronary endothelium, usually due to an atherosclerotic lesion; (2) an active thrombotic system; and (3) a triggering event to create an interaction of factors (1) and (2).

Thrombi usually form at the site of a preexisting atherosclerotic lesion when components of a ruptured plaque, such as collagen fibers, are exposed to platelets, resulting in platelet aggregation and clot formation. The triggering event is usually ill defined but may represent plaque hemorrhage or coronary spasm.

Hypercoagulable states have been recognized in some patients with acute infarcts; however, it is uncertain whether these states are a cause of thrombosis or merely a response to vessel injury.

Irreversible damage, with cellular death, begins within 20 to 40 min of coronary artery occlusion. Ischemia, followed by infarction, develops first in the subendocardial myocardium and expands outward in a wavefront pattern, ultimately becoming transmural. Presumably, the process begins in the subendocardium because this area has the highest myocardial oxygen demand and the most tenuous blood supply.

The term *ischemic cascade* describes the order of events resulting from a coronary occlusion. First, diastolic relaxation of myocardial fibers is impaired; then contractile activity is affected. These changes are followed by ischemic electrocardiographic changes, and, last, by symptoms.

## Recognition

### Clinical Presentation

The immediate recognition of infarction depends on the correct interpretation of the patient's symptoms. Persistent *chest discomfort*, or its equivalent, for over 15 min is usually the presenting complaint. The characteristic chest discomfort associated with a myocardial infarction is retrosternal—pressure, squeezing, or a "heavy" sensation. This pain often radiates into the anterior precordium, the jaw, the medial aspect of the arms, or the elbows.

Up to 30 percent of myocardial infarctions go unrecognized because of the absence of these typical symptoms; however, only about 5 percent of infarcts are truly silent. Unrecognized infarction occurs most commonly in diabetic, hypertensive, and elderly patients.

### Physical Examination

Physical findings during an evolving infarction are very nonspecific. *Restlessness, diaphoresis, and hypertension* occur commonly. Auscultation of the heart may reveal an atrial gallop, reflecting an ischemic, noncompliant ventricle. A ventricular gallop, depending on its location, implies left or right ventricular dysfunction. Physical findings such as hypotension, jugular venous distension, pulmonary rales, or new murmurs are most helpful in identifying the complications of acute infarction.

### Electrocardiography

The progression of electrocardiographic changes in myocardial infarction is as follows:

1. T-wave abnormalities: Symmetrically peaked T waves or inverted T waves suggesting ischemia. (These very early changes are often missed.)
2. ST-segment elevation in the leads overlying the infarction, implying injury to the epicardium.
3. ST-segment elevation with T-wave inversion.
4. Evolution of pathological Q waves, implying cell death.

TABLE 12-1 Localization of Infarct by Electrocardiogram

| Area of infarct | Leads with abnormal Q waves |
|---|---|
| Inferior | II, II, $aV_F$ |
| Lateral | I, $aV_L$, $V_6$ |
| Anteroseptal | $V_1$, $V_2$ |
| Anterior | $V_1$ to $V_6$ |
| Right ventricular | $V_3R$, $V_4R$ |

The sensitivity of the ECG changes in acute myocardial infarction is reduced by the presence of previous infarction, the frequent absence of QRS-complex changes in posterolateral infarctions, and the presence of left bundle branch block. In assessing the patient with new-onset chest pain, the physician must remember that there may be a delay in the appearance of ECG changes.

The specificity of the ECG in recognizing acute infarction is reduced by the presence of electrolyte abnormalities, by ST displacement due to an old aneurysm or pericarditis, and by such normal variants as the early repolarization pattern. The specificity of Q waves as a marker of completed infarction is reduced after the administration of thrombolytic therapy.

### Chest Roentgenography

In an uncomplicated infarct, the chest x-ray is normal. The presence of pulmonary interstitial edema suggests significant left ventricular dysfunction. An enlarged cardiac silhouette implies previous heart disease or pericardial effusion.

### Cardiac Enzymes

Creatine phosphokinase (CPK), lactate dehydrogenase (LDH), and serum glutamic-oxaloacetic transaminase (SGOT) are all released by membrane disruption in dead myocytes. Subfractions specific to cardiac muscle are the CPK–MB band, and the $LDH_1$ isoenzyme.

Serum CPK rises above the normal range about 6 h after a myocardial infarction. Peak loads are reached at approximately 24 h; then the level gradually declines over the next 24 h if myocyte death has stopped. The area under the CPK curve, plotted over time, correlates fairly well with the amount of muscle damage.

If the coronary occlusion reponsible for the infarction spontaneously resolves or is eliminated by thrombolytic therapy, the restoration of blood flow will "wash out" the enzyme released. The peak activity occurs and resolves much sooner with early reperfusion.

For diagnosing infarction more than 48 h beyond the onset of symptoms, the ratio of $LDH_1$ to $LDH_2$ is helpful. ($LDH_1/LDH_2 > 1$ suggests myocardial infarction.)

### Radionuclide Imaging

Isotopes have been developed that identify either "cold spots" of decreased radionuclide uptake due to cell death, or "hot spots" due to foci of labeled inflammatory cells negating to the area of an infarction.

*Thallium-201* ($^{201}$Tl) is a flow marker that produces a defect in an area of infarction regardless of its age. Flow to an infarcted area is absent, due to death of the capillary bed and myocytes in that segment. Persistent $^{201}$Tl images (rest and redistribution scans) can appear as early as 6 h after an arterial occlusion.

Technetium-99m pyrophosphate ($^{99m}$Tc) is an infarct-avid agent that serves as a marker of postnecrotic inflammation. It has little sensitivity until 24 h after infarction, and it requires a significant amount of transmural necrosis before a diagnostic "hot spot" is detected.

Exercise testing and dipyridamole infusion are absolutely contraindicated in the setting of an evolving infarct.

### Echocardiography

Two-dimensional echocardiography can identify akinetic and hypokinetic regions caused by infarction. Segments with compensatory hypercontractility may also be apparent. The primary limitation is the inability of echocardiography to discriminate accurately between new and old infarctions.

Echocardiography is most useful in detecting complications of acute infarction, such as mural thrombi, and coexisting heart disease, such as myocardial hypertrophy and valvular lesions.

## Treatment

The major goals of treatment during an evolving infarct are to alleviate symptoms, to preserve as much myocardium as possible, and to monitor the patient properly for the early recognition and management of possible complications.

### Analgesia

Symptomatic relief is important not only for the patient's comfort, but also to suppress autonomic activity and reduce myocardial oxygen demand. *Opiates and their synthetic derivatives* are the best agents available for reducing pain and anxiety:

• *Morphine*, 4–8 mg IV, while carefully monitoring blood pressure and respiratory rate.
• *Meperidine*, 25–50 mg IV, may cause less vagal stimulation, especially in patients with inferior infarction.

Intravenous *nitroglycerin* can reduce anginal pain by reducing myocardial oxygen demand. This is accomplished by peripheral venous and arterial dilation, resulting in decreased filling pressures and lower wall stress. It may also increase collateral circulation to ischemic myocardium by dilating epicardial coronaries. Dosage should begin at 5 μg/min and increase by 5 μg/min until pain is relieved or blood pressure is lowered more than 10 percent. After 24 to 48 h of intravenous administration, the patient can be put on topical agents if symptoms have not recurred.

*Preservation of Myocardium—Reducing Oxygen Demand*

Altering the demand/supply imbalance that occurs during ischemia may reduce the amount of irreversible myocardial damage. When given as described under "Analgesia," *nitroglycerin* may reduce infarct size.

*Beta blockers* and *calcium antagonists* may also reduce myocardial oxygen demand. There is significant evidence that the early administration of beta blockers reduces infarct size and improves short- and long-term survival. By suppressing sympathetic activity these agents reduce blood pressure, contractility, and heart rate, which contribute to oxygen demand. They may also reduce the frequency of lethal arrhythmias and cardiac rupture following acute infarction. The most widely used agent is *metoprolol* (5 mg IV every 15 min, × 3, then 25 mg PO every 8 h, increasing to 50 mg PO every 8 h). The ultra-short-acting beta blocker *esmolol* can be easily titrated as an intravenous infusion.

*Increasing Myocardial Blood Flow*

Intravenous *heparinization* and oral *aspirin* in the setting of unstable angina or evolving infarction reduce platelet aggregation and the progression of intracoronary thrombus formation. Heparin should be given as a 5000-unit bolus followed by an infusion to keep the PTT at 1 to 2.5 times control. Aspirin is given as a tablet (80 or 325 mg) or dissolved in water. Full heparinization is used for 24 to 48 h following thrombolysis or when lytic therapy is not indicated.

In the setting of right ventricular infarction, *nitroglycerin* may lower right ventricular filling pressures and, as a consequence, drastically reduce left ventricular filling and output.

*Thrombolytic Therapy*

The introduction of thrombolytic agents has significantly reduced mortality and myocardial damage by opening occluded vessels and arresting the progression of cell necrosis in all types of evolving infarcts. The criteria for administering lytic therapy are:

1. Chest pain of 6 hours' duration or less.
2. ST-segment elevation consistent with epicardial injury.
3. No recent surgery (within 2 weeks) or cerebrovascular accident (within 6 months).
4. No active ulcer disease.

Age is only a relative contraindication; clinical trials are now including patients up to 75 years old.

Venipuncture should be limited to easily compressible areas. Arterial puncture should be avoided. Women of childbearing age have been excluded from all thrombolytic trials.

A number of agents have been developed and tested; strepto-kinase and tissue plasminogen activator (tPA) are the most commonly used. Their characteristics are:

- *Streptokinase:* Bacterial product; non-clot-specific; induces a systemic lytic state; premedication with 100 mg hydrocortisone IV and 25 mg Benadryl IV is usually applied; reperfusion rate 45 to 50 percent; relatively inexpensive. Dose: 1.5 million units over 1 h.
- *Tissue plasminogen activator (tPA):* Product of recombinant DNA technology; relatively clot-specific; induces a systemic lytic state; no premedication needed; reperfusion rate about 70 percent; relatively expensive. Dose: 10-mg bolus, 50 mg over first hour, 20 mg over each hour for 2 h.

Lytic therapy should be followed by full heparinization for 24 to 48 h. Tissue plasminogen activator appears to be the more potent lytic agent, with greater efficacy in reperfusing coronary arteries; but it does seem to be associated with a greater likelihood of reocclusion of the infarct-related artery.

### Mechanical Reperfusion—Coronary Angioplasty

In special situations where the facilities of a catheterization laboratory are immediately available, *emergency angioplasty* of the infarct-related coronary artery is a reasonable alternative to thrombolytic therapy. Reperfusion can be achieved in approximately 85 percent of acutely occluded arteries.

Coronary angioplasty immediately following thrombolytic therapy has not proved so successful. If needed at all, it should be delayed for 5 to 7 days after thrombolysis.

### The Role of Coronary Care Units (CCUs)

Every patient with an evolving myocardial infarction should be transferred to a coronary care unit (CCU). Since their introduction, CCUs have reduced the in-hospital mortality due to acute myocardial infarction. This is due mainly to the early detection and treatment of lethal arrhythmias occurring during the first 24 to 48 h after an infarction. In this setting, ventricular tachycardia (VT) and ventricular fibrillation (VF) can occur without warning; there is no arrhythmia that is a reliable harbinger of VT or of VF. The suppression of complex ventricular ectopy in the first 24 to 48 h after an infarction, however, may reduce the incidence of VT and VF. The use of prophylactic intravenous antiarrhythmic drugs is controversial, since these agents have cardiac and noncardiac side effects. In general, *lidocaine* should be considered if PVCs or more complex ventricular ectopic activity are present during this early postinfarction period (75–150-mg IV bolus followed by 1–3 mg/min infusion), but the drug should not be pushed to potentially toxic levels or replaced with another antiarrhythmic agent unless nonsustained or sustained VT or VF develops. (See Table 12-2.)

After 72 h, patients with uncomplicated infarction may be transferred to routine nursing wards. Any CCU patient with (1) anterior myocardial infarction; (2) arrhythmias of pump failure (sinus tachycardia, atrial fibrillation, or atrial flutter); (3) heart block; or (4) congestive failure should be transferred to a step-down unit where telemetry is available. These patients are at risk for late in-hospital sudden death; care in a monitored setting reduces this risk by 50 percent.

## COMPLETED MYOCARDIAL INFARCTION

### Definition

A myocardial infarction is *complete* when necrosis has consumed all the territory made ischemic by occlusion of the coronary artery serving that segment.

### Pathophysiology

The degree of transmural necrosis varies according to the establishment of collateral circulation or to recanalization of the infarct-related artery. The lateral margins of the infarct are determined by the distribution of the infarct-related artery. Myocardial cell death presents in one of two forms: (1) coagulative necrosis occurring in the distribution of arteries that remain completely occluded, and (2) contraction-band necrosis resulting when flow to infarcted tissue is reestablished.

After necrosis is complete the following cellular reaction takes place in the zone of infarction.

- Days 1–3: Edema, polymorphonuclear cell infiltrate, loss of nuclei.
- Days 2–9: Lymphocytic infiltrate, plasma cells appear in region of infarction.
- Days 4–10: Granulation tissue, loss of myocardial fibers.
- Days 9–60: Collagen deposition.

TABLE 12-2 General Measures of Coronary Case Unit (CCU)

Analgesia
    Morphine sulfate 2 mg IV every 10 min until relief is obtained, *or:*
    Meperidine HCl 25–50 mg IV (repeat in 15 min if necessary)
Nasal oxygen therapy
Clear liquid diet for 24 h
Stool softeners; laxative
Bed rest with bedside commode for 24 h
? Role for subcutaneous heparin
Continuous ECG monitoring

Overall contractile activity is inversely related to the size of the infarct. Soon after infarction, unaffected segments become hyper-contractile, and infarcted segments bulge during systole. The noncontracting segment of myocardium also shows changes in its diastolic properties. As cellular infiltration and tissue edema occur, this segment will progressively stiffen. After the healing phase of the infarction is completed, there will be decreased left ventricular compliance due to the remaining fibrous scar.

## Clinical Evidence of Completed Infarction

The diagnosis of a completed acute myocardial infarction is based on the following:

1. Resolution of chest pain or other symptoms that heralded the infarction.
2. Development of pathological Q waves and T-wave inversion. (This is not a specific sign when lytic therapy is used, nor is it sensitive when infarction is limited to the subendocardium.)
3. Enzymatic markers returning to baseline levels.

## Therapy

Patients admitted to the hospital within 48 h after the onset of chest pain should be placed in the CCU. Since the major focus of the CCU is the immediate recognition and expeditious treatment of cardiac arrhythmias, a patient could be transferred from this unit after 48 h without complex ventricular ectopy.

Some patients need more prolonged cardiac monitoring. About one-third of in-hospital deaths occur after discharge from the CCU; half of these are sudden and unexpected. A prime candidate for late in-hospital sudden death shows at least one of the following while in the CCU:

- Arrhythmias of pump failure (sinus tachycardia, atrial flutter, or atrial fibrillation).
- Arrhythmias of electrical instability (VT or VF).
- Acute intraventricular conduction disturbances.
- Circulatory failure (congestive heart failure, pulmonary edema, or significant hypotension).
- Anterior location of infarction.

After discharge from the CCU, the goals of management should be the rehabilitation of the patient—addressing the patient's (and spouse's) psychological needs, risk-factor modification, and activity plan—and the identification of patients at high risk of recurrent infarction or sudden death. The physician should obtain a reasonably accurate assessment of ventricular function, either by echocardiography or by radionuclide or contrast ventriculography. Identification of patients at risk of reinfarction can be based on one of three diagnostic techniques: exercise electrocardiography, exercise thallium scintigraphy, or coronary angiography.

## Acute Complications and In-Hospital Management

### Postinfarction Ischemia

The recurrence of chest pain or ischemic electrocardiographic changes at rest after an infarction suggests the presence of myocardium at risk for further necrosis. This may occur at the border of the infarct zone, or in a distant region, implying multivessel coronary disease.

For patients with postinfarction ischemia one should institute, or intensify, *antithrombotic therapy,* with full heparinization and aspirin; and *antianginal therapy,* including intravenous nitroglycerin, beta blockers, and/or calcium antagonists. These patients should undergo early cardiac catheterization to evaluate the potential of revascularization.

### Pump Failure

Pump failure may be seen with significant necrosis of either ventricle. *Right ventricular infarction* results in inadequate filling of the left ventricle and a marked drop in cardiac output. Right ventricular infarction occurs in at least 33 percent of inferior infarctions but is clinically apparent in only 1 to 2 percent. Significant right ventricular dysfunction can be recognized by jugular venous distension and hypotension without evidence of pulmonary congestion. The echocardiogram or radionuclide ventriculogram will confirm the diagnosis by demonstrating a dilated, noncontractile right ventricle. The diagnosis is usually made without the need for right-sided cardiac catheterization. Initial therapy consists of *volume expansion* with colloids or crystalloids. Low doses of dobutamine or dopamine will improve right ventricular function, but rarely completely correct the hypotension without the use of volume expansion. If bradycardia is present, pacing of the right atrium may prove beneficial.

Pump failure most commonly is secondary to *left ventricular dysfunction* leading to inadequate cardiac output. More than 40 percent of the left ventricular muscle mass must be affected before this state of circulatory inadequacy is reached. Left ventricular pump failure occurs in 10 to 15 percent of all patients with acute myocardial infarction.

The loss of left ventricular contractility and stroke volume triggers an increase in peripheral resistance, tachycardia, and volume retention, which lead to pulmonary congestion and decreased oxygen delivery to tissue. Progressive dysfunction results in systemic hypotension and cardiogenic shock, which carries a mortality of up to 70 percent.

*Invasive monitoring* with pulmonary and intraarterial catheters helps to optimize therapy in these patients. The goals of therapy are:

1. Maintain a cardiac index of at least 2.5 liters/min/m$^2$ with adequate perfusion pressure to vital organs.
2. Reduce pulmonary wedge pressure below 24 mmHg by preload reduction and diuresis.
3. Reduce systemic vascular resistance while maintaining a mean systemic pressure of 60 mmHg or more.

*Nitroprusside infusion* reduces preload and afterload, with maintenance of an adequate blood pressure as the limiting factor. *Nitroglycerin* reduces preload, ischemia, and pulmonary congestion. *Inotropic agents,* such as low-dose dopamine, dobutamine, and amrinone, increase contractility. To correct hypotension, dopamine, in high doses, and specific alpha-receptor agonists are indicated. When pharmacological measures fail to achieve therapeutic goals, *balloon counterpulsation* and *ventricular-assist devices* may stabilize the patient.

### Myocardial Rupture

Rupture of the intraventricular septum, left ventricular free wall, or papillary muscles occurs in up to 15 percent of lethal myocardial infarctions. Free-wall rupture accounts for 85 percent of these ruptures, septal rupture for 10 to 14 percent, and papillary-muscle rupture for the rest.

*Risk factors* for cardiac rupture are hypertension, inferior infarction, advanced age, and diabetes. It occurs most commonly after the first infarction. The size of the infarct is not related to the probability of rupture. Rupture may occur at any time during the first 2 weeks after infarction; the peak incidence is between 5 and 7 days after infarction.

Free-wall rupture occurs most commonly in the posterior lateral segment of the left ventricle; when the site of rupture is sealed by pericardium, a pseudoaneurysm forms. Rupture of the septum results from either anterior or inferior infarction. Rupture of the inferior-posterior papillary muscle occurs more commonly than rupture of the anterior superior muscle, because of the former's single, tenuous coronary arterial supply. Recurrence of chest pain, acute onset of heart failure, development of hypotension, or the emergence of a new murmur suggests rupture.

The *diagnosis* can be made by two-dimensional echocardiography, which can detect septal and free-wall tears, new pericardial effusions, or flail papillary muscles; mitral regurgitation can be documented by Doppler sampling. Right-sided cardiac catheterization detects increases in venous blood oxygen saturation resulting from the intracardiac shunting that follows septal rupture.

The only definitive *treatment* is surgical repair of muscle tears and replacement of the mitral valve. Free-wall tears not sealed by the pericardium require immediate closure. Intensive medical therapy and balloon counterpulsation for ventricular septal defects and papillary-muscle rupture can stabilize the patient in preparation for urgent surgery. Pseudoaneurysms, even in stable patients, should be repaired when discovered, since they are at risk for rupture.

*Electrical Instability—Arrhythmias (See Chapters 3 and 4)*

Coronary occlusion creates areas of electrical instability in the border zone between necrotic and normal tissue. These injured, but viable, cells become partly depolarized, creating a network of slow-conducting fibers that serves as a substrate for reentrant arrhythmias.

After the resolution of early postinfarction edema and inflammation, most border regions either recover completely or fibrose; those that retain abnormal electrical activity take part in the genesis of arrhythmias.

During the first 24 to 48 h, complex ectopy, ventricular tachycardia (VT), and primary ventricular fibrillation (VF) are common. Except for an association between primary VF and increased in-hospital mortality, these early arrhythmias have little long-term prognostic importance. Complex ventricular arrhythmias occurring more than 72 h after infarction are associated with an increased incidence of sudden death in certain groups after infarction.

Supraventricular arrhythmias, such as sinus tachycardia or atrial flutter or fibrillation, suggest that a large mass of ventricular muscle has been infarcted and, therefore, they have earned the name "pump failure arrhythmias."

Accelerated junctional and idioventricular rhythms occur commonly after inferior infarction and have little negative prognostic value. When they occur after an anterior infarction with left ventricular dysfunction the prognosis is worse, usually because of the size of the infarct.

*Electrical Instability—Conduction Blocks*

Infarction of the specialized conduction fibers can block the normal propagation of electrical activity throughout the heart, causing varying degrees of heart block or bundle branch blocks. Parasympathetic reflexes can also create bradycardia and heart block by vagal effects on the proximal portions of the conduction system. Recognizing the type of block that is present is of crucial importance, since conduction disturbances below the AV node can progress to complete heart block and death.

*First-degree AV block* (PR prolongation >0.20 s) is the most common conduction disturbance following an acute myocardial infarction (occurring in 4 to 14 percent of cases). *Mobitz type I second-degree AV block* (progressive PR prolongation followed by a blocked P wave) is second, occurring in 4 to 10 percent of all infarctions. The conduction block in these cases is located proximal to the His bundle. These supra-His blocks occur almost exclusively after inferior infarction, because of stimulation of local parasympathetic fibers of the vagus nerve. First-degree and Mobitz type I AV block respond to the administration of *atropine* (0.6 mg IV) and do not require temporary pacing.

*Mobitz type II block* (blocked P waves not preceded by PR prolongation) occurs essentially only after anterior myocardial infarction. The location of the block is below the His bundle, and progression to high-degree AV block is common (occurring in more than 60 percent of cases). Insertion of a temporary pacemaker is warranted. Patients who progress to *complete heart block,* even if it is transient, require permanent pacing as well. High-degree or complete heart block (AV dissociation with a ventricular rate below 50 beats per minute) with anterior infarction implies that a large amount of myocardial necrosis has occurred. The prognosis is poor because of the size of the infarct.

*Third-degree heart block* can follow an inferior infarction; it commonly results from AV nodal ischemia. The prognosis is not so poor as with anterior infarction, and the block is transient. Temporary pacing is needed only to correct symptomatic bradyarrhythmias or hypotension.

### Bundle Branch Block

The occurrence of bundle branch block after myocardial infarction is significant; it suggests that the infarction may be extensive, and it may be the only warning of impending precipitous complete heart block.

As is suggested by the source of the blood supply to the intraventricular conduction system, bundle branch block is primarily a complication of anteroseptal myocardial infarction. Data on the frequency of progression of various conduction blocks to complete heart block suggests the following:

- Unilateral bundle branch block probably is not an indication for prophylactic temporary pacing.
- Prophylactic temporary standby pacing is indicated in patients with *bilateral bundle branch block* (RBBB with left anterior fascicular block or RBBB with left posterior fascicular block).

- Permanent pacing is indicated if bilateral bundle branch block progresses to *complete heart block*, even if the complete block is transient.

### Systemic Thromboembolism

*Venous thromboembolism* complicates the in-hospital course of 5 to 10 percent of patients with acute myocardial infarction. Risk factors include previous thromboembolism, obesity, cardiogenic shock, and advanced age.

*Arterial embolism* results in cerebral, mesenteric, renal, or peripheral ischemia. The origin is usually mural thrombi in akinetic or dyskinetic ventricular segments.

All patients requiring prolonged bed rest after infarction should receive low-dose *heparin* (5000 units every 8 h) unless they are on full systemic anticoagulation for other reasons.

### Pericarditis

Local inflammation of the pericardium overlying an area of transmural necrosis occurs in 30 to 50 percent of transmural infarctions, but is clinically apparent in only 10 to 15 percent.

A second mechanism of pericardial inflammation (occurring after 2 to 3 percent of myocardial infarctions) is an antibody-mediated response to myocardial antigens released during the infarction. This condition is similar to the postpericardiectomy syndrome that follows open heart surgery, and presents from weeks to months after infarction.

*Symptoms* of pericarditis include chest pain, sometimes pleuritic, which radiates to the shoulder and neck. The ECG shows diffuse ST-segment elevation, except in lead $aV_R$, where ST depression and PR elevation are seen. The white blood cell count and erythrocyte sedimentation rate may be elevated.

*Treatment* consists of either nonsteroidal anti-inflammatory drugs, such as aspirin or indomethacin, or, if symptoms persist, corticosteroids (dexamethasone 8 mg IV or prednisolone 60 mg PO).

## RISK STRATIFICATION

### Prognosis

Prior to the use of thrombolytic therapy, overall in-hospital mortality for myocardial infarction was from 12 to 15 percent, with an additional 3 to 5 percent per year following discharge. Widespread use of lytic agents reduces in-hospital mortality to 8 to 10 percent; post-discharge mortality remains unchanged.

Patients discharged with anterior infarcts are at greater risk for 1-year mortality (10 percent) than those with inferior infarcts (6 percent).

Right ventricular infarction and high-degree AV block increase the in-hospital mortality following inferior infarction, but do not affect long-term survival.

The in-hospital mortality from non-Q-wave infarction is low (under 5 percent), but the 1-year mortality approaches that following transmural infarction. This equilibration in 1-year mortality is due primarily to a higher reinfarction rate with non-Q-wave infarction.

*Resting left ventricular ejection fraction* is the strongest single predictor of survival following infarction. This may be obtained by gated radionuclide blood-pool imaging, echocardiography, or contrast ventriculography.

## Exercise Testing

Symptom-limited exercise stress testing is safe 7 to 10 days after infarction if there are no rest angina, heart failure, or significant ventricular arrhythmias. Some investigators suggest that in uncomplicated infarction following successful thrombolytic therapy, stress testing 48 h after infarction is safe and can select candidates for very early discharge. If pre-discharge stress testing is normal, further exercise testing after discharge adds little prognostic information. It may, however, guide the patient's physical activity during cardiac rehabilitation.

*Exercise-induced ischemia* after infarction is highly predictive of multivessel disease. The presence of exercise-induced angina, ST-segment depression greater than 1 mm, or hypotension suggests that a patient will benefit from early coronary angiography and revascularization.

Adding *thallium-201 scintigraphy* to exercise testing detects underlying ischemia with high sensitivity and specificity in multivessel disease.

[201]Tl imaging is less sensitive in detecting residual ischemia superimposed on infarction in single-vessel disease. It is unclear whether PET imaging offers any improvement.

## Coronary Arteriography

Angiographic evidence of left main coronary artery diameter stenosis greater than 50 percent, significant three-vessel disease with LV dysfunction, or two-vessel disease with tight proximal LAD occlusion is an independent predictor of increased ischemic events and mortality following infarction, despite good medical therapy. Patients with these conditions should proceed to revascularization. Most of these patients are identified by symptoms appearing at rest or on noninvasive tests.

Since the introduction of thrombolytic therapy, the routine use of coronary angiography has become controversial. It used to be that all patients underwent cardiac catheterization. Now there is evidence that groups at low risk for further events can be identified with pre-discharge exercise radionuclide imaging, without the use of coronary arteriography, after successful lytic therapy.

### Predicting Lethal Arrhythmias

Ambulatory ECG monitoring during recovery from myocardial infarction may predict late sudden death from ventricular tachycardia (VT) or ventricular fibrillation (VF). The sensitivity of Holter monitoring is low, because of the unpredictable peak in ectopic activity that may occur up to 6 weeks after infarction.

In patients without bundle branch block, signal-averaged ECG monitoring can detect the presence of late potentials arising from arrhythmogenic foci. These after-depolarizations occur in tissue that may form the slow conducting loops of reentrant pathways. The two most predictive parameters are a prolonged QRS duration (>120 ms) and a root mean square voltage (RMS) of less than 20 mv in the last 40 ms of the QRS. Late potentials occur in up to 35 percent of anterior, and 60 percent of inferior, infarcts.

The absence of late potentials after infarction makes the probability of inducing VT remote (less than 2 percent). The presence of postinfarction late potentials is quite sensitive in predicting the induction of VT, but only moderately specific. The specificity improves significantly (approaching 90 percent) in patients with late potentials and poor left ventricular function (ejection fraction less than 40 percent).

Patients with positive signal-averaged ECGs or clinical sustained VT more than 72 h after infarction should undergo ventricular stimulation to determine whether they have inducible, and subsequently suppressible, VT.

The inability to induce VT is associated with a low probability of sudden death in the first year after infarction.

Before one proceeds with ventricular stimulation, coronary angiography should be performed to exclude active ischemia as a cause of VT and to avoid rapid pacing in the setting of significant coronary stenosis.

## CHRONIC MEDICAL THERAPY

### Nitrates

There are no data to support the use of long-term nitrate therapy following uncomplicated myocardial infarction. If angina recurs, these agents can be used acutely to alleviate symptoms.

## Aspirin

The use of aspirin as an antiplatelet agent reduces the incidence of myocardial infarction in patients with coronary artery disease. Unless an absolute contraindication exists (e.g., active ulcer disease or allergy), every patient should be placed on aspirin after a myocardial infarction. For patients who cannot tolerate 325 mg daily, 80-mg dosages enteric-coated tablets are available.

## Beta Blockers

Long-term trials show that the use of beta blockers without sympathomimetic activity reduces mortality following anterior infarction. The data are less supportive following inferior infarction. Metoprolol (25–100 mg bid), timolol (5–15 mg bid), and atenolol (25–100 mg daily) are all efficacious.

The reduction in mortality acutely and chronically is greater in patients with large infarcts and ventricular dysfunction. So long as congestive failure symptoms are not worsened by beta blockers, a low left ventricular ejection fraction is not a contraindication to their use after infarction.

## Calcium Antagonists

The use of these drugs for routine therapy after transmural myocardial infarction lacks supportive data. Diltiazem may be beneficial after a non-Q-wave infarction in a patient who shows no evidence of left ventricular dysfunction.

## Anticoagulation

Full anticoagulation with warfarin (prothrombin time 1½ to 2 times control) is indicated in patients with demonstrable mobile or pedunculated mural thrombi on echocardiography. Most of the thrombi will develop in the first 48 h after infarction; some will appear as late as 7 days after. Two courses of action seem appropriate in large anterior-apical infarcts: (1) give all of these patients anticoagulation, beginning with heparin on day 1; or (2) treat only those developing mobile or pedunculated mural thrombi. If the latter course is followed, the patient should have echocardiograms on day 2 and day 7, looking for mural thrombi. This latter approach may also reduce thromboembolism in patients with akinetic and dyskinetic segments following large anterior-apical infarcts. Patients with deep-vein thrombosis or pulmonary embolism should also be given oral anticoagulants.

There is no evidence supporting the continued use of anticoagulants beyond 6 months after infarction.

### Digoxin

Chronic treatment with digoxin (0.125–0.375 mg daily) seems beneficial in patients manifesting a ventricular gallop, pulmonary rales, left ventricular ejection fraction below 35 percent, or atrial fibrillation following a myocardial infarction.

### Diuretics

Loop diuretics and thiazides can counteract the overcompensatory volume excess associated with ventricular dysfunction. Hypokalemia must be prevented, since it may trigger dysrythmias in these patients.

### Angiotensin-Converting Enzyme (ACE) Inhibitors

Captopril (6.25 mg to 50 mg tid) reduces left ventricular chamber dimensions after anterior infarction. Trials are under way to see whether survival is also improved. These agents have already proved beneficial in the treatment of chronic congestive failure.

### Antiarrhythmic Agents

#### Supraventricular Arrhythmias

Digoxin and—if tolerated—verapamil, diltiazem, and/or beta blockers can control the rate of AV conduction during atrial fibrillation and atrial flutter. Beneficial conversion to sinus rhythm can be attained by class IA antiarrhythmics (procainamide, quinidine, and disopyrimide). Therapy should be initiated in a monitored setting, since proarrhythmias may occur.

#### Ventricular Arrhythmias

There is no data to support the routine suppression of premature ventricular contractions (PVCs) and couplets following infarction. The proarrhythmic effects of some drugs (encainide, flecainide) may actually increase mortality.

### RISK FACTOR MODIFICATION

Prior to discharge, every patient with an infarct should receive counseling on reducing reversible risk factors, including:

- Smoking: Explain the availability of programs and support groups for discontinuation.
- Hypertension: Urge dietary salt reduction, exercise, and weight loss as well as medical therapy.

- Hypercholesterolemia: The patient should have a consultation with a dietician to begin dietary measures and medical treatment with bile sequestrants (cholestyramine), niacin, gemfibrozil, or a more potent agent (e.g., lovastatin).

## PHYSICAL ACTIVITY AND CARDIAC REHABILITATION

### In-Hospital Guidelines (Uncomplicated Infarction)

| Day | Level of Activity |
|---|---|
| 1 | Bed rest in CCU; may use bedside toilet. |
| 2 | Sitting in chair twice daily. |
| 3–5 | Discharge from CCU; ambulation in room. |
| 6–7 | Ambulation in hallway. |
| 7–10 | Pre discharge exercise testing. |

### Guidelines for Activity After Discharge

| Week | Level of Activity |
|---|---|
| 1 | In-house activities; avoid isometric work. |
| 2–3 | Daily walks of increasing duration. |
| 4 | Resume driving and sexual intercourse. |
| 6–8 | Return to work (half-days for first week). |

Motivated patients may be enrolled in a formal, medically supervised rehabilitation program. Exercise testing can identify patients at high risk for such activity. The benefits of these programs include peer support, improved aerobic metabolism, and increased exercise tolerance.

## SUGGESTED READING

Braunwald E (ed): Symposium on modern thrombolytic therapy. *J Am Coll Cardiol* 10(suppl B):1B–104B, 1987.

Cinitron GB, Hernandez E, Livares E, et al: Bedside recognition, incidence and clinical course of right ventricular infarction. *Am J Cardiol* 47:224–227, 1981.

Conti CR: Myocardial infarction: Rationale for therapy in 1989. *Clin Cardiol* 12:III-1–III-100, 1989.

Harrison DG: Should lidocaine be administered routinely to all patients after acute myocardial infarction? *Circulation* 58:581–584, 1978.

Helfant RH, Klein LW: The Q-wave and non-Q-wave myocardial infarction: Differences and similarities. *Prog Cardiovasc Dis* 29:205–220, 1986.

Hindman MC, Wagner GS, JaRo M, et al: The clinical significance of bundle branch block complicating acute myocardial infarction: Parts I & II. *Circulation* 4:679–688 and 689–699, 1978.

Morris DC, Walter PF, Hurst JW: The recognition and treatment of myocardial infarction and its complications, in Hurst JW et al (eds): *The Heart*, 7th ed. New York, McGraw-Hill, Chap 53C, pp 1054–1078, 1990.

Moss AJ, Bigger JT Jr, Odoroff CL: Post infarct risk stratification. *Prog Cardiovasc Dis* 29:389–412, 1987.

Rotman M, Wagner GS, Wallace AGP: Bradyarrhythmias in acute myocardial infarction. *Circulation* 45:703–722, 1972.

TIMI Study Group: Comparison of invasive and conservative strategies after treatment with intravenous tissue plasminogen activator in acute myocardial infarction. Results of thrombolysis in myocardial infarction (TIMI) phase II trial. *N Engl J Med* 320:618–627, 1989.

# Treatment of Systemic Hypertension

*W. Dallas Hall, M.D.*

## INTRODUCTION

Initial pharmacological therapy for primary (essential) hypertension usually begins with low doses of either a diuretic, a beta blocker, an angiotensin converting enzyme (ACE) inhibitor, or a calcium channel blocker.[1] Disregarding patients' clinical profiles, one finds that approximately 50 percent of compliant patients with mild-to-moderate hypertension respond to monotherapy with any of the above-listed four classes of antihypertensive drugs. This response rate can be improved to about 70 percent by the tailoring of therapy to individual patients. For example, hypertensive blacks generally respond better to initial therapy with diuretics or calcium channel blockers than to initial therapy with ACE inhibitors or beta blockers.[2] Table 13-1 outlines the minimum and maximum dosage range for antihypertensive drugs in common use.

## DIURETICS AS INITIAL THERAPY

Diuretic therapy should begin with low doses, such as the equivalent of 12.5–25 mg daily of chlorthalidone or hydrochlorothiazide, or 2.5 mg daily of indapamide. If the serum creatinine level is normal, there is usually no advantage to beginning therapy with furosemide or bumetanide. If renal function is impaired by 50 to 75 percent or more, however, then the loop diuretics are usually necessary to obtain adequate natriuresis. The usual starting dose of furosemide is 40 mg twice daily; of bumetanide, 0.5 mg daily.

When diuretic therapy is begun in outpatients with uncomplicated essential hypertension, the serum potassium concentration should be measured prior to treatment, again within 4 weeks or less, and once or twice a year thereafter.[3] The development of diuretic-induced hypokalemia relates more closely to the magnitude of the natriuretic response and the increase in aldosterone levels than to the particular agent used. In general, either potassium supplements or a potassium-sparing diuretic (e.g., Maxzide, Dyazide, Aldactazide) should be prescribed when a serum potassium level below 3.5 meq/liter is confirmed in a patient with uncomplicated hypertension. In patients with ventricular ectopy and normal renal function, potassium replacement may be desirable with less severe hypokalemia, particularly if there has been a greater than usual postdiuretic decrease in the serum potassium

**139**

TABLE 13-1 Dosage Range for Antihypertensive Drugs

| Drugs | Minimum initial dose (mg/day) | Maximum dose (mg/day) |
|---|---|---|
| Diuretics | | |
| Thiazide-type | | |
| Bendroflumethiazide | 2.5 | 5 |
| Chlorthalidone | 12.5–25 | 50 |
| Chlorothiazide | 125–250 | 500 |
| Hydrochlorothiazide | 12.5–25 | 50 |
| Indapamide | 2.5 | 5 |
| Metolazone | 1.25–2.5 | 10 |
| Trichlormethiazide | 2 | 4–8 |
| Loop | | |
| Bumetanide | 0.5 | 10 |
| Furosemide† | 40 | 480 |
| Potassium-sparing | | |
| Amiloride | 5 | 10 |
| Spironolactone† | 25 | 100 |
| Triamterene | 50 | 100 |
| Adrenergic inhibitors | | |
| β-Adrenergic blockers | | |
| Acebutolol | 400 | 800–1200 |
| Atenolol | 25 | 100 |
| Metoprolol† | 50 | 300 |
| Nadolol | 40 | 120–320 |
| Penbutolol | 20 | 40 |
| Pindolol† | 10 | 60 |
| Propranolol† | 40 | 480 |
| Timolol† | 20 | 80 |
| Central-acting adrenergic Inhibitors | | |
| Clonidine† | 0.2 | 1.2 |
| Guanabenz† | 8 | 32 |
| Guanfacine | 1 | 3 |
| Methyldopa† | 250 | 2000 |
| Peripheral adrenergic inhibitors | | |
| Guanadrel† | 10 | 150 |
| Guanethidine | 5 | 150 |
| Reserpine | 0.1 | 0.25 |
| $\alpha_1$-Adrenergic blockers | | |
| Prazosin† | 1 | 20 |
| Terazosin | 1 | 20 |
| Combined $\alpha$- and $\beta$-adrenergic blockers | | |
| Labetalol† | 200 | 1200 |
| Vasodilators | | |
| Hydralazine† | 50 | 300 |
| Minoxidil | 2.5 | 60 |

| Angiotensin-converting enzyme inhibitors | | |
|---|---|---|
| Captopril† | 25–37.5 | 150 |
| Enalapril | 5 | 40 |
| Lisinopril | 10 | 80 |
| Calcium channel blockers | | |
| Diltiazem‡ | 120 | 360 |
| Nicardipine‡ | 60 | 90 |
| Nifedipine‡ | 10 | 80 |
| Verapamil† | 240 | 480 |

†This drug is usually given in divided doses, twice daily, unless a long-acting formulation is available.

‡This drug is usually given in divided doses, three or four times daily, unless a long-acting formulation is available.

level (e.g., from 4.8 to 3.8 meq/liter). When hypokalemia is treated with potassium supplements, doses of at least 40 meq daily are typically required. In general, potassium supplements should not be used concomitantly with potassium-sparing diuretics, because of the risk of hyperkalemia.

High dosages of diuretics often cause a modest worsening of serum lipid levels, especially total cholesterol and triglycerides.[4] Hence, high-risk patients with borderline or elevated lipid levels should receive counseling on a low-cholesterol, low-fat diet.[5]

## BETA BLOCKERS AS INITIAL THERAPY

There are several clinical settings in which beta blockers are excellent choices as first-line therapy for hypertension. These include young patients with high-renin essential hypertension or the hyperdynamic beta-adrenergic circulatory state, patients with alcohol-withdrawal hypertension, and, possibly, tachycardia- or anxiety-prone patients with increased adrenergic tone. In addition, the beta blockers are the only class of antihypertensive drugs established as cardioprotective in patients with previous myocardial infarction.

Atenolol, metoprolol, and acebutolol are more cardioselective than nadolol, penbutolol, pindolol, propranolol, and timolol. Pindolol and penbutolol possess intrinsic sympathomimetic activity (ISA).

If one must prescribe a beta blocker for a diabetic patient receiving insulin or for a patient with peripheral vascular disease, the cardioselective agents may be better choices. In contrast, the nonselective beta blockers (i.e., those that possess beta$_2$ receptor–blocking properties) are often more effective when beta blocker therapy is indicated for the treatment of migraine headaches or intention tremors. Once-a-day therapy is advantageous in some patients and is appropriate for atenolol, acebutolol, nadolol, and penbutolol. Like diuretics, the beta blockers can also sometimes be associated with worsening of serum lipid levels, especially lowering of the HDL cholesterol. This effect is not observed, however, in beta blockers with ISA.

## ANGIOTENSIN-CONVERTING ENZYME (ACE) INHIBITORS AS INITIAL THERAPY

ACE inhibitors, such as captopril, enalapril, and lisinopril, are effective first-line drugs in the treatment of Caucasian patients with hypertension. They are also useful in the treatment of diabetic patients, because they do not impair glucose tolerance and can reduce proteinuria.

The starting dose of captopril should be no more than 12.5 mg twice daily. An even lower initial dose (i.e., a 6.25-mg test dose) may be warranted in captopril-sensitive patients with high plasma renin activity—such as those with congestive heart failure and hyponatremia, or accelerated-malignant hypertension—or following acute diuresis. The approximate dosage conversions among enalapril, lisinopril, and captopril are 20, 40 and 100 mg, respectively. Drug interactions are common, especially with nonsteroidal anti-inflammatory agents, which can blunt the antihypertensive efficacy of ACE inhibitors.

Rash is the most frequent adverse effect of ACE inhibitor therapy. A persistent dry, hacking cough can be another bothersome adverse effect. Angineurotic edema is rare but can occur within hours after the initial dose.

## CALCIUM CHANNEL BLOCKERS AS INITIAL THERAPY

The calcium channel blockers, such as diltiazem, nicardipine, nifedipine, and verapamil, are also effective first-line drugs in the treatment of hypertension. They are equally efficacious in blacks and whites. The dihydropyridines (nicardipine and nifedipine) have a predominant effect on peripheral vascular calcium channels, with a lesser effect than diltiazem or verapamil on atrioventricular conduction and cardiac contractility.

Diltiazem and nifedipine have a short half-life and need to be given every 6 hours; nicardipine is given every 8 hours. A longer-lasting form of diltiazem (diltiazem SR) can be given twice daily once the total daily dosage of diltiazem has been established. A sustained-release form of nifedipine (Procardia XL) can be given once daily. Verapamil can be given twice daily, or once a day in the sustained-release form (verapamil SR).

The most common adverse effect of verapamil is constipation, which can be managed with a high-fiber diet and mild laxatives. Caution must be used to avoid precipitation of heart failure or heart block whenever diltiazem or verapamil is used in conjunction with beta-blocker therapy in patients who may have borderline ejection fractions or underlying conduction disturbances. Post-dose flushing and headaches are the most frequent adverse effects of nifedipine. They can sometimes be alleviated by taking the dose with meals (slower absorption), or by converting to the sustained-release nifedipine preparation or an equivalent dosage of nicardipine. Any calcium channel blocker may occasionally produce a severe rash. Peripheral edema can also occur, especially with the dihydropyridines; this is due to a redistribution of intravascular volume, not to retention of salt and water.

One must be aware of certain clinically important drug inter-actions with the calcium channel blockers. For example, cimetidine (but probably not ranitidine) can exaggerate the hypotensive effect of nifedipine. Note especially that verapamil can lead to an increase in the serum level of digoxin. Both diltiazem and verapamil can lead to significant increases in the blood levels of cyclosporine.

## MULTI-DRUG THERAPY FOR OUTPATIENTS WITH SEVERE OR RESISTANT HYPERTENSION[6] (See Table 13-2)

*Severe hypertension* is defined as a diastolic blood pressure of 115 mmHg or more; *resistant hypertension* is a diastolic blood pressure that remains at 100 mmHg or more despite reasonable dosages of three or more antihypertensive drugs.

The most common cause of resistant hypertension is noncompliance with a medication program. Does the patient know all of his or her medications? When was the last dose taken? Has the patient brought all medications with him or her? Is the number of pills left close to the number that should be present after your last prescription? Does the patient often miss appointments?

The second most common cause of resistant hypertension is volume expansion due either to medications or to excessive intake

TABLE 13-2 Factors to Evaluate in Outpatients with Severe or Resistant Hypertension

| |
|---|
| Adherence to therapy |
| Volume expansion |
| Secondary causes |
|    Renovascular disease |
|    Aldosteronism |
|    Pheochromocytoma |
| Pseudohypertension |

of dietary salt. Adding low doses of a diuretic will often control blood pressure in a patient with an incomplete response to one- or two-drug therapy. Increasing the dosage of diuretic is often necessary to control blood pressure in patients receiving therapy with multiple drugs. This is particularly true for obese patients, those with renal insufficiency (i.e., serum creatinine level of 1.7 mg/dl or more), and patients receiving nonsteroidal anti-inflammatory drugs, corticosteroids, dilantin, methyldopa, or minoxidil.

Outpatients with resistant hypertension are good candidates for elective hospital admission. Secondary causes, such as renovascular disease, aldosteronism, and pheochromocytoma, can be excluded by the captopril stimulation test, renal arteriography, saline suppression test, 24-h urinary metanephrine-to-creatinine excretion ratio, and abdominal CT scan. In addition, the patient can be observed for blood-pressure response to his or her usual medication, thus differentiating noncompliance from true resistance to therapy. In selected patients, especially very obese patients and elderly patients with a positive Osler sign, measurement of intraarterial pressure (versus cuff pressure) may be appropriate. A positive Osler's sign is defined as a palpable (i.e., noncollapsed) radial artery despite inflation of the blood pressure cuff above the systolic blood pressure.

## ACUTE THERAPY FOR PATIENTS ADMITTED WITH URGENT, ACCELERATED, OR MALIGNANT HYPERTENSION[7]

*Urgent hypertension* generally refers to diastolic blood pressure between 120 and 160 mmHg without symptoms or acute retinopathy. *Accelerated hypertension* means that retinal hemorrhages or exudates are present; *malignant hypertension* implies papilledema.

Urgent and accelerated hypertension are sometimes treated with oral or sublingual medication, whereas malignant hypertension and hypertensive emergencies (i.e., encephalopathy, intracranial hemorrhage, dissecting aneurysm, acute pulmonary edema, severe chest pain) are generally treated with parenteral therapy (see Table 13-3).

TABLE 13-3 Therapeutic Options for the Acute Management of Patients with Urgent, Accelerated, or Malignant Hypertension

| |
|---|
| Oral and sublingual therapy |
|   Reinstitution of previous medications |
|   Nifedipine |
|   Clonidine loading |
| Parenteral therapy |
|   Sodium nitroprusside or nitroglycerin |
|   Labetalol |
|   Enalaprilat |

## Oral and Sublingual Therapy

Reinstitution of previous antihypertensive therapy (that the patient has not been taking) is often efficacious in reducing severely elevated blood pressure within 4 to 6 h. One must be careful, however, not to "overshoot" and induce hypotension in a patient who has never taken full doses of the prescribed medication. For example, it is wise not to restart initial single doses above 20 mg for nifedipine, 0.2 mg for clonidine, 5 mg for prazosin, and 10 mg for minoxidil. In addition, one must take care to ascertain that a previously prescribed medication is not contraindicated in the new clinical setting. (Beta blockers, for example, should not be used in patients with bradycardia, bronchospasm, or congestive heart failure).

### Nifedipine

Nifedipine capsules have a rapid onset of action, usually within 15 to 30 min. The peak effect occurs within 30 to 90 minutes; the duration is 3 to 8 h. In comatose or intubated patients, one may give it sublingually by squeezing the liquid out of a punctured capsule. Because it is less than 10-percent absorbed sublingually, this is unnecessary in patients who can swallow. Administration of the liquid form (punctured sublingual, bite-and-swallow, or per os) produces an onset of action 5 to 10 min faster than the swallowed capsule; but this very acute effect may not be desirable during initial therapy, because some patients experience excessive hypotension with cardiac complications. The *initial* dose of nifedipine should never exceed 10 mg. In part, this is because the higher the pressure, the greater the fall after therapy with most calcium channel blockers.

### Clonidine Loading

In patients hospitalized with urgent hypertension, it is sometimes appropriate to use the clonidine loading regimen. An oral dose of 0.2 mg is followed by 0.1 mg every hour, for up to 5 h, until diastolic blood pressure is reduced to below 110 mmHg or a total dose of 0.7 mg is reached. This therapy is successful in up to 90 percent of patients with urgent hypertension but may be accompanied by sedation, dry mouth, and, occasionally, orthostatic hypotension.

## Parenteral Therapy

The four most commonly used intravenous therapies for malignant hypertension and hypertensive emergencies are: sodium nitroprusside, nitroglycerin, labetalol, and enalaprilat.

*Nitroprusside and Nitroglycerin*

The starting dose of intravenous sodium nitroprusside is 0.5 μg/kg/min of a solution of 50 mg nitroprusside in 250 ml dextrose and water (i.e., 200 μg/ml). The mixture must be protected from light, and the solution changed every 12 h. The onset of action is immediate; the effects dissipate within 2 to 10 minutes after discontinuation. The rate of administration can be up-titrated to 8 μg/kg/min, but high dosages over several days require monitoring of the serum thiocyanate level, especially in patients with renal impairment. Toxicity usually presents as acidosis, and occasionally as methemoglobinemia if thiocyanate levels exceed 15 to 20 mg/dl. It can be treated by discontinuation of the nitroprusside and administration of the vitamin $B_{12}$ derivative hydroxocobalamin (alphaREDISOL), which binds free cyanide.

When myocardial ischemia is associated with relatively mild degrees of hypertension, nitroglycerin infusion is often preferable to nitroprusside. In patients with more severe elevations of blood pressure, however, nitroprusside or labetalol is more effective for the lowering of blood pressure. The starting dose of nitroglycerin is the same as that for nitroprusside: 0.5 μg/kg/min of a solution of 50 mg mixed into 250 ml dextrose and water. The solution does not need to be shielded from light, but a special nonabsorbing infusion set is required to avoid adherence of nitroglycerin to the plastic or polyvinyl chloride contained in most intravenous lines.

*Labetalol*

The initial dose of labetalol is 20 mg (4 ml of a 20-ml ampule solution containing 5 mg/ml) given intravenously over 2 min. Fifteen minutes after this test dose, a bolus of 40 mg can be given, followed by repeated bolus doses of 40 to 80 mg as needed. The onset of action is usually within 10 to 20 min and the duration is 4 to 6 hours. Once a response is obtained (often after a total dose of 60 to 100 mg), the labetalol can be administered by intravenous infusion of 0.5 to 3.0 mg/min of a mixture containing 100 mg labetalol in 250 ml dextrose and water. Conversion from parenteral to oral therapy is usually accomplished by starting with 100 to 200 mg orally, twice daily.

*Enalaprilat*

Enalaprilat is the active metabolite of enalapril and is available for intravenous administration. A test dose of 0.625 mg (0.5 ml of a 2-ml vial containing 2.5 mg) is infused over 5 min and used initially to avoid exaggerated hypotension. A second dose of 0.625 mg can be repeated after 1 h if there is an inadequate clinical response. The onset of action is usually within 15 min, but the peak effect can be delayed for up to 4 h. In responders, the maintenance dose is usually 1.25 mg intravenously every 6 h for adult patients with serum creatinine levels below approximately 3 mg/dl, and 0.625 mg every 6 hours for those with serum creatinine levels of 3 mg/dl or more.

## REFERENCES

1. The Joint National Committee on Detection, Evaluation, and Treatment of High Blood Pressure: The 1988 Report of the Joint National Committee on Detection, Evaluation, and Treatment of High Blood Pressure. *Arch Intern Med* 148:1023–1038, 1988.
2. Hall WD: Hypertension in blacks, in Wollam GL, Hall WD (eds): *Hypertension Management, Clinical Practice and Therapeutic Dilemmas.* Chicago, Year Book, Chap 3, pp 103–141, 1988.
3. Kaplan NM (ed): *Clinical Hypertension,* 4th ed. Baltimore, Williams and Wilkins, 1986.
4. Lardinois CK, Neuman SL: The effects of antihypertensive agents on serum lipids and lipoproteins. *Arch Intern Med* 148:1280–1288, 1989.
5. National Heart, Lung, and Blood Institute: Report of the National Cholesterol Education Program Expert Panel on Detection, Evaluation, and Treatment of High Blood Cholesterol in Adults. *Arch Intern Med* 148:36–69, 1988.
6. Wollam GL, Hall WD: Treatment of systemic hypertension, in Hurst JW et al (eds): *The Heart,* 7th ed. New York, McGraw-Hill, Chap 59, pp 1171–1190, 1990.
7. Houston UC: Pathophysiology, clinical aspects, and treatment of hypertensive crises. *Prog Cardiovasc Dis* 32:99–148, 1989.

*Robert C. Schlant, M.D.   Hiroshi Kuida, M.D.*

## DEFINITION

*Pulmonary hypertension* (PH) is a pathophysiological condition (not a disease) characterized by elevation of pressure in the pulmonary arterial system above the normal range (12 to 18 mmHg mean pressure at sea level). In most clinical conditions in which it is found there is a plausible underlying pathophysiological basis for pulmonary vascular obstruction; these are considered cases of *secondary pulmonary hypertension*. In rare cases where no identifiable cause can be found, there is a disease of exclusion, presumed to be vasoconstrictive, termed *primary pulmonary hypertension*.

## ETIOLOGY

There are many specific causes of PH, and two or more may coexist in the same patient. The broad generic categories of these are: alveolar hypoxemia-induced pulmonary vasoconstriction (e.g., altitude exposure or hypoventilation); thrombotic, embolic, or vasoactive mediator–induced constrictive occlusion of the pulmonary vasculature; intrinsic pulmonary parenchymal (including vascular) diseases of a wide variety (emphysema being the prototype); disorders leading to elevation of pulmonary veno-capillary pressure (e.g., chronic left heart failure, pulmonary venous occlusion, or mitral stenosis); and congenital heart disease.

## PATHOLOGY

Usually the pathological findings in the pulmonary vasculature ascribable to PH are consistently present only if the PH is severe and/or of long standing. Even then they may be patchy in distribution. Typically there is medial hypertrophy in small pulmonary arteries. Thromboembolic lesions, if present, usually are identifiable as such and distinguishable from the so-called plexiform, fibrinoid necrosis, and onion-skin lesions that are thought to be typical—although not diagnostic—of primary, or unexplained, pulmonary hypertension (PPH).

## CLINICAL MANIFESTATIONS

### History

In the early or mild-elevation stages there are no symptoms attributable to PH *per se*. It is more than likely that symptoms, if present, can be ascribed to the underlying disease process. Moderate-to-severe PH, especially when chronic, is consistently accompanied by dyspnea of a slowly progressive nature and by fatigability. Rarely patients may develop chest pain and/or syncopal attacks. The latter may be prominent in PPH. Some of these symptoms are the same as those of some of the underlying causes of PH. Right ventricular failure secondary to PH can lead to congestive symptoms, such as ankle swelling or right upper quadrant pain due to the capsular stretching from hepatic edema.

### Physical Examination

PH causes increased intensity of the pulmonary component and sometimes narrow splitting of $S_2$, which may be palpable. A decrescendo diastolic murmur of pulmonic valve regurgitation may be present along the left sternal border. If the right ventricle is enlarged and/or has failed, a parasternal lift or heave may be palpable and there will be evidence of elevated jugular venous pressure, with prominent *a* and/or *v* waves present. A holosystolic murmur of tricuspid valve regurgitation may be audible over the lower sternal area. $S_3$ and/or $S_4$ gallop rhythms and systemic fluid retention, in the form of dependent edema or hepatomegaly, may be present.

## USUAL DIAGNOSTIC TESTS

### Chest X-Ray

Excluding findings attributable to underlying diseases, PH typically causes varying degrees of enlargement of the main pulmonary artery. Proximal branches also may be enlarged, while distal ones, in the absence of veno-capillary hypertension, may appear diminished ("pruned"). The right atrium and ventricle may be enlarged.

### Electrocardiogram

The most common ECG finding is right axis deviation in the frontal plane. The P-wave axis also may be shifted rightward due to tall (>2.5 mm) peaked waves in leads II, III, and $aV_F$ of right atrial enlargement. The ECG findings of right ventricular enlargement include a predominant R-wave deflection in precordial lead $V_1$ with ST-T wave changes in leads $V_1$ to $V_3$ of the so-called strain pattern. In secondary PH the underlying disease may independently affect the ECG.

## DIFFERENTIAL DIAGNOSIS

This involves a careful search for the various underlying causes of PH, each of which has its own historical, physical, and routine laboratory manifestations. If none of these is found, it is appropriate to entertain a presumptive diagnosis of PPH.

## SPECIAL DIAGNOSTIC EVALUATION

### Echocardiography

Echocardiography usually demonstrates dilatation of the right ventricle and right atrium, paradoxical motion of the ventricular septum, and abnormal motion of the pulmonary valve leaflets suggestive of PH. There may be evidence of underlying cardiac disease, such as mitral valve disease.

### Cardiac Catheterization

Cardiac catheterization allows direct measurement of the pulmonary artery pressure and of the pulmonary capillary (wedge) pressure. The latter is elevated if the PH is secondary to left-sided heart disease, but normal otherwise. Pulmonary angiography may demonstrate pulmonary emboli, though the procedure has an increased risk in the presence of marked PH.

### Arterial Blood Gas Studies

Arterial blood gas studies may document arterial hypoxemia.

### Pulmonary Function Tests

Pulmonary function tests may reveal changes from chronic lung disease or changes from chronic congestive heart failure. Acute pulmonary embolism is usually associated with an arterial $P_{O_2}$ of less than 90 mmHg, together with respiratory alkalosis.

### Ventilation-Perfusion Lung Scans

Ventilation-perfusion lung scans may reveal evidence of pulmonary thromboembolism.

### Venography

Venography may reveal evidence of venous disease in a lower extremity as a source of pulmonary emboli.

## Prognosis

The prognosis is generally very poor when chronic PH is present from any cause except living at high altitude.

## TREATMENT

The treatment consists of treating the underlying cardiac or pulmonary disease, if one is identified. Patients who develop acute PH at high altitude should be given oxygen and moved promptly to a lower altitude, *especially if they also have acute pulmonary edema*. Patients with recurrent pulmonary emboli should be kept on chronic anticoagulation with warfarin and considered for insertion of a filter in the inferior vena cava. There is no clear evidence that therapy with any particular vasodilator produces consistent long-term benefit in patients with PPH. On the other hand, it is often appropriate to try therapy with a calcium channel blocker, such as nifedipine, and to follow the patient with careful clinical and hemodynamic monitoring. Chronic anticoagulation is often employed in patients with PPH, but there is little objective evidence of clear benefit. Chronic oxygen therapy, especially at night, may be useful in patients whose pulmonary artery pressure is demonstrated to decrease during oxygen inhalation.

### Heart-Lung Transplantation

This is still an experimental procedure for far-advanced cases, and should be restricted to major centers gathering research data from protocols. The morbidity and mortality are clearly greater than for heart-only transplantation.

## SUGGESTED READING

Dalen JE, Alpert JS: Pulmonary Embolism, in Hurst JW et al (eds): *The Heart,* 7th ed. New York, McGraw-Hill, Chap 61, pp 1205–1219, 1990.

Fishman AP, Turino GM, Bergofsky EH: The syndrome of alveolar hypo-ventilation. *Am J Med* 23:333–339, 1957.

Fuster V, Steele PM, Edwards WD, et al: Primary pulmonary hypertension: Natural history and the importance of thrombosis. *Circulation* 70:580–587, 1984.

Glanville AR, Burke CM, Theodore J, et al: Primary pulmonary hypertension. Length of survival in patients referred for heart-lung transplantation. *Chest* 91:675–681, 1987.

Heath D, Edwards J: The pathology of hypertensive pulmonary vascular disease. *Circulation* 18:533–547, 1958.

Hughes JD, Rubin LJ: Primary pulmonary hypertension: An analysis of 28 cases and a review of the literature. *Medicine* 65:56–72, 1986.

Hultgren HN, Lopez CE, Lundberg E, et al: Physiologic studies of pulmonary edema of high altitude. *Circulation* 29:393–408, 1964.

Kuida H: Primary and secondary pulmonary hypertension: Pathophysiology, recognition, and treatment, in Hurst JW et al (eds): *The Heart,* 7th ed. New York, McGraw-Hill, Chap 60, pp 1191–1204, 1990.

Newman JH, Ross JC: Chronic cor pulmonale, in Hurst JW et al (eds): *The Heart,* 7th ed. New York, McGraw-Hill, Chap 62, pp 1220–1229, 1990.

Penaloza D, Sime F, Banchero N, et al: Pulmonary hypertension in healthy men born and living at high altitude. *Am J Cardiol* 11:150–157, 1963.

Rich S, Brundage BH, Levy PS: The effect of vasodilator therapy on the clinical outcome of patients with primary pulmonary hypertension. *Circulation* 71:1191–1196, 1985.

## 15 | Infective Endocarditis

*David T. Durack, M.B., D. Phil.*

## DEFINITIONS

*Infective endocarditis* (IE) is caused by microbial infection of the endothelial lining of the heart. The characteristic lesion is a vegetation, which usually develops on a heart valve. *Acute bacterial endocarditis* (ABE) is caused by virulent organisms and runs its course over days to weeks. *Subacute bacterial endocarditis* (SBE) is caused by organisms of low virulence and runs its course over weeks to months. Sterile vegetations are called *nonbacterial thrombotic endocarditis* (NBTE).

## THE SUSCEPTIBLE HOST

IE can occur at any age, but today is most common in older adults. The median age of onset is about 50 years. The male/female ratio is approximately 2:1 overall, but is higher in elderly patients. Most patients who develop IE have a preexisting cardiac condition that affects the valves. The lesions pose different degrees of risk for development of IE (Table 15-1). Intravenous drug abusers are at high risk for IE; they have a high frequency of tricuspid valve infection caused by *Staphylococcus aureus*.

## PATHOGENESIS AND PATHOLOGY

Figure 15-1 shows the pathogenesis of IE. NBTE may develop on heart valves in a wide variety of clinical conditions. Small aggregates of platelets have been found occasionally on normal valves, but they occur frequently on the surfaces of valves damaged by congenital or rheumatic disease or by previous infective endocarditis. The common factor leading to platelet deposition is endothelial damage. This exposes subendothelial connective tissue containing collagen fibers, which in turn causes platelets to aggregate at the site. These microscopic platelet thrombi may harmlessly embolize away, or they may be stabilized by fibrin to form NBTE. The vegetations of NBTE are friable masses, usually situated along the lines of valve closure. They vary greatly in size, frequently being rather large and causing infarctions when they embolize. There is little inflammatory reaction at the site of attachment. Histologically, the vegetations of NBTE consist of degenerating platelets interwoven with strands of fibrin.

The essential event leading to infective endocarditis is attachment of microorganisms circulating in the bloodstream onto an endocardial surface, especially NBTE. Once lodged on the endocardium, bacteria multiply rapidly. The vegetation provides an ideal environment for the growth of microbial colonies. The presence of bacteria stimulates further thrombosis; layers of fibrin are deposited around growing bacteria, causing the vegetations to enlarge. Histologically, colonies of microorganisms are found embedded in a fibrin-platelet matrix. Although the inflammatory reaction at the site of attachment may be extensive, even progressing to form a frank abscess, the vegetations themselves characteristically contain relatively few leukocytes. Even these few are prevented from reaching bacteria by layers of fibrin, which form protective barriers around colonies.

Formation of an abscess is one of the most important complications of valvular infection. Abscesses often develop by direct extension of valvular infection into the fibrous cardiac skeleton supporting the valves. From here, abscesses can extend further into the adjacent myocardium. Abscesses are uncommon in SBE unless a valvular prosthesis is present. They occur more often in ABE, and are found in the majority of patients who die with active

TABLE 15-1 Estimates of the Relative Risk for Infective Endocarditis Posed by Various Cardiac Lesions

| Relatively High Risk | Intermediate Risk | Very Low or Negligible Risk |
|---|---|---|
| Prosthetic heart valves | Mitral valve prolapse | Atrial septal defects |
| Aortic valve disease | Mitral stenosis without insufficiency | Arteriosclerotic plaques |
| Mitral insufficiency ± stenosis | Tricuspid valve disease | Coronary artery disease |
| Patent ductus arteriosus | Pulmonary valve disease | Syphilitic aortitis |
| Ventricular septal defect | Asymmetrical septal hypertrophy | Cardiac pacemakers |
| Coarctation of the aorta | Calcific aortic sclerosis | Surgically corrected cardiac lesions (without prosthetic implants, more than 6 months after operation) |
| Marfan syndrome | Hyperalimentation or pressure-monitoring lines that reach the right atrium | |
| Cyanotic congenital heart disease | Nonvalvular intracardiac prosthetic implants | |
| Previous infective endocarditis | | |

*Source:* Adapted from Hurst JW et al (eds). *The Heart*, 7th ed, New York, McGraw-Hill, 1990, Chap 63, p 1332, with permission of the publisher.

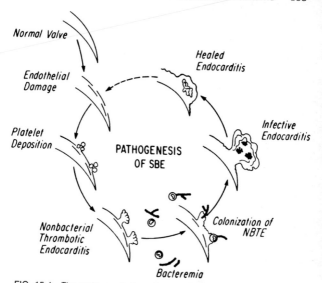

FIG. 15-1 The main events in pathogenesis of nonbacterial thrombotic endocarditis (NBTE) and subacute bacterial endocarditis (SBE).

prosthetic valve infection (PVE). Because valve-ring abscesses are located close to the conduction system, they can cause conduction disturbances and arrhythmias.

## ETIOLOGIC ORGANISMS

Many different species of microbes can cause infective endocarditis, but gram-positive cocci predominate. Streptococci or staphylococci cause more than 80 percent of IE on native valves. Among the streptococci, α-hemolytic (viridans) streptococci from the mouth cause most cases of SBE. The approximate frequencies of the main organisms causing IE are shown in Table 15-2.

## CLINICAL MANIFESTATIONS

The clinical and laboratory manifestations of infective endocarditis can be grouped under three headings (see Table 15-3):

- Manifestations of a systemic infection.
- Manifestations of an intravascular lesion.
- Manifestations of an immunologic reaction to infection.

TABLE 15-2 Frequencies of Various Microorganisms That Cause Infective Endocarditis

|  | NVE (%) | IV drug abusers (%) | Early PVE (%) | Late PVE (%) |
|---|---|---|---|---|
| *Streptococcus* spp. | 60 | 15 | 10 | 35 |
| viridans, α-hemolytic | 35 | 5 | <5 | 25 |
| *S. bovis* (group D) | 15 | <5 | <5 | <5 |
| *S. fecalis* (group D) | 10 | 8 | <5 | <5 |
| Other streptococci | <5 | <5 | <5 | <5 |
| *Staphylococcus* spp. | 20 | 50 | 50 | 30 |
| Coagulase-positive | 20 | 50 | 20 | 10 |
| Coagulase-negative | <5 | <5 | 30 | 20 |
| Gram-negative aerobic bacilli | <5 | 15 | 20 | <5 |
| HACEK* group | 5 | <1 | <1 | <5 |
| Other organisms | <5 | 5 | 5 | 5 |
| Culture-negative endocarditis | 5 | <5 | <5 | <5 |

* HACEK: *Haemophilus* spp., *Actinobacillus* spp., *Corynebacterium* spp., *Eikenella* spp., *Kingella* spp. NVE = native valve endocarditis; PVE = prosthetic valve endocarditis.

*Source:* Adapted from Hurst JW et al (eds). *The Heart,* 7th ed, New York, McGraw-Hill, Chap 63, 1990, p 1233, with permission of the publisher.

The symptoms of SBE can develop insidiously, and with great variability. Fevers, chills, rigors, night sweats, general malaise, anorexia, fatigue, and weakness are typical. The patient often loses weight. Headaches and musculoskeletal complaints, including myalgias, arthralgias, and back pain, are common. This symptom complex is often described by the patient or physician as a "flu-like illness." Symptoms usually persist over several weeks, worsening intermittently, before the diagnosis is made. In ABE, the symptoms are both accelerated and accentuated in severity. Patients experience hectic fevers, rigors, and prostration, usually leading to admission to hospital within a few days.

Evidence of an intravascular lesion is provided by symptoms of left- or right-sided heart failure and by such manifestations of embolization as focal neurological injury, chest pain, flank pain, left upper quadrant pain, hematuria, or ischemia of an extremity. Symptoms of cardiac failure may develop or worsen suddenly in either acute or subacute disease, because of mechanical complications such as perforation of a valve leaflet, rupture of chordae tendineae, or development of functional stenosis from obstruction of blood flow by large vegetations. Alternatively, heart failure may develop insidiously, or preexisting chronic heart failure may worsen because of progressive damage to the valves or associated structures. Myocardial infarction due to coronary artery embolism may contribute to heart failure.

IE should be considered in any patient who presents with the classic triad of *fever, anemia, murmur*. Important physical signs of IE include new or changed murmurs (especially if they indicate aortic or mitral insufficiency), heart failure, splenomegaly, signs of embolization, and peripheral signs (see Tables 15-3 and 15-4).

## DIAGNOSTIC TESTS

### Usual Diagnostic Tests

The *chest x-ray* may be normal, or may reveal congestive heart failure or other manifestations of valvular heart disease. Multiple small, patchy opacities can be due to septic pulmonary emboli from tricuspid valve vegetations. *Electrocardiography* may show evidence of hypertrophy, or of myocardial infarction due to emboli. AV block indicates the possibility of a valve-ring abscess near the conduction system. Pericarditis is unusual in IE, except in patients with renal failure.

*Anemia* and an elevated *erythrocyte sedimentation rate* are usual, but nonspecific, findings. The *white blood cell count* may be normal or elevated, and is seldom helpful in the diagnosis of IE. *Urinalysis* can reveal microscopic hematuria and proteinuria due to microemboli, or gross hematuria due to embolic infarction. Immune-complex glomerulonephritis is a common complication of IE that can produce red cell casts, white cell casts, and proteinuria in the urine.

The antigenic stimulus due to organisms in the vegetation can result in positive *rheumatoid factor* in about 30 percent of SBE; also circulating immune complexes, and false positive tests for syphilis.

*CT scanning* can reveal cerebritis, embolic infarction, or hemorrhage in the brain, and infarcts or abscess formation in the spleen or at other sites.

### Blood Culture

This is the most important test in the diagnosis of IE. In more than 90 percent of cases, three sets of blood cultures suffice to yield the infecting organisms. These should be drawn several hours apart, before antibiotic therapy is started. If the clinical setting indicates that antibiotic therapy must be started immediately, the three sets can be drawn with minimal delay.

### Echocardiography

Echocardiography is extremely useful in the diagnosis and assessment of IE. It can detect vegetations, valve leaflet rupture, chordal

TABLE 15-3 Summary of the Major Clinical Manifestations of Infective Endocarditis

| | History | Examination | Investigations |
|---|---|---|---|
| Manifestations of systemic infection | Fever, chills, rigors, sweats, malaise, weakness, lethargy, delirium, headache, anorexia, weight loss, backache, arthralgia, myalgia<br>Portal of entry:<br>  Oropharynx, skin<br>  Urinary tract<br>  Drug abuse<br>  Nosocomial bacteremia | Fever<br>Pallor<br>Weight loss<br>Asthenia<br>Splenomegaly | Anemia<br>Leukocytosis (variable)<br>Raised ESR<br>Blood cultures positive<br>Abnormal CSF |
| Manifestations of intravascular lesion | Dyspnea, chest pain, focal weakness, stroke, abdominal pain, cold and painful extremities | Murmurs<br>Signs of cardiac failure<br>Petechiae—skin, eye, mucosae<br>Roth spots, Osler's nodes<br>Janeway lesions<br>Splinter hemorrhages<br>Stroke<br>Mycotic aneurysm<br>Ischemia or infarction of viscera or extremities | Hematuria<br>Chest x-ray<br>Echocardiography<br>Arteriography<br>Liver-spleen scan<br>Lung scan, brain scan, CT scan<br>Histology, culture of emboli |

| Manifestations of immunologic reactions | Arthralgia, myalgia, tenosynovitis | Arthritis<br>Signs of uremia<br>Vascular phenomena<br>Finger clubbing | Proteinuria, hematuria, casts, uremia, acidosis<br>Polyclonal increases in gamma globulins<br>Rheumatoid factor, decreased complement, and immune complexes in serum<br>Antistaphylococcal teichoic acid antibodies |

*Source:* Adapted from Hurst JW et al (eds) *The Heart,* 7th ed, New York, McGraw-Hill, Chap 63, 1990, p 1240, with permission of the publisher.

TABLE 15-4 Characteristics of Some Peripheral Signs of Infective Endocarditis

| | Petechiae | Splinter hemorrhages | Roth spots | Osler's nodes | Janeway lesions | Clubbing |
|---|---|---|---|---|---|---|
| Appearance | Tiny red hemorrhagic spots | "Splinters" under nails; red when fresh, then brown or black | Small bright red patches with white centers | Pea-sized red or purplish nodules | Red macules | Curvature of the nails in two planes, with swelling of the terminal phalanges |
| Distribution | Anywhere, especially above clavicles, in mouth, and in conjunctivae | Distal third of nails | Retinae | Fingers and toes; occasionally on hands and feet | Palms and soles; occasionally on flanks, forearms, ankles, feet, ears | Fingers and/or toes |
| Incidence | Common, in both SBE and ABE | Common, in both SBE and ABE | Infrequent; usually in SBE | Infrequent; usually in SBE | Infrequent; usually in ABE | Rare; in SBE only |

| | | | | | | |
|---|---|---|---|---|---|---|
| Pathology | Increased capillary permeability; microemboli | Blood in avascular squamous epithelium under nail; due to microemboli or increased capillary fragility | Inflammation and hemorrhage | Intracutaneous local vasculitis; bacteria rarely found; occasional abscess formation; probably embolic in origin | Origin uncertain; possibly embolic or allergic in origin | Soft-tissue proliferation; occasionally periosteal new-bone formation |
| Pain | None | None | None | Mild to moderately severe | None | Usually none; sometimes painful |
| Duration | Days | Weeks | Days | Days | Several hours to days | Weeks to months |
| Diagnostic significance | Nonspecific; also found in septicemia, after cardiac surgery, and in many other disorders | Nonspecific; found in up to 10% of normal people and up to 40% of patients with mitral stenosis | Strongly suggestive of endocarditis but not diagnostic | Almost pathognomonic for endocarditis | Suggestive of endocarditis | Nonspecific; found in many cardiopulmonary disorders; can be congenital |

*Source:* Adapted from Hoeprich PD, Jordan MC (eds): *Infectious Diseases*, 4th ed. Philadelphia, JB Lippincott, 1989, Chap 144, p 1245, with permission of the authors and publisher.

rupture, valve-ring abscess, and myocardial abscess. Two-dimensional echocardiography combined with a Doppler flow study is particularly useful in evaluating endocarditis, especially if a transesophageal sensor is used. Two-dimensional echocardiography is 80- to 90-percent sensitive for larger vegetations, but cannot detect very small vegetations; therefore, a negative echocardiogram does not rule out IE. It is somewhat more difficult to assess IE echocardiographically when the tricuspid valve, the pulmonic valve, or prosthetic valves are involved. Serial echocardiograms may be helpful in assessing cardiac function and the need for valve replacement. The persistence or disappearance of vegetations on echocardiograms following treatment is not a reliable criterion for the success or failure of antibiotic therapy.

## Cardiac Catheterization

Cardiac catheterization is generally well tolerated and safe during IE. It can define anatomic abnormalities, such as valvular lesions, congenital defects, coronary artery disease, asymmetrical septal hypertrophy, coarctation of the aorta, or mycotic aneurysm, and provide physiological measurements that aid management. It is especially useful when surgery is being considered, or when antibiotic treatment seems to be failing.

## Microbiological Tests

The etiologic organism should be accurately identified. Then, if possible, the minimal inhibitory and bactericidal concentrations (MIC, MBC) of appropriate antibiotics for the organism should be determined. The results will guide the choice of an appropriate antibiotic. Measurement of serum inhibitory and bactericidal titers (SIT, SBT) for the organism while the patient is being treated is not essential in routine management of IE. It can provide useful information in unusual or complex cases, even though the test is difficult to perform and standardize.

## DIFFERENTIAL DIAGNOSIS

Because the clinical manifestations of endocarditis are numerous and often nonspecific, the differential diagnosis of this disease is very wide. ABE shares many clinical features with primary septicemias due to *Staph. aureus, Neisseria,* pneumococci, and gram-negative bacilli. Pneumonia, meningitis, brain abscess, stroke, malaria, acute pericarditis, vasculitis, and disseminated intravascular coagulation may cause diagnostic confusion. SBE must be considered during the workup of every patient with fever of unknown origin. Its manifestations can mimic those of rheumatic fever, osteomyelitis, tuberculosis, meningitis, intraabdominal infections, salmonellosis, brucellosis, glomerulonephritis, myocardial infarction, stroke, endocardial thrombi, atrial myxoma, connective tissue diseases, vasculitis, occult malignancy (especially lymphomas), chronic cardiac failure, pericarditis, and even psychoneurosis.

## NATURAL HISTORY AND PROGNOSIS

IE is almost always fatal if untreated. Optimal treatment regimens can give cure rates of 95 percent or better for streptococcal native-valve endocarditis and for *Staph. aureus* IE in intravenous drug abusers. However, cure rates are much lower when unfavorable prognostic factors are present. Heart failure is the most important adverse prognostic factor. Others include gram-negative or fungal infection, prosthetic valve infection, development of abscesses in the valve ring or myocardium, old age, renal failure, and culture-negative IE.

Eradication of the etiologic organisms (microbiological cure) can be achieved in a high proportion of patients with bacterial endocarditis. However, both early and long-term mortality rates remain significant because of preexisting disease and because of damage done before the infection is eradicated. Survival curves after admission with IE show a significant number of late deaths over time, despite microbiological cure.

## RECURRENCE

*Recurrent endocarditis* is a general term that includes both *relapses* and *reinfections*. Occasional relapses occur even after optimal treatment, so follow-up clinical evaluation, including blood cultures, should be meticulously performed. Most relapses occur within a few weeks of the end of treatment. Reinfection is a new episode of endocarditis occurring after cure of a previous episode. Patients remain permanently at risk of reinfection after cure of infective endocarditis, because of residual valve scarring (see Fig. 15-1). Further episodes are fairly common, being recorded in from 5 to 30 percent of cases. This wide variation in reported incidence of recurrence is partly due to variable duration of follow-up. Intravenous drug abusers and patients with severe periodontitis are at highest risk for reinfection. Some patients have suffered three or more separate episodes of IE. Patients who have previously had native-valve endocarditis are at higher risk for prosthetic valve infection, for reasons not yet understood.

## TREATMENT

*Antibiotic therapy* should be started immediately after blood cultures have been drawn if the patient has ABE or is deteriorating rapidly. If the patient has SBE and is stable, antibiotics may be

TABLE 15-5 Treatment Regimens for Infective Endocarditis Caused by Gram-Positive Cocci

| Organism | Regimen | Duration, weeks | Comments |
|---|---|---|---|
| Alphahemolytic (viridans) streptococci; Strep. bovis | 1. Penicillin G 4 million units IV every 6 h plus gentamicin 1.0 mg/kg every 12 h IV or | 2 | Standard regimen, for patients less than 65 years old without renal failure, eighth-nerve defects, or serious complications |
| | 2. Penicillin G 4 million units IV every 6 h plus gentamicin 1.0 mg/kg every 12 h IV (for first 2 weeks only) or | 4 | For patients with complicated disease—e.g., CNS involvement, shock, moderately penicillin-resistant streptococci; failed previous treatment |
| | 3. Penicillin G 4 million units IV every 6 h IV, or | 4 | For patients more than 65 years old, with renal failure or eighth-nerve defects |
| | 4. Ceftriaxone 2g IV once daily or | 4 | For patients allergic to penicillins |
| | 5. Vancomycin 10 mg/kg IV every 12 h | 4 | For patients allergic to penicillins and cephalosporins |
| Strep. fecalis and other penicillin-resistant streptococci | 1. Ampicillin 2 g IV every 4 h plus gentamicin 1.0 mg/kg IV every 8 h; or | 4–6 | 4 weeks should be adequate for most cases with symptoms present for less than 3 months. |
| | 2. Vancomycin 15 mg/kg IV every 12 h IV plus gentamicin 1.0 mg/kg IV (not to exceed 80 mg) every 8 h | 4–6 | For patients allergic to penicillins; 4 weeks should be adequate for most cases. Serum levels should be monitored. |

| _Staph. aureus_ | 1. Nafcillin 1.5 g IV every 4 h, or | 4–6 | Standard regimen |
| | 2. Nafcillin as above, _plus_ gentamicin 1.0 mg/kg IV every 8 h for the first 3–5 days only, or | 4–6 | For patients with severe disseminated staphylococcal disease, synergy may be advantageous during early stages of treatment. |
| | 3. Cefazolin 2 g IV every 8 h, or | 4–6 | For patients allergic to penicillins |
| | 4. Vancomycin 15 mg/kg IV every 12 h | 4–6 | For patients allergic to penicillins and cephalosporins; for methicillin-resistant strains |
| HACEK* group | 1. Ampicillin 2 g IV every 4 h _plus_ gentamicin 1.0 mg/kg every 12 h IV, or | 4 | Gentamicin may be discontinued if the organism is fully sensitive to ampicillin. |
| | 2. Ceftriaxone 1–2 g IV once daily | 4 | For patients allergic to penicillins; suitable for home therapy after stabilization in hospital. |

* HACEK: _Haemophilus_ spp., _Actinobacillus_ spp., _Corynebacterium_ spp., _Eikenella_ spp., _Kingella_ spp.
_Source_: Adapted from Hurst JW et al (eds) _The Heart_, 7th ed, New York, McGraw-Hill, Chap 63, 1990, p 1248, with permission of the publisher.

withheld for 1 to 2 days while investigations and blood cultures are in progress. Appropriate empirical treatment for SBE is ampicillin 2.0 g IV every 4 h *plus* gentamicin 1.0 mg/kg IV every 8 h. For ABE, *add* nafcillin 1.5 g IV every 4h.

*Standard treatment regimens* for the most common organisms causing IE are given in Table 15-5. The choice of treatment regimens for gram-negative ABE, fungal IE, and other uncommon forms of endocarditis requires specialist consultation.

*Surgical treatment* usually consists of removal of the infected native valve and insertion of a prosthetic valve. Clear indications should be present before one proceeds with valve replacement for IE, because prosthetic valves cause significant long-term morbidity. When surgery is indicated, however, it should not be delayed, because the patient's condition may deteriorate rapidly. Valve replacement can be successful even if the duration of antimicrobial therapy has been too short to kill the organisms. Other procedures include excision of vegetations, valvuloplasty, valve repair, and closure of an abscess cavity. Indications for surgery include moderate or severe heart failure not responding to medical therapy, presence of a valve-ring abscess, valvular obstruction, unstable prosthesis, repeated major emboli, and failure of antimicrobials to control infection. Surgical intervention may be indicated for management of major systemic emboli, removal of splenic abscess, or treatment of mycotic aneurysms.

## PREVENTION

*Antibiotics* may prevent IE if given just before dental and other procedures that can cause transient bacteremia. This is appropriate when both the preexisting cardiac lesion and the procedure seem to pose significant risk for IE—e.g., tooth extraction in a patient with a bicuspid aortic valve. Suggested regimens are listed in Tables 15-6 and 35-2. Antibiotic prophylaxis for IE is unnecessary for many low-risk procedures such as diagnostic cardiac catheterization, pacemaker insertion, intubation, flexible bronchoscopy, uncomplicated gastrointestinal diagnostic procedures, dental fillings above the gum line, and adjustment of orthodontic appliances.

## SUGGESTED READING

Bisno AL, Dismukes WE, Durack DT, et al: Antimicrobial treatment of infective endocarditis due to viridans streptococci, enterococci, and staphylococci. *JAMA* 261:1471–1477, 1989.

Durack DT: Infective and noninfective endocarditis, in Hurst JW et al (eds): *The Heart,* 7th ed. New York, McGraw-Hill, Chap 63, pp 1230–1255, 1990.

Durack DT: Prophylaxis of infective endocarditis, in Mandell GL, Douglas RG Jr, Bennett JE (eds): *Principles and Practice of Infectious Diseases,* 3d ed. New York, Churchill Livingstone, Chap 63, pp 716–721, 1990.

TABLE 15-6 Regimens for Prophylaxis of Infective Endocarditis

| Standard regimen | For dental procedures; oral or upper respiratory tract surgery; minor GI or GU tract procedures | Amoxicillin, 3.0 g orally 1 h before, then 1.5 g 6 h later |
|---|---|---|
| Special regimens | Oral regimen for penicillin-allergic patients (oral and respiratory tract only) | Erythromycin 1.0 g orally 1–2 h before, then 0.5 g 6 h later |
| | Parenteral regimen for high-risk patients; also for GI or GU tract procedures | Ampicillin 2.0 g IM or IV, *plus* gentamicin 1.5 mg/kg IM or IV, 0.5 h before |
| | Parenteral regimen for penicillin-allergic patients | Vancomycin, 1.0 g IV slowly over 1 h, starting 1 h before; *add* gentamicin; 1.5 mg/kg IM or IV, if GI or GU tract involved |
| | Cardiac surgery including implantation of prosthetic valves | Cefazolin, 2.0 g IV, at induction of anesthesia, repeated 8 and 16 h later *or* vancomycin, 1.0 g IV slowly over 1 h, starting at induction, then 0.5 g IV 8 and 16 h later |

*Source:* Adapted from Hurst JW et al (eds). *The Heart,* 7th ed, New York, McGraw-Hill, 1990, Chap 63, p 1251, with permission of the publisher.

Magilligan DJ Jr, Quinn EL (eds): *Endocarditis. Medical and Surgical Management.* New York, Marcel Dekker, 1986.

Scheld WM, Sande MA: Endocarditis and intravascular infections, in Mandell GL, Douglas RG Jr, Bennett JE (eds): *Principles and Practice of Infectious Diseases,* 3d ed. New York, Churchill Livingstone, Chap 61, pp 670–706, 1990.

Threlkeld MG, Cobbs CG: Infectious disorders of prosthetic valves and intravascular devices, in Mandell GL, Douglas RG Jr, Bennett JE (eds): *Principles and Practice of Infectious Diseases,* 3d ed. New York, Churchill Livingstone, Chap 62, pp 706–715, 1990.

## 16 | Myocarditis and Dilated Cardiomyopathy

*Nanette Kass Wenger, M.D.*

## MYOCARDITIS

### Definition

*Myocarditis* is an inflammatory process involving the myocardial wall, attributed to a wide variety of infectious agents.

### Etiology

Myocarditis may be caused by any bacterial, viral, rickettsial, spirochetal, mycotic, or parasitic organism. The prevalence of etiologic agents varies with age, geographic location, prevalence of infectious illness, and the specific patient's associated diseases or therapies; most cases of myocarditis in the United States and Europe are caused by viruses. It is not known whether the myocarditis represents direct invasion and tissue damage by the infectious agent or, instead, a toxic, allergic, or immunologic response to that agent.

### Pathology

Myocarditis is characterized by extravasated leukocytes in the myocardial interstitium in association with myofiber necrosis (in the absence of coronary artery occlusion). Stainable microorganisms reinforce the diagnosis.

Most patients diagnosed clinically as having myocarditis survive the acute episode; examination of the myocardium in cases where death occurs long after the acute episode typically discloses only increased fibrosis of the myocardial interstitium. Certain infections have fairly predictable effects on the myocardium—e.g., the apical thinning and bulging of Chagas' disease, the hydatid cysts of echinococcosis, the granulomas of histoplasmosis, etc.

### Clinical Manifestations

#### History

Fatigue, decreased exercise tolerance, dyspnea, and palpitations are common. Occasionally there is precordial discomfort. Typically these features appear during convalescence from an infectious illness. Myalgia has been thought to warn of cardiac involvement in viral infections.

The presentation may vary from no symptoms to fulminant heart failure, associated pericarditis with effusion, or arrhythmia leading to syncope or sudden death.

### Physical Examination

Tachycardia is common, usually disproportionate to the fever. The heart is enlarged, neck veins distended, and hypotension may be evident with a narrow pulse pressure. With severe disease, the $S_1$ is soft and there are atrial and ventricular gallop sounds as well as murmurs of mitral and/or tricuspid regurgitation, pulmonary congestion, hepatomegaly, and peripheral edema. Pericardial rubs, arrhythmias, and pulmonary or systemic embolization may occur.

Alternatively, the evidence of myocarditis may be so mild that it is overshadowed by the manifestations of the acute infectious illness.

### Electrocardiogram

ECG abnormalities are frequent, nonspecific, and often transitory: they include arrhythmias, conduction defects, low voltage, and ST-T wave changes. Both these and the clinical presentation may mimic myocardial infarction.

### Chest X-Ray

Cardiac enlargement may be due to cavity dilatation, pericardial effusion, or both. Interstitial pulmonary edema and pleural effusion signify severe myocardial involvement.

## Specific Diagnostic Evaluation

### Routine Blood Tests

The erythrocyte sedimentation rate is usually elevated. There may be leukocytosis or eosinophilia, depending on the specific infection. Elevated levels of cardiac serum enzymes reflect the extent of myocardial necrosis.

### Other Tests for Infective Agents

Blood cultures, acute and convalescent serum antibody titers, and other appropriate studies can identify specific infective agents. Throat washings, urine, and feces should be cultured for viruses. Skin testing may be helpful, as for tuberculosis.

### Echocardiography

This procedure is valuable in identifying chamber size, ventricular function, and pericardial effusion initially and serially. There is usually global biventricular hypokinesis, but regional wall motion abnormalities may simulate myocardial infarction. Doppler studies can assess mitral and/or tricuspid regurgitation.

### Nuclear Imaging of the Heart

Radionuclide ventriculography can also provide the data cited above. Myocardial imaging with technetium-99m, gallium-67, or indium may identify diffuse or focal myocardial necrosis or inflammation, but the findings are nonspecific. Thallium-201 perfusion scintigraphy may be abnormal due to faulty myocyte uptake, mimicking myocardial infarction. The use of myosin-specific monoclonal antibodies remains investigational.

### Exercise Testing

This procedure is contraindicated during acute myocarditis. After recovery, exercise testing can document functional impairment and define recommended activity levels.

### Ambulatory ECG Recording

In patients with symptoms suggesting arrhythmia, this may identify the problem and assess response to therapy.

### Cardiac Catheterization and Coronary Angiography

This is rarely indicated except to exclude other remediable disease.

### Endomyocardial Biopsy

Myocyte necrosis or degeneration in proximity to an interstitial inflammatory infiltrate is considered diagnostic of myocarditis on biopsy. However, the sensitivity and specificity of this technique remain unknown, and there is high interobserver variability in diagnosis. Its role remains controversial.

## Abnormal Physiology

Myocardial damage and dysfunction may be due to direct invasion by, or toxic effects of, the microorganism. An autoimmune, cellular, or humoral response, either to the microorganism or to the damaged myocyte, may occur. The different mechanisms at different stages of the disease may explain the variably beneficial and harmful responses described to immunosuppressive therapy.

There is impaired myocardial contractility, with elevated ventricular diastolic volumes and pressures.

Specific etiologies of myocarditis may have characteristic pathophysiological alterations—e.g., the neurotoxic properties of diphtheria toxin and of *Trypanosoma cruzi* (Chagas' disease) affecting conduction tissue.

## Natural History and Prognosis

Most adult patients with mild acute myocarditis recover spontaneously. The percentage of cases that blend into "idiopathic dilated cardiomyopathy" (see below) is uncertain.

A few patients succumb to the acute illness, and some have recurrent or chronic myocarditis. The roles of genetic susceptibility and immunologic responses are under investigation. The prognostic value of endomyocardial biopsy is controversial. Acute myocarditis is a cause of sudden death in young adults.

## Differential Diagnosis

Myocarditis must be differentiated from other causes of myocardial ischemia or necrosis, heart failure, and arrhythmia: acute myocardial infarction, dilated cardiomyopathy, pericarditis with effusion, the myocardial necrosis of collagen vascular disease or other noninfectious etiology, and, at times, valvular heart disease.

## Treatment

Initial medical management should be in the hospital; patients with hypotension or shock, pericardial effusion, cardiac rhythm abnormalities, heart failure, or evidence of myocardial ischemia should have *intensive-care surveillance.*

*Medical management* involves specific therapy for the underlying infection (if known), general measures to reduce cardiac work (modified bed rest, antipyretic agents, supplemental oxygen), and control of the complications of myocarditis: heart failure, cardiogenic shock, arrhythmias or heart block, and thromboembolism.

The initially promising results of immunosuppressive therapy with corticosteroid hormones and/or azathioprine have been increasingly challenged, as adverse effects have been described in humans and in animal models.

*Heart failure* can be managed with dietary sodium restriction, digitalis, and diuretic and vasodilator drugs. For patients with low cardiac output, dobutamine may provide inotropic enhancement with limited vasoconstriction and arrhythmogenic effects. Intraaortic balloon counterpulsation or temporary cardiac-assist devices may provide a bridge to cardiac transplantation.

Temporary or permanent *cardiac pacing* may be lifesaving; *anticoagulation* is advisable, to prevent thromboembolic complications.

## DILATED CARDIOMYOPATHY (DC)

### Definition

The predominant feature of *dilated cardiomyopathy* (DC) is cardiomegaly with ventricular dilatation; myocardial mass is also increased. Characteristically, systolic dysfunction is present and there is no valvular or ischemic heart disease. This is the most common type of cardiomyopathy.

### Etiology

Although no etiology is evident for DC, a number of conditions have been suggested as potentiating or causal: alcohol abuse, systemic arterial hypertension, microvascular spasm, pregnancy and the puerperium, immunologic disorders, viral infections, genetic predisposition, nutritional deficiencies, and a number of potentially toxic chemical and physical agents.

### Pathology

Biventricular dilatation is the major morphological feature of DC; the left ventricle is usually more severely affected. Although heart weight is increased, the ventricular free wall and septum may not be thickened, because of marked cavity dilatation. Ventricular dilatation causes relative stasis of blood in the apical portions, with resultant intracavitary thrombosis; thrombi are also frequent in the atria as a consequence of poor atrial emptying. Intracardiac thrombi give rise to pulmonary and systemic emboli.

There is variable interstitial myocardial fibrosis, usually inadequate to explain the poor contractility. Some myocardial cells are hypertrophied, others atrophied. Other changes are nonspecific. The cardiac valves are usually normal, with valvular regurgitation due to papillary muscle dysfunction and/or annular dilatation. The coronary arteries are normal.

### Clinical Manifestations

#### History

The insidious onset of left ventricular failure progresses from exertional dyspnea to resting dyspnea, nocturnal dry cough, and pulmonary edema. Symptoms of right-sided congestive heart failure may follow. Chest pain may be due to subendocardial ischemia, pulmonary emboli, or pericarditis.

#### Physical Examination

The physical findings are those of heart failure: breathlessness, tachycardia with a small pulse volume, pulsus alternans with advanced disease, and an elevated jugular venous pressure, often with a prominent systolic regurgitant wave. The blood pressure usually remains normal because of peripheral vasoconstriction. The apex impulse is displaced laterally and enlarged; often a presystolic impulse is present. The pulmonic valve closure sound is accentuated when pulmonary hypertension is present. Gallop sounds are characteristic, and the systolic murmurs of mitral and tricuspid regurgitation typically diminish in intensity with treatment. Lung rales and hepatomegaly are frequent, with a pulsatile liver reflecting tricuspid regurgitation. There are pleural and pericardial effusions, peripheral edema, and ascites.

### Electrocardiogram

Sinus tachycardia is characteristic, with atrial abnormalities and, often, lowered QRS voltage. There may be evidence of left ventricular hypertrophy. Arrhythmias and conduction abnormalities are frequent; Q waves may mimic myocardial infarction.

### Chest X-Ray

Cardiomegaly is due to biventricular and biatrial dilatation. There are pulmonary venous hypertension, pleural effusion, and changes of pulmonary infarction. The "water-bottle heart" of pericardial effusion may be present.

## Special Laboratory Studies

### Echocardiography

Biventricular dilatation and global hypokinesis are characteristic, often with paradoxical septal motion. However, segmental wall motion abnormalities may mimic myocardial infarction. The mitral apparatus is displaced posteriorly, with decreased mitral leaflet separation. Ventricular and atrial mural thrombi and pericardial effusion may be evident. Pulsed Doppler studies can quantitate the valvular regurgitation.

### Ambulatory ECG Recording

High-grade or frequent ventricular ectopic activity has been described as identifying patients with a reduced ejection fraction at high risk for sudden death.

### Programmed Electrical Stimulation (PES)

PES-induced ventricular arrhythmias correlate poorly with those seen on ambulatory ECG; neither these nor endocardial late potentials appear to predict sudden death.

### Radionuclide Imaging Techniques

Blood-pool imaging can confirm the ventricular dilatation and global hypokinesis, and serial examinations can assess the response to therapy. Perfusion defects on thallium-201 scintigraphy occur with DC, so the test cannot reliably distinguish DC from ischemic cardiomyopathy. Positron emission tomography seems better able to differentiate ischemic from nonischemic DC. Regional wall motion abnormalities may reflect localized fibrosis.

### Cardiac Catheterization

Coronary arteries usually are widely patent. The ventricles are enlarged, globular, and hypokinetic, at times with filling defects due to intracavitary thrombi.

### Endomyocardial Biopsy

Although this procedure is relatively safe and widely available, histopathological and electron-microscopic findings are nonspecific, with high interobserver variability. Rarely, specific muscle disease such as hemochromatosis or amyloidosis can be identified. This remains an investigational technique.

## Pathophysiology

Ventricular dilatation and diminished contractility result in a low ejection fraction and high end-systolic volume. This limits atrial emptying, leading to high atrial end-diastolic volumes with resulting atrial dilatation.

In the early stages, tachycardia compensates for the reduced stroke volume to maintain cardiac output. Exercise capacity correlates poorly with the functional status of the ventricle.

In the late stages cardiac output is decreased, and increased pulmonary venous pressure causes symptoms of pulmonary venous congestion; ultimately, pulmonary arterial hypertension and right-sided heart failure may occur.

Decreased renal perfusion stimulates the renin-angiotensin-aldosterone system; this and increased sympathetic activity increase intravascular volume, but may increase peripheral vascular resistance as well. This vicious circle further reduces cardiac output.

Decreased coronary vasodilator reserve or microvascular abnormalities may cause subendocardial ischemia and chest pain.

## Natural History and Prognosis

The course of DC is usually steadily downhill, with death common between 6 months to a few years after symptoms appear. Severity of left ventricular dysfunction is the main determinant of prognosis; left bundle branch block and malignant ventricular arrhythmias are also adverse prognostic indicators, the latter predicting sudden death. Nevertheless, about 20 percent of patients have a more favorable course.

Systemic and pulmonary embolism are common complications; warfarin therapy is reported to increase the survival rate.

Energetic treatment of heart failure often produces remission, but symptoms recur after a variable interval; recurrent episodes of heart failure become increasingly difficult to control.

### Differential Diagnosis

DC must be distinguished from other causes of congestive heart failure: principally, coronary atherosclerotic heart disease, hypertensive cardiovascular disease, valvular heart disease, heart muscle disease secondary to specific systemic disorders, and heart failure secondary to diastolic dysfunction (as with hypertrophic cardiomyopathy).

Chest pain, ECG abnormalities, focal myocardial wall motion abnormalities, and myocardial perfusion defects on thallium imaging may mimic myocardial infarction.

### Treatment

*Medical treatment* remains that of heart failure, with activity restriction, avoidance of alcohol, a nutritious sodium-restricted diet, digitalis (with care to avoid toxicity), diuretics, and anticoagulation to reduce thromboembolic complications—even in patients with sinus rhythm. Pregnancy is inadvisable.

Corticosteroid hormones and immunosuppressive therapy remain controversial and entail potential risk. Reduction of resistance to left ventricular ejection with *vasodilator drugs*—nitrates, hydralazine, and angiotensin-converting enzyme inhibitors—may dramatically improve symptoms, and has improved the rate of survival. Their use is recommended unless specific contraindications are present.

The use of *parenteral positive inotropic agents* such as dopamine and dobutamine is promising; oral preparations with both positive inotropic and vasodilator properties have improved symptoms and exercise capacity, but have not altered survival.

The role of antiarrhythmic therapy remains to be defined, because of the risk of proarrhythmic effects. Both automatic implanted cardioverter/defibrillators and permanent pacemakers may be lifesaving. The use of low-dose selective beta-adrenergic blockade is likewise controversial.

The only *surgical treatment* of DC is *cardiac transplantation.* Temporary mechanical support devices may improve the rate of survival while awaiting transplantation.

## SUGGESTED READING

Aretz HT, Billingham ME, Edwards WD, et al: Myocarditis. A histopathologic definition and classification. *Am J Cardiovasc Pathol* 1:3–14, 1986.

Borow KM, Lang RM, Neumann A, et al: Physiologic mechanisms governing hemodynamic responses to positive inotropic therapy in patients with dilated cardiomyopathy. *Circulation* 77:625–637, 1988.

Griffin ML, Hernandez A, Martin TC, et al: Dilated cardiomyopathy in infants and children. *J Am Coll Cardiol* 11:139–144, 1988.

Keogh AM, Freund J, Baron DW, et al: Timing of cardiac transplantation in idiopathic dilated cardiomyopathy. *Am J Cardiol* 61:418–422, 1988.

Nakayama Y, Shimizu G, Hirota Y, et al: Functional and histopathologic correlation in patients with dilated cardiomyopathy: an integrated evaluation by multivariate analysis. *J Am Coll Cardiol* 10:186–192, 1987.

Weinstein C, Fenoglio JJ: Myocarditis. *Hum Pathol* 18:613–618, 1987.

Wenger NK, Abelmann WH, Roberts WC: Myocarditis, in Hurst JW et al (eds): *The Heart,* 7th ed. New York, McGraw-Hill, Chap 64, pp 1256–1277, 1990.

Wenger NK, Abelmann WH, Roberts WC: Cardiomyopathy and specific heart muscle disease, in Hurst JW et al (eds): *The Heart,* 7th ed. New York, McGraw-Hill, Chap 65, pp 1278–1347, 1990.

## 17 | Hypertrophic Cardiomyopathy

*Nanette Kass Wenger, M.D.*

### DEFINITION

The cardinal feature of *hypertrophic cardiomyopathy* (HC) is a considerable increase in myocardial mass, with no ventricular dilatation. Cavity size may be normal or decreased, and systolic function is preserved.

### ETIOLOGY

The etiology of HC is not known, though a familial incidence is often noted. Genetically determined abnormalities of catecholamine function and vascular and myocardial abnormalities secondary to elevated cytosolic calcium levels have been suggested as causes.

### PATHOLOGY

Characteristic abnormalities at necropsy include ventricular septal thickening greater than that of the left ventricular free wall, small or normal-sized right and left ventricular cavities, a fibrous endocardial mural plaque on the left ventricular outflow tract in apposition to the anterior mitral leaflet, mitral valvular thickening, atrial dilatation, abnormal intramural coronary arteries with thick walls and narrow lumina, and myofiber disorganization in the ventricular septum.

The posterobasal left ventricular free wall is the thickest portion of the free wall with obstructive HC. In the patient with a resting left ventricular outflow gradient, the left ventricular free wall is thickest midway between the left ventricular apex and the base of the posterior mitral leaflet. The posterobasal left ventricular free wall is thinner than normal with nonobstructive HC, and is often pointed like a bird's bill. Apical HC and midventricular obstruction are also described.

### CLINICAL MANIFESTATIONS

#### History

Dyspnea and chest pain are the main symptoms. Dyspnea is due to abnormal ventricular compliance and resultant increased pulmonary venous pressure, and is accentuated by tachycardia. Angina may reflect relative ischemia of the hypertrophied myocardium or may be due to intramural coronary artery abnormalities. Palpitations, dizziness, and syncope may reflect ventricular underfilling or may be caused by arrhythmia.

### Physical Examination

The three dominant physical findings when a systolic pressure gradient is present include: a spindle-shaped systolic murmur along the left sternal border that radiates to the apex, at times with a thrill, that decreases with squatting and handgrip and is intensified after a premature ventricular contraction, with standing, and with the Valsalva maneuver; an abrupt upstroke to the arterial pulse, at times with a bisferiens configuration of an initial brisk percussion wave and a subsequent tidal wave; and an ill-sustained bifid apical systolic impulse, often preceded by a powerful presystolic impulse giving a triple-beat character to the apex impulse. An *a* wave in the jugular venous pulse and a prominent $S_4$ at the cardiac apex are common.

## USUAL DIAGNOSTIC TESTS

### Electrocardiogram

A normal ECG virtually excludes significant HC. Increased QRS voltage and ST-T wave abnormalities of left ventricular hypertrophy are common. Left anterior hemiblock, inferior Q waves due to massive septal hypertrophy (that may simulate infarction), and left atrial abnormality are common. A delta wave of preexcitation may be present, and ventricular arrhythmias are common. Giant T-wave inversion is seen with apical HC.

### Chest X-Ray

The cardiac silhouette is often normal, though left atrial enlargement and interstitial pulmonary edema may be present.

## SPECIAL DIAGNOSTIC EVALUATION

### Echocardiography

The two-dimensional echocardiogram is the most valuable noninvasive diagnostic technique. Echocardiographic diagnosis of HC is based on disproportionate septal thickness (asymmetric septal hypertrophy or ASH) with a septal-to-free-wall ratio of more than 1.5; poor septal contractility with vigorous contraction of the left ventricular free wall; decreased end-systolic cavity dimension; displacement of the anterior mitral leaflet anteriorly toward the septum; a reduced rate of mitral valve closure; and (when a gradient is present) systolic anterior motion (SAM) of the anterior mitral leaflet and midsystolic (premature) closure of the aortic valve. Doppler flow studies can evaluate the diastolic dysfunction, the dynamic characteristics of the outflow pressure gradient, and the severity of mitral regurgitation.

### Ambulatory Electrocardiography

This procedure best detects the frequent ventricular arrhythmias. Supraventricular arrhythmias may also be present.

### Radionuclide Imaging Techniques

Technetium-99m labeling of the blood pool and gated blood pool scanning can define anatomy, small cavity size, increased ejection fraction, and response to therapy. Myocardial perfusion imaging with thallium 201 may show reversible perfusion defects.

### Cardiac Catheterization and Angiography

Angiocardiography is indicated when surgery is considered to relieve severe outflow obstruction; and when one needs to define ventricular volumes, outflow gradient, response to maneuvers, or status of the coronary arteries. A slit-like ventricular cavity is typical at end-systole, with gradients more common in the middle than at the apex of the left ventricle.

### Endomyocardial Biopsy

There is no clinical indication for endomyocardial biopsy. The procedure may be hazardous because of the disordered septal geometry.

## ABNORMAL PHYSIOLOGY

The predominant functional abnormality in HC is a decrease in ventricular compliance with impedance to diastolic filling, presumably due to the chaotic myofibrillar architecture and resultant incoordination of myocardial contraction and relaxation. Impaired ventricular filling compromises cardiac function.

Abnormalities of systolic function result in a dynamic outflow gradient that is augmented by a premature ventricular beat, inotropic stimulation, decreased ventricular volume, and/or lowered aortic diastolic pressure. An initial vigorous ventricular contraction expels most of the stroke volume; the decreased end-systolic volume displaces the anterior mitral leaflet toward the hypertrophied septum.

## NATURAL HISTORY AND PROGNOSIS

The natural history varies from long life with few symptoms to a rapidly progressive fatal illness. About half of all patients die suddenly. Younger age onset is associated with more severe obstruction, heart failure, and sudden death. The disease appears more benign in the elderly.

Severe left ventricular hypertrophy and serious ventricular arrhythmias increase the risk of sudden death, but there is little relation between the outflow gradient and sudden death. The onset of atrial fibrillation, with loss of the atrial contribution to ventricular filling, usually causes severe clinical deterioration with heart failure and, at times, systemic embolism.

HC is a common cause of sudden death in young athletes; its cause may be mechanical (increased outflow gradient) or arrhythmic.

Ventricular dilatation may occur after myocardial necrosis or septal resection. Infective endocarditis is also a hazard. Pregnancy usually is well tolerated.

## DIFFERENTIAL DIAGNOSIS

The murmur of HC can mimic that of aortic stenosis (AS), pulmonic stenosis, ventricular septal defect (VSD), or mitral regurgitation (MR).

The pronounced presystolic impulse of HC is not present with VSD or MR, and the arterial pulse is not sustained due to left ventricular "runoff." The slowly-rising small volume pulse of AS, at times with an ejection click, is not seen with HC, where the murmur begins later and is often shorter. Heavy calcific deposits on the aortic valve virtually exclude HC; although mitral anular calcium is common in elderly patients with HC. HC with right ventricular outflow obstruction may mimic PS.

Chest pain may mimic coronary heart disease, and the abnormal ECG may suggest myocardial infarction.

## TREATMENT

There is no known prevention. Violent exercise, tachycardia, sudden decrease in blood pressure or blood volume, and positive inotropic and vasodilator drugs all enhance outflow obstruction and should be avoided to minimize the risk of sudden death. Improvement in ventricular compliance, with beta blockers or calcium antagonists, and control of ventricular arrhythmias may improve prognosis. Antibiotic prophylaxis is indicated to avert infective endocarditis.

*Asymptomatic patients* with mild disease may not need specific therapy, though a definite family history of HC probably warrants propranolol or verapamil to attempt to retard disease progression.

*Angina* and *dyspnea* commonly respond to large doses of beta blockers; propranolol (noncardioselective) is the drug of choice and may also control tachyarrhythmias. Amiodarone may be added if ventricular arrhythmias persist with maximally tolerated doses of beta blockers.

Verapamil reduces symptoms and improves exercise capacity with both obstructive and nonobstructive HC, presumably by enhancing diastolic filling. Verapamil and beta blockers used concomitantly require caution to avert pulmonary congestion and conduction abnormalities.

Amiodarone, despite considerable systemic toxicity, effectively controls ventricular arrhythmias, but should not be given if atrioventricular block is present. The onset of *atrial fibrillation (AF)* is a medical emergency requiring DC cardioversion. Anticoagulation is indicated with persistent AF. Pacemaker therapy is indicated for unacceptable bradycardia and for heart block. Vasodilator and diuretic drugs should be avoided in treating concomitant hypertension. Digitalis may increase the outflow gradient.

*Surgical treatment* with partial septal resection and/or incision is advised for severely symptomatic patients with an outflow gradient of at least 50 mmHg. The gradient and the mitral regurgitation are generally reduced or abolished, and symptoms relieved. There is no firm evidence for prolonged survival or decreased sudden death; recent reports suggest a smaller operative risk than the 8 percent previously described.

Mitral valve replacement is rarely indicated except for severe mitral regurgitation, as from infective endocarditis.

## SUGGESTED READING

Brigden W: Hypertrophic cardiomyopathy. *Br Med J* 58:299–302, 1987.

Maron BJ, Bonow RO, Cannon RO III, et al: Hypertrophic cardiomyopathy: interrelations of clinical manifestations, pathophysiology, and therapy. *N Engl J Med* 316:780–789, 844–852, 1987.

ten Cate FJ (ed): *Hypertrophic Cardiomyopathy: Clinical Recognition and Management.* New York, Marcel Dekker, 1985.

Wenger NK, Abelmann WH, Roberts WC: Cardiomyopathy and specific heart muscle disease, in Hurst JW et al (eds): *The Heart,* 7th ed. New York, McGraw-Hill, Chap 65, pp 1278–1347, 1990.

Wigle ED: Hypertrophic cardiomyopathy: a 1987 viewpoint. *Circulation* 75:311–322, 1987.

## 18 | Restrictive Cardiomyopathy

*Nanette Kass Wenger, M.D.*

### DEFINITION

*Restrictive (obliterative) cardiomyopathy* (RC) is impairment of ventricular filling by endocardial or myocardial disease or both, producing hemodynamic and clinical responses similar to those of constrictive pericarditis. The hallmark is an abnormality of diastolic function. Obliterative cardiomyopathy is primarily an endocardial disease, and ventricular cavity size is often reduced.

### ETIOLOGY

Endomyocardial fibrosis (EMF) is the most common cause of RC in the tropics. In temperate zones, RC may be due to Loeffler's endomyocardial fibrosis with eosinophilia or to idiopathic myocardial fibrosis. Amyloid heart disease often results in a restrictive physiology, as may hemochromatosis, sarcoid heart disease, Fabry's disease, neoplasms, scleroderma, and radiation heart disease.

### PATHOLOGY

Endocardial fibrosis and mural endocardial thickening of one or both ventricles, with variable eosinophilia, is characteristic of EMF and Loeffler's endomyocardial fibrosis. An acute necrotic stage, a thrombotic stage, and a late fibrotic stage have been documented by endomyocardial biopsy. When fibrosis involves the papillary muscles and chordae tendineae, atrioventricular valvular regurgitation occurs. In the late stage, ventricular cavity obliteration may ensue. In the specific heart muscle diseases listed above, the characteristic morphological infiltrative abnormalities are evident at microscopic examination.

### CLINICAL MANIFESTATIONS

#### History

Tiredness and abnormal swelling (ascites) are common with right-sided EMF. Progressive dyspnea and cough occur when left-sided disease predominates.

#### Physical Examination

Sinus tachycardia is a common finding, as compensation for the almost fixed stroke volume. Episodic atrial fibrillation may occur.

The arterial pulse is small and decreases with inspiration. With right ventricular involvement, elevation of the jugular venous column reflects the high mean right atrial pressure; a large systolic wave is common. The steep $x$ and $y$ descents of the jugular venous pulse are evidence of restriction to filling. Hepatomegaly and ascites are present, but edema is rare; the murmur of tricuspid regurgitation is usual with right-sided disease. Lung rales and the murmur of mitral regurgitation are evidence of left-sided disease, and an $S_3$ is common.

## USUAL DIAGNOSTIC TESTS

### Electrocardiogram

Low QRS voltage is frequent on the ECG, with right ventricular hypertrophy, left ventricular hypertrophy, or both reflecting the predominant ventricular involvement. Right axis deviation may be present with predominant right ventricular disease. The comparable atrial abnormality (P wave) is also present, and there are nonspecific T-wave abnormalities.

### Chest X-Ray

The cardiac silhouette is typically enlarged, in part because of pericardial effusion. Pleural effusions are common. Linear calcium deposition may be evident at the obliterated right or left ventricular apex. Left atrial enlargement and pulmonary venous congestion are evidence of left ventricular dysfunction, and right atrial enlargement and lung underfilling occur with predominant right ventricular disease.

## SPECIAL DIAGNOSTIC EVALUATION

### Eosinophilia

Eosinophilia in the blood is frequent in EMF and Loeffler's endomyocardial disease, and the eosinophils are often immunologically abnormal. Degranulated peripheral blood eosinophils suggest the need for diagnostic endomyocardial biopsy.

### Echocardiography and Radionuclide Imaging

Echocardiography may show prominent bright echoes from the increased endocardial collagen. Apical obliteration or thrombus, at times with calcium deposition, is present. Preserved ventricular contractility and atrial dilatation are prominent. *Doppler studies* can define the hemodynamic abnormalities, including the diastolic mitral and tricuspid regurgitation. Echocardiography and radionuclide imaging can aid in differentiation from dilated cardiomyopathy by defining the normal-to-diminished ventricular cavity size.

### Endomyocardial Biopsy

Endomyocardial biopsy may help differentiate RC from constrictive pericarditis and prevent unnecessary thoracotomy. Endomyocardial biopsy may diagnose one of the specific heart muscle diseases mentioned above as responsible for a restrictive physiology.

### Magnetic Resonance Imaging

Magnetic resonance imaging may show a prominent atrial signal in all phases of the cardiac cycle, reflecting stasis of atrial blood secondary to elevation of ventricular diastolic pressure. It can define normal pericardial thickness and distinguish between constrictive pericarditis and RC.

### Angiocardiography

At angiocardiography, the ventricular cavity size is reduced and the endocardium is thickened. Apical blunting is evident, and ventricular contractile function is characteristically preserved. Ventricular cavity distortion by fibrosis and thrombosis helps in differentiation from constrictive pericarditis. Pericardial effusion and mitral and tricuspid regurgitation can be identified.

## ABNORMAL PHYSIOLOGY

Diastolic ventricular volume and stretch are impaired by endocardial fibrosis and/or progressive cavity obliteration by fibrous tissue and thrombus. This limits ventricular filling and leads to increased filling pressures. Rapid ventricular filling occurs early in diastole, and the noncompliant ventricle abruptly limits late diastolic filling. The cardiac output is decreased. The sharp early diastolic dip and high end-diastolic plateau in the right ventricle mimics the "dip-and-plateau" of constrictive pericarditis. The inspiratory increase in venous pressure (Kussmaul's sign) and decrease in arterial pressure are less pronounced than in constrictive pericarditis.

## NATURAL HISTORY AND PROGNOSIS

Heart failure is progressive and poorly responsive to usual therapy. Systemic emboli may complicate the clinical course. Surgery (see below) has effected short-term success in the treatment of EMF.

## DIFFERENTIAL DIAGNOSIS

Differentiation from *constrictive pericarditis* is most important. Helpful features are the similarity of diastolic pressure in both ventricles in constrictive pericarditis, but not in RC; also pulmonary hypertension is common in RC, when there is predominant left ventricular involvement and mitral regurgitation, but is not present in constrictive pericarditis.

Differentiation from dilated cardiomyopathy has been described above ("Echocardiography and Radionuclide Imaging"). Occasional differentiation is required from hypertrophic cardiomyopathy, hypertensive cardiovascular disease, right atrial myxoma, and the like.

## TREATMENT

The medical treatment of the congestive heart failure is largely unsatisfactory, and the clinical course is that of progressive deterioration. Digitalis (except when atrial fibrillation is present) and vasodilator drugs are of little help, and excessive use of diuretic drugs may worsen the clinical problem.

Surgical resection of the obliterating endocardial tissue, with repair or replacement of the regurgitant mitral and tricuspid valves, has been described as effecting short-term success. Laser photoablation has been suggested. Cardiac transplantation should be considered for end-stage disease.

Thromboembolic complications and documented ventricular thrombus should be treated with anticoagulation. Corticosteroid and immunosuppressive drugs have each occasionally produced improvement in patients with endomyocardial fibrosis.

## SUGGESTED READING

Metras D, Coulibaly AO, Ouattara K: The surgical treatment of endomyocardial fibrosis: results in 55 patients. *Circulation* 72(suppl 2):274–279, 1985.

Olsen EGJ, Spry CJF: Relation between eosinophilia and endomyocardial disease. *Prog Cardiovasc Dis* 27:241–254, 1985.

Presti C, Ryan T, Armstrong WF: Two-dimensional and Doppler echocardiographic findings in hypereosinophilic syndrome. *Am Heart J* 114:172–175, 1987.

Schoenfeld MH, Supple EW, Dec GW Jr, et al: Restrictive cardiomyopathy versus constrictive pericarditis: role of endomyocardial biopsy in avoiding unnecessary thoracotomy. *Circulation* 75:1012–1017, 1987.

Wenger NK, Abelmann WH, Roberts WC: Cardiomyopathy and specific heart muscle disease, in Hurst JW et al (eds): *The Heart,* 7th ed. New York, McGraw-Hill, Chap 65, pp 1278–1347, 1990.

*Ralph Shabetai, M.D.*

## ACUTE VIRAL AND IDIOPATHIC PERICARDITIS

The inflammation is fibrinous, and pericardial effusion is sometimes present. The illness presents with malaise, fever, and chest pain which may be either pleuritic or retrosternal and crushing. The pain is sometimes relieved by sitting up. Trapezoid ridge radiation is characteristic. The leukocyte count and erythrocyte sedimentation rate are elevated.

Pericardial friction rub is the diagnostic sign. It is superficial, scratchy or creaky, and best appreciated using firm pressure with the stethoscope.

Diffuse ST-segment elevation is the classic ECG finding. The ST is depressed in a $V_R$ and $V_1$. The T wave remains upright. PR depression is specific but insensitive.

### Treatment

The illness is usually brief and responsive to nonsteroidal anti-inflammatory agents. The patient must be observed for increasing pericardial effusion (echocardiogram) and tamponade.

## RECURRENT PERICARDITIS

In some patients an immunological abnormality develops that causes violent attacks of pericarditis, with or without effusion, to recur over many months or years.

### Treatment

Attempt to treat recurrences with nonsteroidal anti-inflammatory agents. When that is not possible prednisone should be given, usually starting at 60 mg per day, supplemented with an anti-inflammatory agent, such as ibuprofen. Azathioprine can also be used as an adjunct. Colchicine may be effective. Relapses may recur for many years. Try to prevent steroid dependency in such patients. Pericardiotomy should be considered only when the patient is dependent upon steroids and has side effects.

## PERICARDIAL EFFUSION

### Etiology

The common causes are acute viral or idiopathic pericarditis, and neoplasm—most commonly bronchogenic, mammary, or lymphomatous. Drugs such as procainamide can also cause pericardial effusion.

### Diagnosis

There are no specific symptoms; physical examination is helpful only when there is tamponade. Whenever pericardial effusion is a reasonable possibility, it is essential to obtain an echocardiogram. It is important to assess cardiac function as well, so as to rule out underlying cardiac dysfunction.

### Nature of the Fluid

Pericardial fluid is quite often bloody, almost regardless of the cause. Pericardiocentesis for diagnosis has a remarkably low yield and should be avoided. Pericardiocentesis indicated for treatment, paradoxically, has a significant diagnostic yield. Thus, in patients who undergo the procedure for cardiac tamponade or persistence of a large effusion, diagnosis of the underlying cause is often possible.

## THE PERICARDIAL COMPRESSIVE SYNDROMES

*Cardiac tamponade* and *constrictive pericarditis* share important features, but also have a number of important differentiating features. The pathophysiology in both is impaired diastolic filling. In both, systemic and pulmonary venous pressures are elevated, cardiac output may be low, and there is equalization of left and right ventricular diastolic pressure.

In *tamponade* the raised venous pressure is characterized by respiratory variation and a dominant *x* descent, coincident with the carotid pulse. In *constrictive pericarditis* the characteristic rapid *y* descent of venous pressure is out of phase with the carotid pulse.

*Pulsus paradoxus* occurs in moderate and severe cardiac tamponade, but not in mild tamponade. Pulsus paradoxus is less common in constrictive pericarditis, except in elastic constrictive pericarditis, in which the pericardium can stretch a little.

### Cardiac Tamponade

Common causes include trauma (which may be iatrogenic), neoplasm, and viral or idiopathic pericarditis.

In the acute form, often due to trauma, the heart is small, the venous pressure is extremely high, and hypotension is prominent. The effusion may be small, because the pericardium cannot be stretched fast enough to accommodate a large effusion. Pulsus paradoxus is often prominent.

In medical cases, effusion usually develops more slowly and the effusions are usually larger. In moderately severe cases, cardiac output is reduced about 25 percent, but arterial blood pressure is maintained at or near normal. Venous pressure is elevated.

As cardiac tamponade worsens, hypotension occurs, cardiac output is considerably lower, and pulsus paradoxus is usually evident. Venous pressure is high and the *x* descent prominent. A pericardial friction rub may be present, and the ECG may not show signs of acute pericarditis but may show pulsus alternans.

### Echocardiography

This is a singularly helpful examination. The diagnosis cannot be entertained if the echocardiogram does not confirm pericardial effusion. Right atrial compression and right ventricular diastolic collapse are highly sensitive and specific signs of early-to-moderate tamponade. These echocardiographic signs appear before hypotension or pulsus paradoxus and when the reduction of cardiac output is modest. If untreated, tamponade progresses to the decompensated state marked by hypotension, low cardiac output, oliguria, and altered consciousness.

### Preexisting Heart Disease

Preexisting heart disease may alter the manifestations of cardiac tamponade. Particularly important is elevation of left ventricular end-diastolic pressure, as may occur in patients receiving hemodialysis. In these cases, pulsus paradoxus characteristically is absent. Pulsus paradoxus is also absent in aortic regurgitation and atrial septal defect.

### Treatment

In mild cases, especially idiopathic or viral, it may be unnecessary to remove pericardial fluid. Such cases should be observed frequently and monitored by serial echocardiograms while undergoing anti-inflammatory treatment. If the pericardial effusion becomes smaller and signs of cardiac tamponade diminish, the patient usually will not require pericardiocentesis. Failure of such resolution is an indication for removal of pericardial fluid.

Other cases, including all with significantly compromised hemodynamics, must undergo pericardiocentesis or open drainage. Pericardiocentesis, except in drastic emergencies, should always be preceded by echocardiography.

Administering isoproterenol, or a vasodilator, and volume infusions are improvising measures that precede pericardiocentesis and are not substitutes for removal of fluid.

## Constrictive Pericarditis

### Etiology

The common causes are neoplasm, radiation, and infection. Tuberculosis is less common in recent series. Many cases are idiopathic, and some posttraumatic. A small number are complications of cardiac surgery.

### Symptoms

The symptoms are indistinguishable from those of severe right-sided heart failure, but there may be a history of pericarditis. Dyspnea, fatigue, weight gain, edema, and ascites are the principal features.

### Physical Examination

Signs suggesting congestive heart failure without apparent etiology should raise the possibility of constrictive pericarditis. The venous pressure is elevated and dominated by a prominent y descent. The apex beat may be impalpable, or systolic retraction may be evident. A third heart sound, the pericardial knock, is fairly common. The electrocardiogram usually shows nonspecific ST- and T-wave changes.

### Hemodynamics

Cardiac output may be low. The atrial pressure shows a deep y descent corresponding with the early diastolic dip of ventricular pressure. The left and right ventricular diastolic pressures show a dip and plateau (square root) configuration, and the two plateaus are equal.

## Effusive Constrictive Pericarditis

This syndrome occurs when there is not just pericardial effusion, often causing cardiac tamponade, but also pericardial *pathology*. When pericardial fluid is removed, the classic clinical and hemodynamic findings of cardiac tamponade give way to those of constrictive pericarditis. The syndrome should be suspected in cases of tamponade when right atrial pressure does not return to normal after removal of pericardial fluid.

### Differential Diagnosis

The syndrome is sometimes mistaken for *cirrhosis of the liver* because of edema, ascites, and hepatic dysfunction. In cirrhosis, however, venous pressure is normal or only slightly elevated.

*Tricuspid valve disease* may simulate right-sided heart failure or constrictive pericarditis. Patients should be auscultated for the systolic murmur of tricuspid regurgitation or the diastolic rumble of tricuspid stenosis, both of which become louder during inspiration. Doppler echocardiographic studies of the tricuspid valve are helpful.

*Right ventricular infarction* may also simulate right-sided heart failure or constrictive pericarditis. In right ventricular infarction, however, there are usually other features of ischemic heart disease.

*Restrictive cardiomyopathy* simulates constrictive pericarditis. The differential diagnosis can be straightforward or difficult. Prior pericarditis or calcification of the pericardium favors constrictive pericarditis. ST-T wave changes favor cardiomyopathy. The finding of equal diastolic pressures in the ventricles is consistent with either diagnosis, but left ventricular diastolic pressure considerably above the right favors cardiomyopathy. A thickened pericardium by CT or NMR imaging is helpful, but a normal-appearing pericardium does not rule out constrictive pericarditis. If doubt still remains, endomyocardial biopsy should be performed. In the very small minority of cases that remain undiagnosed, exploratory thoracotomy is justified.

### Other Syndromes of Constrictive Pericarditis

*Occult constrictive pericarditis* may be disclosed by infusion of a large volume of fluid, which causes the previously normal right atrial and pulmonary wedge pressures to become equal and develop the waveform of constrictive pericarditis.

*Localized constrictive pericarditis* can occur, especially in postoperative cases.

#### Treatment

The usual treatment is *pericardiectomy*. Venous pressure below 7 or 8 mmHg can be followed. With the availability of cardiopulmonary bypass, surgical mortality has been greatly reduced. Heavily calcific constrictive pericarditis still poses a surgical risk, in the range of 5 to 10 percent. When constriction is by the visceral pericardium, it is difficult to separate the planes; the operation is risky, and it is seldom possible to perform a complete pericardiectomy.

### SOME SPECIFIC PERICARDIAL DISORDERS

#### Dialysis-Related and Uremic Pericardial Disease

Pericarditis is a late finding in *untreated chronic renal disease* and often predicts short survival.

Patients undergoing *hemodialysis* are subject to pericarditis at lower levels of nitrogen retention. This may take the form of pericardial effusion, or a friction rub. Effusions frequently lead to cardiac tamponade.

Diagnosis is difficult; the venous pressure is often high, because these patients retain fluid. Therefore, the combination of a pericardial effusion by echocardiogram and raised venous pressure may or may not indicate cardiac tamponade. These patients do not have pulsus paradoxus. Right atrial pressure may be lower than pulmonary wedge pressure. Thus, cardiac tamponade develops when pericardial pressure becomes equal to right atrial pressure but is not as high as pulmonary wedge pressure. This difference is the reason for the absence of pulsus paradoxus. The echocardiogram should be scanned for right atrial compression or right ventricular collapse.

In some hospitals, a large persistent pericardial effusion, and certainly cardiac tamponade, is an indication for subxyphoid drainage of the pericardial fluid. In others the policy is less aggressive. The patient with effusion but without tamponade may respond to intensification of dialysis. Pericardiocentesis is done in some dialysis units for early cardiac tamponade, but not in others, where surgical drainage is preferred. Mortality from cardiac tamponade in dialysis patients is considerable.

### Pericardium and Myocardial Infarction

*Pericardial friction rub* is common in the first day or two of acute myocardial infarction. It is not an indication to stop anticoagulants or thrombolytic treatment.

*Asymptomatic pericardial effusion* is common in the course of acute myocardial infarction.

*Dressler's syndrome* is probably an autoimmune response to myocardial injury. There may be an infective component, as suggested by the epidemiology, which shows swings from frequent occurrence to long periods when it is not encountered.

### Post-Pericardiotomy Syndrome

This is a syndrome of fever, leukocytosis, chest pain, and, frequently, pericardial effusion in patients who have undergone operation involving the opening of the pericardium. The syndrome may appear a week or two after operation or may be delayed. Sometimes it exhibits features of recurrence. Treatment should be with nonsteroidal anti-inflammatory drugs, but if the syndrome cannot be suppressed, prednisone is needed.

### Neoplastic Pericardial Disease

The most common neoplasms are secondaries, from the lung or from breast lymphoma, and leukemia. Mesothelioma is the most common primary tumor.

Neoplasm is an important cause of pericardial effusion. Cardiac tamponade and constrictive pericarditis are fairly frequent. When a long remission or cure has not been secured, treatment should be directed toward the patient's comfort. Patients in whom the outlook from the neoplasm is favorable can be treated more radically.

### Radiation-Induced Pericardial Disease

Radiation of the mediastinum can produce both constrictive pericarditis and restrictive cardiomyopathy. The onset may be early, but can be delayed several years. Endomyocardial biopsy is useful in deciding whether the patient would improve with pericardiectomy.

### Hypersensitivity and Collagen Vascular Pericardial Disorders

*Rheumatoid arthritis* can cause subacute constrictive pericarditis and be associated with other abnormalities such as heart block and valve disease. Pericardiectomy is often required.

Pericardial disease develops in nearly all patients with *lupus erythematosus* when life is prolonged by steroid treatment. The usual lesion is fibrinous pericarditis, but a large pericardial effusion may develop. Late complications include cardiac tamponade and constrictive pericarditis.

### Drug-Induced Pericardial Disease

Pericardial abnormalities may develop in response to hydralazine, procainamide, and isoniazid.

### Infectious (Nonviral) Pericarditis

#### Tuberculous Pericarditis

This disease is now quite uncommon, though it is encountered in patients with impaired immunological status—e.g., in AIDS patients and in the hemodialysis population. Tuberculosis should be suspected if no other etiology is readily apparent, if pericardial disease does not subside spontaneously or respond readily to antiinflammatory treatment, or if pericardial disease occurs in a patient who has had immunosuppression.

Tuberculous pericarditis is usually treated with a triple drug regimen such as rifampin 600 mg, isoniazid 300 mg daily, and ethambutol 50 mg per kg body weight.

#### Bacterial Pericarditis

Infectious pericarditis has become less common. However, it is a life-threatening disease with a high mortality. Staphylococcus can affect the pericardium, especially in the elderly and in the immunocompromised. Most frequently, treatment is by open surgical drainage.

## SUGGESTED READING

Leimgruber PP, Klopfenstein HS, Wann LS, et al: The hemodynamic derangement associated with right ventricular diastolic collapse in cardiac tamponade. *Circulation* 68:612–620, 1983.

Schoenfeldt MH, Supple EW, Dec GW, et al: Restrictive cardiomyopathy versus constrictive pericarditis. *Circulation* 75:1012–1017, 1987.

Shabetai R: Diseases of the pericardium, in Hurst JW (ed): *The Heart,* 7th ed. New York, McGraw-Hill, Chap 66, pp 1348–1374, 1990.

Shabetai R, Fowler NO, Guntheroth WG: The hemodynamics of cardiac tamponade and constrictive pericarditis. *Am J Cardiol* 26:480–489, 1970.

Spodick DH: Acoustic phenomena in pericardial disease. *Am Heart J* 81:114–124, 1971.

Spodick DH: Diagnostic electrocardiographic sequences in acute pericarditis. *Circulation* 48:575–580, 1973.

# Traumatic Heart Disease

*Panagiotis N. Symbas, M.D.*

## DEFINITIONS

The third leading cause of death in the United States, and in most other industrialized nations, is trauma. Injury to the heart or great vessels is the cause of death in a major number of trauma victims. The most common causes of traumatic injuries to the heart are penetrating injuries, from missiles and knives, and blunt injuries, from direct compressing or decelerating forces to the chest—usually suffered in vehicular accidents. Other types of cardiac injury include the iatrogenic injuries occurring during angioplasties, cardiac catheterization, cardiopulmonary resuscitation, and insertion of various catheters and pacemaker electrodes, and injuries due to ionizing radiation and electrical currents.

Penetrating wounds of the heart usually are due to penetrating wounds of the thorax. These wounds may cause injury to any of the cardiac structures—the cardiac wall, the atrial or ventricular septum, the cardiac valves, the coronary arteries, and/or the pericardium. Penetrating injury to the heart commonly causes cardiac tamponade or massive blood loss. In addition, such injury may lead to structural defects, such as the formation of aneurysms, septal defects, and fistulas between heart chambers and great vessels. Valvular and papillary muscle injury may result in acute valvular regurgitation; injury to coronary vessels may cause myocardial infarction, coronary arteriovenous fistula, or coronary artery aneurysm.

Pericardial wounds may cause serofibrinous (usually), suppurative (occasionally), and constrictive (very rarely) pericarditis. Foreign-body or thrombotic embolic events may occur, and rhythm and conduction disturbances are not uncommon.

Nonpenetrating trauma also may cause injury to any of the cardiac structures, resulting in a variety of pathophysiological changes. Contusion of the heart is the most common blunt injury. It can cause rhythm or conduction disturbances and can evolve to subsequent rupture of the free cardiac wall or septum, or to aneurysm formation. Rupture of the cardiac valves, the free cardiac wall, or the cardiac septa may also result from nonpenetrating trauma.

## CLINICAL MANIFESTATIONS

The initial clinical presentation and the course of cardiac injury depend on the type and site of injury and the degree of damage sustained. This may vary from no symptoms—particularly in patients sustaining blunt trauma—to immediate death, usually from cardiac tamponade or massive blood loss, from laceration or penetration of the free cardiac wall or coronary vessels, or from rhythm disturbances usually seen in blunt trauma. Delayed or residual sequelae, such as ventricular and atrial septal defects, shunts between cardiac chambers or great vessels, valvular regurgitation, endocarditis, and embolic phenomena, should be suspected and sought so that they can be recognized promptly and managed appropriately. Symptoms of angina or congestive heart failure, or symptoms associated with arrhythmias, may occur. The physical examination varies, depending on the type of trauma and the time lapsed since the injury. Careful assessment of the vital signs should be made during the immediate postinjury period; this includes a search for evidence of hemodynamic instability and its causes. The cardiovascular examination should include a thorough search for evidence of cardiac tamponade, bleeding or congestive failure resulting from myocardial damage, or valvular regurgitation. During the later postinjury period, the physical examination should be directed toward the detection of signs of residual damage from the cardiac injury—e.g., of valvular dysfunction, various shunts, or pericarditis.

## DIAGNOSTIC EVALUATION

More than the usual diagnostic evaluation may be warranted. The extent of the evaluation depends on the patient's clinical condition and the time elapsed since the injury. It should include an echocardiogram, which often is very helpful in determining the presence of myocardial or valvular damage and in helping to document and quantify pericardial effusions. Measurements of cardiac isoenzymes should be routinely obtained in cases of suspected contusion. Occasionally, cardiac catheterization may be necessary for full assessment of the extent of damage before surgical repair can be undertaken. Patients exposed to major decelerating forces, such as occur in a motor vehicle accident, should be examined for aortic rupture. The blood pressure should be measured in both upper and lower extremities to help detect aortic injury. Chest x-rays can prove very helpful in suspected rupture of the aorta, by demonstrating alteration of the mediastinal silhouette; aortography should be performed in all patients with such alteration.

## NATURAL HISTORY AND PROGNOSIS

Unprecedented numbers of patients with traumatic injuries to the heart are now reaching the hospital alive, thanks to improved emergency facilities. About one-half of victims of stab wounds to the heart survive long enough to reach the hospital, but the outlook for projectile injuries is much more ominous. Advances in resuscitative and surgical techniques now allow repair in a relatively large proportion of patients who reach the hospital alive. The long-term outlook for a given patient depends not only on the nature and degree of acute injury but also on the detection and appropriate management of the residual, or delayed, sequelae of the trauma.

## TREATMENT

The care of these patients must be individualized according to the nature of the injury. For penetrating wounds, prompt diagnosis of the clinical situation, with appropriate resuscitative and surgical intervention, is necessary. For myocardial contusion, the treatment is usually symptomatic and basically like that for myocardial infarction, with appropriate periods of bed rest and gradual ambulation. Monitoring for arrhythmias is mandatory in the early stages, with pharmacological therapy given when necessary.

## SUGGESTED READING

Symbas PN: *Cardiothoracic Trauma.* Philadelphia, Saunders, 1989.
Symbas PN, Arensberg D: Traumatic heart disease, in Hurst JW et al (eds): *The Heart,* 7th ed. New York, McGraw-Hill, Chap 67, pp 1375–1381, 1990.

# 21 | Neoplastic Diseases of the Heart

*Robert J. Hall, M.D.*

Tumors of the heart are uncommon, but they present in protean ways and challenge the acumen of the physician. Cardiac tumors may be primary in origin (see Table 21-1) or secondary from proximate or remote sites, and they are expressed in a limited number of ways. The general manifestations of these tumors are listed in Table 21-2, by site of cardiac involvement.

## PRIMARY TUMORS OF THE HEART

### Cardiac Myxomas

*Intracardiac myxoma* is the most common benign tumor of the heart. Approximately 75 percent of atrial myxomas are located within the left atrium and arise from the interatrial septum. Usually they are pedunculated and prolapse through the mitral valve during diastole. Myxomas occur most commonly in women from 30 to 60 years of age. Patients generally present with symptoms from a triad of manifestations—constitutional, embolic, and obstructive. *Systemic manifestations,* which are noted in 90 percent of patients, consist of weight loss, fever, anemia, elevated sedimentation rate, and elevated immunoglobulin concentration (usually IgA).

In 50 percent of patients *systemic emboli* occur, involving the brain (half of all emboli), heart, kidneys, extremities, and the aortic bifurcation. Histological examination of all surgically removed emboli should be performed in order to confirm a diagnosis of myxoma. Emboli should arouse suspicion of myxoma in young patients, especially when they are in sinus rhythm. With left atrial myxomas, *obstruction* of either the mitral valve or the pulmonary veins may occur, producing pulmonary venous and arterial hypertension with secondary right-sided heart failure. Symptoms include dyspnea, orthopnea, manifestations of acute pulmonary edema, hemoptysis, dizziness, and syncope; occasionally, sudden death occurs. Change of the patient's position may also produce symptoms.

In the physical examination of a patient with a left atrial myxoma, the electrocardiographic and radiographic findings resemble those seen with mitral valve disease; however, sinus rhythm is usually present. Auscultation reveals a loud $S_1$ and an accentuated $S_2$, followed by an early diastolic sound. This sound, the "tumor plop," is produced by prolapse of the tumor through the mitral

TABLE 21-1 Most Common Tumors and Cysts of the Heart and Pericardium

| Benign | Percentage | Malignant | Percentage |
|---|---|---|---|
| Myxoma | 24.4 | Angiosarcoma | 7.3 |
| Pericardial cyst | 15.4 | Rhabdomyosarcoma | 4.9 |
| Lipoma | 8.4 | Mesothelioma | 3.6 |
| Papillary fibroelastoma | 7.9 | Fibrosarcoma | 2.6 |
| Rhabdomyoma | 6.8 | Lymphoma | 1.3 |
| Fibroma | 3.2 | Others | 3.7 |
| Hemangioma | 2.8 | | |
| Teratoma | 2.6 | | |
| Mesothelioma of the AV node | 2.3 | | |
| Bronchogenic cyst | 1.3 | | |
| Others | 1.5 | | |

*Source:* McAllister HA Jr, Fenoglio JJ Jr: *Tumors of the Cardiovascular System.* Washington, DC, Armed Forces Institute of Pathology, 1978.

valve. An apical diastolic or systolic murmur, or both, is usually present. The two-dimensional echocardiogram is diagnostic and demonstrates the location, origin, and movement of the intracardiac mass. Because cardiac catheterization and angiography increase the risk of tumor embolization, they are indicated only for diagnosis

TABLE 21-2 Manifestations of Cardiac Tumors (Classification by Site of Involvement)

Pericardial Involvement
    Pericarditis, pain
    Pericardial effusion
    Cardiac enlargement on chest x-ray
    Arrhythmias (predominantly atrial)
    Tamponade (usually with bloody fluid)
    Cardiac constriction

Myocardial Involvement
    Arrhythmias, both atrial and ventricular
    Electrocardiographic changes (usually nonspecific)
    Conduction defects and AV block
    Cardiac enlargement on chest x-ray
    Congestive heart failure
    Coronary involvement: angina, infarction

Intracavitary Involvement
    Cavity obliteration
    Valvular obstruction or insufficiency, or both
    Embolic phenomena: systemic, neurological, coronary
    Constitutional symptoms: fever, weight loss

of concomitant cardiac disease. Treatment for left atrial myxoma consists of prompt surgical resection of the tumor, together with a generous portion of the atrial septum from which it arises.

*Right atrial myxomas* occur with one-fifth the frequency of left atrial myxomas and are characterized by manifestations of systemic venous hypertension: a prominent jugular *a* wave, hepatomegaly, ascites, and edema. There is a loud early systolic sound at the lower sternal border, and systolic and diastolic murmurs at the tricuspid valve area may mimic a pericardial friction rub. As in cases of left atrial myxoma, echocardiography is applied in the diagnosis, and surgical treatment is recommended.

## Other Benign Primary Cardiac Tumors

*Rhabdomyoma,* which is the most common cardiac tumor in children, frequently accompanies tuberous sclerosis. Located in the myocardium, rhabdomyomas usually cause arrhythmias and obstructive manifestations. *Fibromas* may cause sudden death and, like *lipomas,* may grow to a large size.

## Malignant Primary Tumors of the Heart

Almost all primary malignant tumors of the heart are *sarcomas*—most frequently *angiosarcomas,* which usually originate in the right atrium or pericardium. One-fourth of all angiosarcomas produce valvular obstruction and manifest right-sided heart failure and pericardial tamponade with hemorrhagic pericardial fluid. Tumor excision, radiation therapy, and chemotherapy may offer some relief of symptoms.

## Tumors of the Pericardium

Since 75 percent of all *pericardial cysts* are asymptomatic, these tumors are usually found coincidentally on chest x-ray. They most often reside in the right cardiophrenic angle and are distinguished from solid tumors by echocardiography and by computed tomography (CT) scanning. *Mesothelioma,* a malignant tumor of the pericardium, may mimic several conditions, including pericarditis, constrictive pericardial disease, and vena caval obstruction. Aspiration and histological examination of the usually bloody pericardial fluid is often diagnostic. The prognosis for patients with mesothelioma is poor, and surgical excision is rarely possible.

## SECONDARY TUMORS OF THE HEART

Metastatic tumors of the heart or pericardium occur 20 to 40 times more frequently than primary tumors. Tumor invasion of the heart may occur by direct contiguous growth from adjacent structures, or along the vena cava or pulmonary veins. Metastatic invasion may also take place by hematogenous or lymphatic channels. The heart is the site of metastatic tumor in 2 to 20 percent of patients with malignant tumors; bronchogenic and breast carcinoma are the most common sources. Cardiac involvement is also common in patients with leukemia and the lymphomas and is seen with Kaposi's sarcoma in some patients with acquired immunodeficiency syndrome (AIDS).

Secondary tumors of the heart may be located in the pericardium, myocardium, endocardium, valves, or coronary arteries. *Pericardial involvement* results in pleuritic pain and a pericardial friction rub. Cardiac enlargement, signs of tamponade, and reduced QRS amplitude in the electrocardiogram may be evident. Electrical alternans may be present with serious tamponade. The echocardiogram will reveal pericardial effusion; diastolic collapse of the right atrium and ventricle is highly specific for significant tamponade. CT scanning is usually necessary to detect a pericardial tumor mass. *Myocardial involvement* results in ST and T wave changes in the electrocardiogram and often arrhythmias, including atrial flutter and fibrillation, ventricular ectopic rhythms, conduction disturbances, and even complete heart block. Widespread myocardial involvement may produce congestive heart failure, but cardiac damage and myocardial failure may also result from the effects of radiotherapy and chemotherapy. *Coronary artery involvement* can result from tumor embolization or external compression, as well as from the consequences of radiotherapy. *Intracavitary tumor* may be seen when there is extension of a primary tumor, such as renal cell carcinoma, hepatocellular carcinoma, or uterine leiomyoma, any of which may spread along the inferior vena cava and into the right atrium, or bronchogenic carcinoma, which may extend into the left atrium. Successful surgical resection of intracavitary tumors has been reported.

## DIAGNOSIS

Diagnosis of tumor involvement of the heart is fostered by a strong index of clinical suspicion. Cardiac enlargement, arrhythmias, chest pain, or features of congestive heart failure in any patient with a malignancy should arouse suspicion of cardiac metastases. Two-dimensional transthoracic and transesophageal echocardiography, CT scanning, and magnetic resonance imaging provide highly diagnostic information. Cytological examination of pericardial fluid and endomyocardial biopsy specimens may establish a histological diagnosis.

## TREATMENT

Depending on cytological type, the treatment of choice for cardiac tumors is *radiation therapy,* with or without *systemic chemotherapy.* Pericardial effusion with tamponade requires urgent *pericardiocentesis,* either by needle aspiration or by limited subxiphoid surgical drainage. Malignant pericardial effusions respond to intrapericardial administration of various agents such as fluorouracil, radioactive gold, nitrogen mustard, and tetracycline. Persistent reaccumulation of pericardial fluid may require surgical creation of a *pericardial window.* Surgical removal of intracavitary obstructing secondary tumors may ameliorate symptoms and prolong life.

## SUGGESTED READING

DeLoach JF, Haynes JW: Secondary tumors of the heart and pericardium. Review of the subject and report of one hundred thirty-seven cases. *AMA Arch Intern Med* 91:224–249, 1953.

Fine G: Neoplasms of the pericardium and heart, in Gould SE (ed): *Pathology of the Heart and Blood Vessels.* Springfield, IL, Charles C Thomas, pp 851–883, 1968.

Hall RJ, Cooley DA, McAllister HA Jr, et al: Neoplastic diseases of the heart, in Hurst JW (ed): *The Heart,* 7th ed. New York, McGraw-Hill, Chap 68, pp 1382–1403, 1990.

Hurst JW, Hall RJ, Becker AE, et al: Neoplastic disease of the heart, in Hurst JW (ed): *Atlas of the Heart.* New York, McGraw-Hill, pp 13.1–13.14, 1988.

Kralstein J, Frishman W: Malignant pericardial diseases: Diagnosis and treatment. *Am Heart J* 113:785–790, 1987.

Lung JT, Ehman RL, Julsrud PR, et al: Cardiac masses: Assessment by MR imaging. *AJR* 152(3):469–73, 1989.

McAllister HA Jr: Primary tumors and cysts of the heart and pericardium. *Curr Probl Cardiol* 4(2):1–51, 1979.

McAllister HA Jr, Fenoglio JJ Jr: *Tumors of the Cardiovascular System.* Fascicle 15, Second Series, *Atlas of Tumor Pathology.* Washington, DC, Armed Forces Institute of Pathology, 1978.

McAllister HA Jr, Hall RJ, Cooley DA: Surgical pathology of tumors and cysts of the heart and pericardium, in Waller BF (ed): *Contemporary Issues in Surgical Pathology,* vol 12. New York, Churchill Livingstone, 1988.

Press OW, Livingston R: Management of malignant pericardial effusion and tamponade. *JAMA* 257:1088–1092, 1987.

## 22 | Diseases of the Aorta

*Joseph Lindsay, Jr., M.D.*

### DEFINITION

Aneurysm, dissection, or rupture of the aorta may result from weakening of its wall by either acquired disease or congenital anomalies. Less commonly, such processes narrow the aorta or the origin of one of its branches. Because of the uncomplicated nature of the structure and function of this vital conduit, a relatively limited number of clinical syndromes results from diverse disease processes.

### ETIOLOGY

*Atherosclerosis* of the aorta accompanies aging in most individuals in the western world, but the process varies in severity from subject to subject. It is characteristically accelerated by diabetes, hypercholesterolemia, hypertension, and smoking. Because atherosclerosis is most severe in the abdominal aorta, its most frequent clinical manifestations are aneurysm and obstruction of the abdominal aorta below the renal arteries.

*Medial degeneration* also accompanies aging. As a consequence, the aorta becomes elongated, tortuous, and inelastic. Severe medial degeneration is the characteristic cardiovascular abnormality in the Marfan syndrome. In the absence of other manifestations of that syndrome, medial degeneration may be severe enough to result in clinical disease in individuals who seem otherwise normal, as well as in some with aortic coarctation, biscuspid aortic valve, polycystic kidneys, or the Turner syndrome. Unlike atherosclerosis, medial degeneration is most severe in the proximal aorta. As a consequence, aneurysm of the proximal aorta, including the sinuses of Valsalva, is the most frequent manifestation.

*Infectious aortitis* may result from extension of aortic valve endocarditis to the adjacent wall; less commonly, it may occur by direct extension from infection of periaortic structures. Bloodborne infection may invade an aortic intima damaged by atherosclerosis or another process. The late effects of syphilitic aortitis (aneurysm and aortic regurgitation) are still encountered.

*Nonspecific aortitis*, often associated with evidence of an "autoimmune" process, has been termed *Takayasu's aortitis*. A *nonspecific aortitis of the proximal aorta* often accompanies ankylosing spondylitis and Reiter syndrome, the HLA-B27 arthropathies.

Common congenital anomalies encountered after early childhood include aortic coarctation and aneurysms of the sinuses of Valsalva.

*Penetrating or nonpenetrating trauma* that is not immediately fatal may result in false aneurysm formation.

## CLINICAL MANIFESTATIONS

Most aortic aneurysms are asymptomatic and are first detected in the course of a routine examination or an examination directed at another organ. Typically, physical examination, x-ray study, or another imaging technique reveals their presence. Some produce discomfort by impinging on, or eroding, adjacent structures. For example, an aneurysm of the aortic arch may produce hoarseness or dysphagia. It is a good clinical rule of thumb to regard any symptoms of recent onset that are referable to aneurysm as signs of expansion and impending rupture.

*Rupture of an aneurysm* is life-threatening and demands immediate operative treatment. Sudden onset of abdominal discomfort in a patient with an abdominal aneurysm or of chest pain in one with an aneurysm in the thoracic aorta heralds such events. Evidence of blood loss usually accompanies the pain and alerts the examiner to the vascular nature of the illness.

*Aortic regurgitation* commonly results from congenital or acquired proximal aortic disease. The most frequently encountered etiology is anuloaortic ectasia, attributable to medial degeneration of the aortic tissue. The resulting dilatation of the aortic sinuses, ascending aorta, and aortic valve ring eventuates in an incompetent aortic valve. Aortitis due to syphilis or to the HLA-B27 arthropathies may also produce aortic regurgitation. When a regurgitant valve is the initial manifestation of aortic root disease, the underlying process may not be suspected until echocardiography is performed.

*Aortic dissection*—longitudinal cleavage of the medial fibers—produces a dramatic clinical syndrome characterized by the abrupt onset of severe midline chest, back, or abdominal pain or, less commonly, by sudden syncope.

*Obstruction* of the origin of one or more of the major branches of the arch of the aorta, a consequence of aortitis or of atherosclerosis, may produce ischemic symptoms of the central nervous system or of an upper extremity. The Leriche syndrome—exertional discomfort of the low back, buttocks, or thighs, together with impotence in males—usually reflects atherosclerotic obstruction of the terminal aorta. Sudden occlusion of the aortic bifurcation by a saddle embolus or aortic dissection results in bilateral lower-extremity ischemia, which may be accompanied by weakness or frank paralysis.

## Physical Examination

Detection of a murmur of aortic regurgitation or of diminished carotid, radial, or femoral pulses may direct the examiner's attention to the possibility of aortic disease, or may add supporting data when its presence has been suggested by other observations. Moreover, every abdominal examination should include a search for the expansile mass of an abdominal aneurysm. The presence of a tracheal tug or of a lift of either sternoclavicular joint may reflect aneurysm or dissection of the aortic arch.

One should be particularly alert for evidence of aortic disease in individuals whose body habitus suggests either the Marfan or Turner syndrome.

## Usual X-Ray Studies

The aortic silhouette on the chest x-ray is usually, but not invariably, distorted in the presence of disease of the thoracic aorta. The findings are seldom specific and, when aortic disease is confined to the intrapericardial aorta, may be entirely absent. Notching of the underside of the ribs is virtually pathognomonic of aortic coarctation.

Abdominal x-rays, particularly when proper techniques are employed, frequently disclose the calcified outline of an abdominal aneurysm. A "cross-table lateral" may be rewarding.

## DIFFERENTIAL DIAGNOSIS

As might be supposed from the data outlined, the differential diagnosis for aortic disease is often broad. It may manifest itself as pain, suggesting myocardial infarction or an acute abdominal illness. At times the manifestations of an infectious or an autoimmune process may seem to dominate. The mass of an aneurysm may lead to the suspicion of a neoplastic process.

## SPECIAL DIAGNOSTIC EVALUATION

Aortography, using selective contrast-medium injection through a catheter, is the most definitive way to image the aorta. In experienced hands it carries only a small risk. Almost as much information can be gained about aneurysm or dissection by means of ultrasound or computed tomography (CT). Transesophageal echocardiography allows visualization of the descending thoracic aorta. These modalities also allow serial examinations of a lesion. Magnetic resonance imaging (MRI) provides remarkably detailed images of the aorta. When it becomes widely available, the need for aortography will be greatly reduced.

## NATURAL HISTORY AND PROGNOSIS

Rupture and dissection of the aorta are acute, highly lethal emergencies. Survival for more than a few days is exceptional unless surgical repair is possible.

Aortic aneurysms tend to enlarge gradually. The greater their size, the more likely they are to rupture. An aneurysm 6 cm or more in diameter is considered large; with such an aneurysm the possibility of rupture is an important consideration. Smaller aneurysms also rupture, but less often. One should bear in mind that advanced age or associated illness may be more threatening to a patient's well-being than his or her aneurysm.

Aortic regurgitation and aortic branch obstruction also tend to be progressive.

## TREATMENT

*Surgical repair* of aortic lesions is now usually possible in suitable patients, and is the only definitive approach in most cases. For rupture of an aneurysm or for dissection of the proximal aorta, surgical treatment is the life-saving option. *Medical treatment* generally is supportive or is aimed at preventing progression of a demonstrated lesion. For example, the patient with medial degeneration and anuloaortic ectasia may receive a beta-blocking agent, or other antihypertensive drugs, to reduce wall stress and the severity of aortic regurgitation.

Aggressive reduction of blood pressure has a special role in many cases of acute aortic dissection. In a patient whose dissection begins beyond the aortic arch, chronic antihypertensive therapy may be preferable to surgery.

## SUGGESTED READING

Goldman AP, Katler MN, Scanlon MH, et al: Complementary role of magnetic resonance imaging, Doppler echocardiography, and computed tomography in the diagnosis of dissecting thoracic aneurysms. *Am Heart J* 111:970–981, 1986.

Hall S, Ban W, Lie JT, et al: Takayasu arteritis. *Medicine* 64:89–99, 1986.

Lindsay J Jr, DeBakey ME, Beall AC Jr: Diseases of the aorta, in Hurst JW et al (eds): *The Heart,* 7th ed. New York, McGraw-Hill, Chap 70, pp 1408–1423, 1989.

Lindsay J Jr, Hurst JW: *The Aorta.* New York, Grune and Stratton, 1979.

Pyeritz RE, McKusick VA: The Marfan syndrome: Diagnosis and management. *N Engl J Med* 300:772–779, 1979.

Savunen T: Anuloaortic ectasia—a clinical, structural, and biochemical study. *Scand J Thorac Cardiovasc Surg* 37(suppl):1–45, 1986.

## 23 | Cerebrovascular Disease and Neurological Manifestations of Heart Disease

*Kari E. Murros, M.D.*
*James F. Toole, M.D.*

## ATHEROSCLEROTIC CEREBROVASCULAR DISEASE

### Asymptomatic Carotid Stenosis

Carotid bifurcations are among the sites of predilection for atherosclerosis in cervical arteries. Patients with asymptomatic carotid stenosis have an increased risk of both cerebral and myocardial infarction. Bruits over carotid arteries suggest local stenosis, but they may be transmitted from cardiac valvular disease, or may be due to turbulent flow caused by hemodynamic changes. On the other hand, bruits may be absent despite significant carotid stenosis.

### Transient Ischemic Attacks (TIAs)

TIAs are transient episodes of neurological dysfunction resulting from disturbed blood flow in a specific arterial distribution. Though they occasionally persist as long as 24 h, most TIAs resolve within 1 h. This restitution of normal function does not necessarily mean that infarction has not occurred. The pathogenic mechanisms of TIA (especially artery-to-artery embolism) are the same as in cerebral infarction.

### Cerebral Infarction

Cerebral infarction may be manifest as a sudden transient or permanent neurological deficit, or it may be asymptomatic. *Progressing cerebral infarction* is a generic term describing the progression of neurological signs over hours and days. Old age, hypertension, cigarette smoking, diabetes, hyperlipidemia, ischemic and valvular heart disease, asymptomatic carotid stenosis, and TIAs increase the risk of cerebral infarction. The pathogenic mechanisms include local atherothrombosis, artery-to-artery emboli (especially from carotid bifurcations to distal cerebral arteries), cardiogenic emboli, local vasospasm due to migraine or subarachnoid hemorrhage, and hematologic disorders.

## Clinical Manifestations of Focal Cerebral Ischemia

Motor and/or sensory symptoms in the extremities and the face on the same side of the body suggest a carotid distribution disturbance, as does transient blindness of one eye (amaurosis fugax) or dysphasia. Bilateral motor and/or sensory symptoms, diplopia, vertigo, dystaxia, bulbar symptoms (dysarthria and dysphagia), and an altered consciousness suggest a vertebrobasilar insufficiency. An occlusion of the posterior cerebral artery (supplied in one-third of people by the carotid, and in two-thirds by the vertebrobasilar system) usually leads to homonymous visual field defect.

Cerebral infarction is often accompanied by mild to moderate headache. The frequency of significant cardiac arrhythmias in the setting of acute cerebral infarction is approximately 5 to 10 percent.

## Diagnostic Evaluation

### Ultrasound

Real-time ultrasound (B-mode) and Doppler flow-velocity measurements are superior methods of noninvasive evaluation of carotid arteries.

### Echocardiography

Echocardiography is indicated in most cases where focal cerebral ischemia is suspected. Cardiogenic embolism accounts for about 15 to 20 percent of all cerebral infarctions.

### Cranial Computed Tomography (CCT)

CCT should be a routine procedure for every patient with TIAs or a cerebral infarction.

### Magnetic Resonance Imaging (MRI)

MRI is superior to CCT in detecting cerebral infarcts at early stages, small infarcts, and infratentorial infarcts.

### Angiography

Angiographic studies are indicated in patients who are potential candidates for carotid endarterectomy and in patients in whom aneurysms, arteriovenous malformations, inflammatory arteriopathies, or venous occlusions are suspected.

**Management**

*Asymptomatic Carotid Stenosis and TIAs*

The first step is reduction of known risk factors. The value of platelet antiaggregant therapy in asymptomatic carotid stenosis is not known. Aspirin therapy (e.g., 325 mg daily) probably reduces the risk of cerebral infarction in patients with TIAs. Another approach for TIA patients is to start with warfarin for up to 6 months and then shift to antiplatelet therapy. The value of carotid endarterectomy is unproven in patients with asymptomatic carotid stenosis. Carotid endarterectomy is accepted in patients with TIAs and a hemodynamically significant carotid stenosis. When both carotid endarterectomy and coronary bypass procedure are considered, priority is usually given to the coronary bypass procedure.

**Cerebral Infarction**

The mainstays of treatment are good nursing care, nutritional support, early ambulation, and risk-factor reduction. The use of anticoagulants is controversial for progressing cerebral infarction, and it is contraindicated in hemorrhagic infarction. A rapid lowering of blood pressure may be hazardous. Subcutaneous low-dose heparin (5000 I.U. three times a day) may be effective in preventing deep venous thrombosis of the paralyzed leg in bedridden patients when instituted within the first 2 days.

**CEREBRAL EMBOLISM**

Cardiogenic embolism accounts for about 15 to 20 percent of cerebral infarctions. The differential diagnosis of cardiogenic embolism versus atherothrombosis is often difficult, and in some cases impossible. An embolic etiology is favored by a young age of patient, symptoms from multiple anatomic regions, hemorrhagic infarction on CCT, and minimal atherosclerotic changes in ultrasound or angiographic studies.

**Etiology**

*Rheumatic heart disease* is associated with systemic embolization in up to 20 percent of patients. Rheumatic mitral stenosis, especially with atrial fibrillation, and rheumatic mitral regurgitation account for most of the emboli.

*Nonvalvular atrial fibrillation* increases the risk of embolic stroke. Embolism is more likely to occur when the atrial rhythm changes during cardioversion or spontaneously.

*Sick sinus syndrome with arrhythmias* is associated with an increased risk of cerebral embolism.

*Prosthetic heart valves* predispose to cerebral embolism. Patients with artificial valves carry a higher risk of embolism than those with tissue valves.

*Mitral valve prolapse, calcific aortic stenosis, and bicuspid aortic valves* may be sources of emboli, but other etiologies should be excluded before one attributes cerebral infarction to any of these rather common disorders.

*Paradoxical embolism* may occur in patients with patent foramen ovale, atrial and ventricular septal defects, or pulmonary arteriovenous fistula. Cerebral infarction in patients with deep venous thrombosis and pulmonary embolism should raise the suspicion of paradoxical cerebral embolism.

*Dilated cardiomyopathy* is associated with both poor systolic wall motion and rhythm disorders, either of which may predispose to thrombus formation and subsequent embolism.

*Atrial myxoma* presents with cerebral emboli in one-quarter of patients. Tumor fragments may cause cerebral infarction either by occluding the vascular lumen or by invading the arterial wall, in which case they may cause an arterial rupture or obstruction.

Patients with *debilitating illness* may have nonbacterial thrombotic endocarditis with sterile vegetations on the heart valves, which may be the source of cerebral emboli.

*Libman-Sacks endocarditis* in systemic lupus erythematosus may produce cerebral emboli.

*Septic endocarditis* carries up to a 30-percent risk of cerebral embolism. In addition to occlusion of intracranial arteries, mycotic aneurysms may develop and rupture into the brain parenchyma or subarachnoid space, leading to meningoencephalitis, brain abscess, and/or hemorrhage.

### Clinical Manifestations and Diagnostic Evaluation

In addition to the routine procedures for all patients with cerebral infarction, *echocardiography* should usually be performed when cardiogenic emboli are suspected. A normal ECG with normal heart auscultation does not rule out a cardiogenic etiology. *Continuous ECG monitoring* and *cardiac catheterization* may be needed. CCT may show multiple or hemorrhagic infarcts. *Angiography* may show not atherosclerotic changes but, rather, multiple filling defects in cerebral arteries, especially in the middle cerebral artery. In case of endocarditis or myxoma, arterial aneurysms may be seen.

### Management

Because 10 percent of patients with cerebral embolism suffer recurrence during the first 2 weeks, *early anticoagulation with warfarin* is often indicated. The use of heparin is very controversial. Uncontrolled hypertension and hemorrhagic infarction are contraindications to anticoagulants. The potential for hemorrhagic transformation of a pale infarct, which usually occurs within 48 h after the ictus, should be kept in mind.

The treatment of *septic endocarditis* includes appropriate *antibiotics*. Anticoagulant therapy is usually contraindicated, but is usually necessary for patients with infective prosthetic valve endocarditis.

## OTHER OCCLUSIVE VASCULAR DISORDERS

*Inflammatory angiopathies*—such as Takayasu's disease, polyarteritis nodosa, systemic lupus erythematosus, Wegener's granulomatosis, Behçet's disease, hypersensitivity vasculitis, and angitis secondary to infections and toxins—may cause cerebral infarcts.

*Fibromuscular dysplasia,* a nonatheromatous, noninflammatory disease, causes stenosis and dilatation of the large cervical arteries. The diagnosis is made arteriographically. The findings may be incidental, with no correlation to clinical symptoms.

*Dissections of cervical arteries,* either spontaneous or traumatic, may cause TIAs or cerebral infarcts.

*Moyamoya disease* is a nonatheromatous, noninflammatory intracranial arteriopathy with occlusions of basal arteries and extensive collaterals.

*Thrombosis of a cerebral vein or sinus* may occur postoperatively, during pregnancy, or in patients with malignancies, hematological disorders, or local infections.

*Binswanger's disease* is a subcortical arteriosclerotic encephalopathy with periventricular lacunar infarcts and ischemic demyelination of subcortical white matter. The main clinical features are dementia and strokes.

## HYPERTENSIVE CEREBROVASCULAR DISEASE

Hypertension accelerates atherosclerosis (see "Atherosclerotic Cerebrovascular Disease," above) and may cause lacunar infarctions, intracerebral hemorrhages, and hypertensive encephalopathy.

*Lacunar infarction* results from occlusion of a small penetrating arteriole in deep cerebral structures. The most common manifestations of lacunar infarction are pure motor and pure sensory hemisyndromes, but there may be no symptoms. CCT may not show small lacunar infarcts.

*Intracerebral hemorrhage* is usually caused by rupture of a small penetrating cerebral artery weakened by hypertension, atherosclerosis, systemic diseases, or emboli from bacterial endocarditis.

Rupture of an arterial aneurysm may cause—in addition to subarachnoid hemorrhage—intracerebral bleeding, especially in the temporal regions. Involvement of basal structures, including the internal capsule, is common and may result in acute hemiplegia, headache, and deterioration of consciousness. Deviation of the eyes toward the side of the hemorrhage is common. *Emergency surgery* should be considered in some cases—e.g., in patients with cerebellar hemorrhage presenting with symptoms of brain stem compression or obstructive hydrocephalus. *Mannitol* may have some therapeutic effect in reducing brain edema.

Patients with hypertensive encephalopathy usually have headache, altered mental status, and convulsions. Hypertensive retinopathy and papilledema are usually present. *CCT or MRI* is needed to rule out other etiologies, such as intracerebral or subarachnoid hemorrhage. *Sodium nitroprusside* is effective treatment, but its use requires close monitoring.

## SUBARACHNOID HEMORRHAGE

Spontaneous subarachnoid hemorrhage is usually caused by rupture of a congenital berry aneurysm in the region of the circle of Willis. Rare etiologies include arteriovenous malformations, blood dyscrasias, inflammatory arteriopathies, neoplastic conditions, and endocarditis. A sudden, severe headache is the leading symptom. In addition, about one-half of patients present with altered consciousness. Strict *bed rest,* adequate doses of *analgesics* that do not increase bleeding tendency, and *sedatives* are required. *Surgical treatment* of congenital aneurysms and arteriovenous malformations is usually indicated. *ECG changes* may occur in up to 70 percent of patients with either subarachnoid or intracerebral hemorrhage. The most common ECG changes include flat or inverted T waves, depressed or elevated ST segments, prolonged QT intervals, Q waves, U waves, and arrhythmias. Various arrhythmias may be an important cause of sudden death in patients with subarachnoid hemorrhage. Because sympathetic overactivity is likely to induce these arrhythmias, the use of beta-blocking agents should be considered in the treatment.

## CEREBRAL HYPOPERFUSION

Decreased cardiac output may cause cerebral hypoperfusion with diffuse, focal, transient, or permanent cerebral manifestations. Syncopal attacks and dizziness are the most common symptoms. In some patients, cerebral hypoperfusion may lead to seizures. The etiology of syncopal attacks can usually be determined by history, physical examination, and ECG.

Cerebral hypoperfusion may be caused by:

- *Dysrhythmias* such as ventricular and supraventricular tachycardias and bradyarrhythmias can lead to cerebral symptoms. Conversely, it should be remembered that a central nervous system lesion may be the primary cause of cardiac arrhythmias and myocardial damage.
- *Myocardial dysfunction* in severe cardiac heart failure or shock.
- *Valvular and mechanical dysfunction* in aortic valvular stenosis, hypertrophic obstructive cardiomyopathy, atrial myxoma, primary pulmonary hypertension, or pulmonary embolism.
- *Vagal reflex bradycardia* or *heart standstill* due to a hypersensitive carotid sinus, at times associated with micturition, defecation, or swallowing, or in response to severe pain.
- *Orthostasis* induced by drugs, such as diuretics and vasodilators, or by CNS disorders.

## COMPLICATIONS OF CARDIAC CATHETERIZATION AND HEART SURGERY

The overall serious complication rate during cardiac catheterization is less than 1 percent. An *embolism from the catheter surface* may result in hemiparesis and focal seizures. Patients with right-to-left shunt have an increased risk of cerebral embolism.

*Cerebral complications, mental symptoms, stroke, and/or seizures* occur in about 4 percent of patients having coronary artery bypass surgery. The risk of complications is even higher in valve repair. These complications may be due to various kinds of emboli such as air, cell aggregates, particles from calcified valves, atheromatous debris, thrombi, fat, and silicone. Mental symptoms may also be caused by hypoxia or other metabolic disturbance, but these cases usually end in complete recovery. *Intracranial bleedings* are rare complications of cardiac surgery. Cardiac transplantation is associated with complications similar to those of other cardiac surgery. *Invasion of the CNS with an opportunistic organism,* due to immunosuppressive therapy, is a possible delayed complication of cardiac transplantation.

## CONGENITAL HEART DISEASE

*Neurological complications* of congenital heart disease include episodes of cerebral hypoperfusion, cerebral infarction due to arterial or venous thrombosis, and cerebral lesions due to emboli from bacterial endocarditis. Syncopal attacks are common; they are often induced by exertion. Cerebral infarction may be caused by paradoxical embolism, but cerebral venous thrombosis is often found to be the primary cause of cerebral infarction in patients with cyanotic congenital heart disease and polycythemia. *Medical treatment* of cerebral complications is often unsatisfactory. Correction of hyperviscous blood by phlebotomy and/or volume replacement may be needed. Anticoagulant therapy usually is not indicated. Since a sudden neurological deficit may be caused by septic embolism, immediate antibiotic therapy should be considered for any patient with congenital heart disease who has a suspected stroke.

## SUGGESTED READING

Cerebral Embolism Task Force: Cardiogenic brain embolism. The second report of the Cerebral Embolism Task Force. *Arch Neurol* 46:727–743, 1989.

Grotta JC: Current medical and surgical therapy for cerebral vascular disease. *N Engl J Med* 317:1505–1516, 1987.

Rem JA, Hachinski VC, Boughner DR, et al: Value of cardiac monitoring and echocardiography in TIA and stroke patients. *Stroke* 16:950–956, 1985.

Talman WT: Cardiovascular regulation and lesions of the central nervous system. *Ann Neurol* 18:1–12, 1985.

Toole JF, Murros KE: Cerebrovascular disease and neurologic manifestations of heart disease, in Hurst JW et al (eds): *The Heart,* 7th ed. New York, McGraw-Hill, Chap 72, pp 1446–1454, 1990.

Toole JF: *Cerebrovascular disorders.* New York, Raven Press, 1984.

## 24

Vascular Disease of the Digestive System

*W. Scott Brooks, Jr., M.D.*


## DEFINITION, ETIOLOGY, AND PATHOLOGY

Ischemic disease of the intestines may manifest itself acutely or chronically. Occlusion of a mesenteric artery or vein presents acutely with abdominal pain, often progressing to infarction of the small intestine before the clinician can appreciate the severity of the event. Occlusion may be due to embolism, occasionally seen after cardiac catheterization, or to thrombosis. Nonocclusive ischemia, due to hypoperfusion, occurs less frequently and is seen in the clinical setting of cardiac dysfunction. Recurrent mesenteric ischemia, often called "abdominal angina," is a chronic condition of poor arterial flow to the intestines, which becomes symptomatic with pain after meals. The term "abdominal angina" suggests that nitroglycerin would be helpful, but in fact nitroglycerin reduces flow through a stenotic mesenteric artery; hence this term should not be used.

## CLINICAL MANIFESTATIONS

### History

Acute thrombosis should be suggested by the sudden onset of severe mid-abdominal pain in a patient with a history of atherosclerotic vascular disease. Embolism presents the same clinical picture, but a history of recent arterial manipulations may suggest the diagnosis. Ischemic colitis presents with left-sided pain. Diarrhea, often bloody, may occur with either condition in the acute setting.

Recurrent postprandial pain and food avoidance, with weight loss, are seen with recurrent ischemia. Most of these patients are smokers with histories of significant vascular disease.

### Physical Examination

The patient is usually very restless when the pain is acute, but characteristically there are no abdominal findings: no tenderness, no guarding, and normal bowel sounds. In the setting of acute pain, this lack of findings is so peculiar that the diagnosis of an acute ischemic event should come quickly to mind. This uncommon picture occurs because the initial ischemic event affects only the mucosa and not the serosal surfaces; thus peritoneal signs are not seen early. With progression of the ischemia over time, transmural infarction develops and the picture becomes that of the typical acute abdomen. Ischemic colitis, however, often does not progress to full infarction, although some abdominal findings do develop. In the patient with recurrent pain due to ischemia, a bruit can usually be heard.

## USUAL DIAGNOSTIC TESTS

Blood studies in the acute situation often show hemoconcentration, with elevation of the hemoglobin and hematocrit. A twofold elevation of the serum amylase is not uncommon. Blood, occult or visible, is present in the stool of the acute patient, and occasionally in that of the patient with recurrent ischemia.

## DIFFERENTIAL DIAGNOSIS

Other diagnoses to be considered are those of the acute abdomen. Acute pancreatitis is often mistaken for ischemic disease of the intestines, because of the elevated amylase. Patients with ischemic disease more often are elderly, without risk factors for pancreatitis, and with pain more apparent than abdominal findings. Ischemic colitis is often confused with diverticulitis, but bloody diarrhea is uncommon with the latter. Recurrent ischemia is a diagnosis of exclusion, with symptoms mimicked by gallstone disease or virtually any anatomic abnormality of the gastrointestinal tract, but weight loss is uncommon with other benign diseases.

## SPECIAL DIAGNOSTIC EVALUATION

Acute ischemia requires rapid diagnosis before infarction. Not only is *mesenteric angiography* diagnostic, but it may help in planning treatment. Ischemic colitis may not show angiographic changes, but on *colonoscopy* it shows a characteristic dusky, ulcerated appearance. Recurrent ischemia requires angiography to demonstrate the lesion; often all three abdominal vessels are involved.

## NATURAL HISTORY, PROGNOSIS, AND TREATMENT

Acute small bowel ischemia, be it venous or arterial, requires surgical correction, and is associated with a 55-percent hospital mortality rate under the best of circumstances. Untreated, the ischemia progresses to infarction and death from sepsis. Ischemic colitis often does not progress to infarction; supportive therapy and antibiotics may be sufficient, but late strictures may occur. Recurrent ischemia may progress to acute thrombotic occlusion if not diagnosed in time for revascularization or percutaneous angioplasty.

## SUGGESTED READING

Borden EB, Scott JB: Early diagnosis of acute mesenteric ischemia. *J Crit Ill* 1(9):17–24, 1986.

Brooks WS Jr: Vascular disease of the digestive system, in Hurst JW et al (eds): *The Heart*, 7th ed. New York, McGraw-Hill, Chap 73, pp 1454–1464, 1990.

## 25

Diseases of the Peripheral Arteries
and Veins

*Mark T. Stewart, M.D.*
*Robert B. Smith, III, M.D.*

## PERIPHERAL ARTERIAL DISEASE

### Definition

*Peripheral arterial diseases* are abnormalities that impair the ability of the circulatory tree to transmit blood or weaken its intrinsic strength resulting in aneurysmal dilatation.

### Etiology

*Atherosclerosis* is the most common cause of arterial disease. Risk factors for its development include male gender, smoking, hypertension, diabetes mellitus, lipid abnormalities, and family history of atherosclerosis. *Inflammatory arteriopathies and autoimmune diseases* such as giant cell arteritis. Takayasu's disease, polyarteritis nodosa, lupus erythematosus, and thromboangiitis obliterans (Buerger's disease) can result in either aneurysmal degeneration or arterial obstruction. *Vasoactive drugs, emboli, trauma, or systemic shock* can also compromise blood supply to the extremity.

### Clinical Manifestations

#### History

Chronic obstruction of arterial flow to an extremity causes exercise-related fatigue and cramping (intermittent claudication) of the muscles distal to the obstruction. If collateral circulation around the obstruction is inadequate, the symptoms of reduced blood supply will become evident even without exercise. More severe chronic obstruction eventually results in pain at rest—a severe burning discomfort located in the most distal portion of the extremity—or actual tissue necrosis. Acute ischemia with inadequate collateral circulation produces severe pain associated with diminished tactile sensation and motor paresis.

#### Physical Examination

Diminished peripheral pulses are found in the presence of significant arterial obstruction. Severe chronic ischemia may also cause dependent rubor, thickened nails, absent hair, and thin, shiny skin. The extremity often is cool and pale, and may have gangrenous changes. In acute ischemia the limb may show pulselessness, pain, pallor, paresthesia, and paralysis.

## Special Diagnostic Evaluation

### Plain X-Ray

Plain x-rays are not often helpful, but may show calcified blood vessels and evidence of chronic osteomyelitis.

### Doppler Pressures and Arterial Plethysmography

These vascular laboratory studies are useful to confirm the clinical suspicion of arterial obstruction and to quantify its severity.

### Angiography

Contrast arteriography is seldom required to demonstrate the presence and severity of arterial disease, which usually can be determined by the noninvasive methods listed above; but it is necessary for planning the method of arterial reconstruction.

## Differential Diagnosis

The differential diagnosis includes all causes of peripheral circulatory disease plus the whole spectrum of disorders responsible for nonvascular pain of the lower extremities.

## Natural History and Prognosis

Atherosclerotic obstruction is characterized by slow progression in the degree and extent of disease. Individuals complaining of symptoms of intermittent claudication have a relatively favorable course with an amputation rate at five years of only 5 to 10 percent. On the other hand, patients with severe restriction of blood supply who have rest pain or gangrene face a very high rate of limb amputation if not revascularized. Similarly, patients with acute limb ischemia and inadequate collateral blood supply face imminent limb loss if flow is not promptly restored. Peripheral aneurysms rarely rupture but often cause severe ischemia through the mechanism of sac thrombosis or distal embolization.

## Treatment

### Medical

*Cessation of smoking* is critical for patients with atherosclerotic occlusive disease or thromboangiitis obliterans. Excellent *foot care* is also mandatory to avoid development of a nonhealing lesion on the foot. The hemorrheologic agent pentoxifylline benefits some patients with intermittent claudication (usual dose: 400 mg PO tid). Vasodilators are occasionally helpful for vasospastic disorders, and corticosteroids may be beneficial in individuals with inflammatory arteriopathies.

### Interventional and Surgical

Optimal treatment for arterial occlusion consists of *removal of the intraluminal obstruction* or *revascularization* by means of a bypass graft. Therapy of patients with non-limb-threatening ischemia is elective and, in many cases, not indicated. Limb-threatening blockage should be treated, if the patient can tolerate the required procedure. *Catheter techniques* of balloon angioplasty, atherectomy, laser-assisted balloon angioplasty, and transarterial thrombolytic therapy may be applicable for patients with limited disease. Patients with more extensive lesions or advanced ischemic changes usually must be treated *surgically* with bypass, endarterectomy, or thromboembolectomy. Sympathectomy is occasionally useful in patients with ischemic ulceration and rest pain, or in vasospastic disorders; it is not effective for intermittent claudication. Primary amputation is reserved for nonreconstructible problems or life-threatening sepsis.

## DEEP VENOUS THROMBOSIS

### Definition

*Deep venous thrombosis* is clotting that develops in the deep veins of the lower extremity or pelvis.

### Etiology

Stasis of blood, vessel wall injury, and increased coagulability are the triad of etiologic factors described by Virchow as precipitating venous thrombosis. *Stasis of blood* results from conditions that reduce venous return, such as surgical procedures, prolonged sitting or bed rest, limb paralysis, and congestive heart failure. *Vessel wall injury* may be caused by surgical operations, penetrating or blunt trauma, or venous catheterization. *Increased coagulability* is associated with disorders such as thrombocytosis, erythrocytosis, malignant tumors (lung, pancreas), severe trauma, postpartum status, exogenous estrogen administration, and deficiencies of serum proteins (protein C, protein S, antithrombin III).

### Clinical Manifestations

#### History

The presence of deep venous thrombosis is often asymptomatic. Local complaints, when present, are usually pain and swelling of the extremity, but the first indication of the condition may be sudden pulmonary embolism.

### Physical Examination

*Clinical findings* include edema and tenderness, rarely erythema. Palpable cords caused by thrombosis of a vein are unusual except in superficial venous thrombosis. A positive *Homans' sign*—resistance to passive dorsiflexion of the foot—may be present, but is nonspecific for venous disorders. If the venous occlusion is extremely severe, compromised arterial flow may occur (phlegmasia cerulea dolens).

## Differential Diagnosis

The differential diagnosis includes any condition that can be responsible for pain, swelling, or tenderness of the lower extremity: myositis, cellulitis, muscle trauma, ruptured Baker's cyst, lymphedema, etc.

## Special Diagnostic Evaluation

Objective confirmatory studies in the vascular laboratory or the radiology department are necessary in suspected deep venous thrombosis, because clinical criteria for the diagnosis result in only 50-percent accuracy.

### Doppler Ultrasound

The hand-held Doppler device allows the examiner to evaluate blood flow in the deep and superficial veins of the lower extremities. Experienced examiners using this method can achieve an accuracy in detection of venous thrombosis in the range of 90 percent.

### Venous Capacitance/Venous Outflow

*Venous capacitance* is the percent increase in size of the calf in response to inflation of a venous tourniquet on the thigh; *venous outflow* is a measurement of the initial rate of decrease in the volume of the leg after release of the tourniquet. These parameters can be measured by impedance or strain-gauge plethysmography; these tests are commonly available in the vascular laboratory. They have an accuracy of 90 percent for the detection of occlusive thrombi located above the knee, but are less sensitive for calf-vein clots.

### Duplex Scanning

This technique, which combines ultrasound imaging and Doppler analysis, is a very accurate noninvasive method for identification of venous occlusion of the popliteal and femoral veins; it is less useful for calf and pelvic veins.

*Contrast Phlebography*

This most accurate of tests for the detection of deep venous thrombosis is available almost universally and is easily interpreted. It requires administration of a radiographic contrast medium.

*Radionuclide Phlebography*

Radionuclide phlebography utilizes technetium 99m-labeled macroaggregates of albumin injected into a vein on the dorsum of each foot to outline the deep venous system. It has the advantage of avoiding allergic reactions such as may happen in contrast phlebography, but is less accurate than standard radiographic phlebography and does require invasive injections.

## Natural History

The majority of venous thrombi begin in the veins of the calf muscles and propagate proximally into the thigh and pelvic veins. Untreated, 30 percent of patients with calf-vein thrombosis experience spontaneous resolution and 50 percent remain unchanged, but 20 percent have proximal extension of the clot into larger veins. Nontreatment carries the risk not only of pulmonary embolism but also of probable venous insufficiency of the lower extremity related to venous obstruction or to venous valvular incompetence. The latter conditions may lead to chronic venous hypertension with pain, edema, and stasis ulceration. Patients with free-floating thrombus in the inferior vena cava are at high risk of pulmonary embolism even if treated with anticoagulation.

## Treatment

Most patients with deep venous thrombosis are treated by *bed rest, leg elevation, and anticoagulation* with an intravenous infusion of heparin for 7 to 10 days. (Partial thromboplastin time [PTT] should be 2.0 times control.) *Prolonged anticoagulation* with oral warfarin (Coumadin) should be continued for at least 3 months. (Prothrombin time [PT] should be 1.5 times control.) Knee-length elastic *support stockings* are prescribed for use during ambulation for 6 months. Surgical thrombectomy should be considered in the rare case where medical treatment of phlegmasia cerulea dolens fails. Vena caval interruption may be indicated: (1) in patients suffering from recurrent pulmonary embolism despite adequate anticoagulation, (2) when there is an inability to anticoagulate the patient, (3) if a severe complication of anticoagulation develops, or (4) prophylactically in individuals who are identified as being at high risk for fatal pulmonary embolism. Cardiopulmonary bypass and pulmonary artery embolectomy should be reserved for the patient with proven pulmonary embolism who is not responding to maximal therapeutic measures.

## SUPERIOR VENA CAVA SYNDROME

### Definition

Obstruction of the superior vena cava may result in a syndrome characterized by increased venous pressure, resulting in upper body cyanosis, massive edema, and difficult breathing.

### Etiology

Extrinsic compression from tumors, most likely of the lung, or from mediastinal fibrosis can obstruct venous flow in the mediastinum. Thrombosis of the superior vena cava may also result from complications related to indwelling venous devices.

### Clinical Manifestations

*History and Physical Examination*

Symptoms are due primarily to massive facial and laryngeal edema, which may be severe enough to obstruct the airway. Evidence of increased intracranial pressure as a result of cerebral edema may also be present, with headache, blurred vision, and lethargy. Cyanosis and prominent superficial veins on the neck, shoulders, and chest are also seen.

### Differential Diagnosis

The presence of severe right-sided congestive heart failure, massive fluid overload, or tricuspid regurgitation should be excluded.

### Special Diagnostic Evaluation

Plain radiographs of the chest may demonstrate a centrally located lung tumor. Computed tomography (CT) may be useful to examine the mediastinal structures. Phlebography usually is not required for diagnosis, but may be indicated for the planning of therapy.

### Natural History

The natural history is a function of the underlying disease process. Epithelial malignancies in this location are not curable, but lymphomas may respond to treatment.

### Treatment

Radiation therapy or chemotherapy may palliate patients with malignant tumors. Acute venous thrombosis can be treated with thrombolytic agents or heparinization. Transluminal balloon dilatation and intravascular stents have been effective for both benign and malignant obstructions. Surgical bypass is also an option in highly selected patients.

## SUGGESTED READING

Bernstein EF (ed): *Noninvasive Diagnostic Techniques in Vascular Surgery*, 3rd ed. St. Louis, CV Mosby Co, 1985.

Rutherford RB (ed): *Vascular Surgery*, 2nd ed. Philadelphia, WB Saunders Co, 1984.

Sasahara AA (ed): Symposium on deep vein thrombosis. *Am J Surg* 150(4A):1–70, 1985.

Smith RB III: Diseases of the peripheral arteries and veins, in Hurst JW (ed): *The Heart*, 7th ed. New York, McGraw-Hill, Chap 71, pp 1423–1445, 1990.

Stewart MT: Thrombophlebitis of the lower extremity, in Hurst JW (ed): *Medicine for the Practicing Physician*. Stoneham, MA, Butterworth Publishers, Chap 49, pp 1094–1096, 1988.

## 26 | Heart Disease and Pregnancy

*John H. McAnulty, M.D.*
*James Metcalfe, M.D.    Kent Ueland, M.D.*

Heart disease in a pregnant woman directly affects the health of two individuals. When planning treatment, one must consider the well-being of both. However, if the reader is to come away from this chapter with one thing in mind, it is that the health of the mother has highest priority. If there is a safer alternative to some diagnostic procedure or therapy that threatens to affect the fetus adversely, then that alternative should be used; but any diagnostic study, medication, or surgery that is *necessary* to the mother's well-being should be used regardless of possible effects on the fetus.

Further, some cardiovascular abnormalities make pregnancy so dangerous to the mother that their presence is a reason to advise prospective parents against pregnancy—and, if pregnancy does occur, to recommend interruption. (See Table 26-1.)

## CARDIOVASCULAR CHANGES DURING NORMAL PREGNANCY

The changes that take place in the cardiovascular system during normal pregnancy are so remarkable that it is not surprising that certain maternal cardiac abnormalities are not well tolerated. Total body water increases steadily throughout pregnancy, by 6 to 8 liters; most of this is extracellular. Plasma volume begins to increase as early as 6 weeks after conception, approaches its maximum in the second trimester, and is one and one-half times normal by the time of delivery.

An increase in resting cardiac output begins in the first trimester and reaches levels 30 to 50 percent above nonpregnant values by the twentieth week. The cardiac output may stay high throughout the rest of the pregnancy, but it is sensitive to changes in body position that affect venous return to the heart. The compression of the inferior vena cava by the enlarged uterus is more severe in certain body positions; this can result in decreased venous return and a fall in cardiac output. In a few women, maintenance of the supine position may result in an alarming hypotension and bradycardia—a vasovagal syndrome that has been labeled the *supine hypotension syndrome of pregnancy*. It can cause syncope. The treatment is avoidance of the supine position. The changes in cardiac output are accompanied by a continuous rise in resting

TABLE 26-1 Cardiovascular Abnormalities Placing a Mother and Infant at Extremely High Risk

Advise avoidance or interruption of pregnancy for:
  Pulmonary hypertension
  Dilated cardiomyopathy with congestive failure
  Marfan syndrome with dilated aortic root
  Cyanotic congenital heart disease
  Symptomatic obstructive lesions
Give Pre-pregnancy Counseling and Close Clinical Follow-up for:
  Prosthetic valve
  Coarctation of the aorta
  Marfan syndrome
  Dilated cardiomyopathy in asymptomatic women
  Obstructive lesions

heart rate (generally to a level below 100 beats per minute) and by a progressive fall in systemic vascular resistance.

Uterine blood flow is vulnerable. When redistribution is required in order to serve the mother, uterine blood flow falls. Prolonged excitement, heat, exercise, and falls in venous return have all been shown to reduce uterine flow and should be avoided by women with heart disease.

## CLINICAL EVALUATION OF THE PREGNANT WOMAN

The recognition and definition of heart disease is difficult at any time; this is especially true during pregnancy. There are symptoms and physical findings, however, that should arouse suspicion of heart disease. (See Table 26-2.)

When diagnostic procedures are required, the potential risks to the mother and the fetus should be considered. Unless the normal changes of the pregnancy are recognized, the findings may be misinterpreted. Electrocardiography is safe. Cardiac ultrasound is a particularly useful diagnostic study and is safe for the mother and fetus. All x-ray procedures should be avoided if possible, especially in the early stages of pregnancy. They are associated with an increased risk of abnormal fetal organogenesis and of subsequent malignancy. Radionuclides generally stay in the intravascular space; but if they fail to remain bound to maternal plasma components, or if there is a placental tear, the fetus may be exposed to them.

## CARDIOVASCULAR DISEASE IN PREGNANCY

Other chapters of this book address the abnormalities to be discussed below. The present discussion will address these abnormalities as potential complications of pregnancy, describing their

TABLE 26-2 Indicators of Heart Disease
_____

Symptoms
  Severe or progressive dyspnea
  Progressive orthopnea
  Paroxysmal nocturnal dyspnea
  Hemoptysis
  Syncope with exertion
  Chest pain related to effort or emotion
Signs
  Cyanosis
  Clubbing
  Persistent neck-vein distension
  Systolic murmur greater than grade 3/6 in intensity
  Diastolic murmur
  Cardiomegaly, general or localized
  Documented sustained arrhythmia
  Split $S_2$, persisting unchanged during expiration
  Criteria for pulmonary hypertension
    Left parasternal lift
    Loud $P_2$
_____

demonstrated and known risks to mother and fetus and their management during pregnancy.

**Pulmonary Hypertension**

Pulmonary hypertension, whether primary or secondary (i.e., due to prolonged left-to-right shunting, drug abuse, or recurrent pulmonary emboli), results in maternal mortality rates approaching 50 percent. This abnormality heads our discussion because it is so dangerous that *no matter what the cause, it is a contraindication to pregnancy*. Death most often occurs late in gestation or in the postpartum period. Fetal mortality approaches 50 percent even when the mother survives. If pregnancy occurs in a woman with pulmonary hypertension, interruption should be recommended. If this recommendation is not accepted, aggressive attempts to prevent hypovolemia are essential, especially during and after delivery.

**Valve Disease**

Each lesion must be considered individually, but one caution applies to all: Once valve disease has been recognized, *antibiotic prophylaxis against endocarditis* is required at the time of dental or surgical procedures. While not the recommendation of the American Heart Association, antibiotic prophylaxis at the time of labor and delivery *is* recommended by most physicians who care for pregnant women with heart disease. It should be started at the time of labor and continued for 24 h after delivery.

*Mitral Stenosis*

Symptoms occur in 25 percent of patients with mitral stenosis during pregnancy. Maternal death, from pulmonary edema due to severe stenosis, has occurred. Conversely, sudden death may also occur with the other extreme—a relative hypovolemia causing a decline in left atrial pressure and a consequent dramatic fall in cardiac output.

When severe mitral stenosis is identified prior to pregnancy, *surgical mitral commissurotomy or balloon valvuloplasty* should be performed before conception. An asymptomatic woman with mitral stenosis can do well during pregnancy. *Digitalis* should be started to prevent a fast ventricular response if the patient develops atrial fibrillation. If a pregnant woman with mitral stenosis has symptoms that are unremitting despite medical therapy and limitation of activity, balloon valvuloplasty or surgical commissurotomy can be performed. If thrombotic complications develop, the patient must be given instruction in subcutaneous heparin administration.

*Mitral Regurgitation*

Mitral regurgitation generally is well tolerated during pregnancy. If the hemodynamic alterations of a normal pregnancy overwhelm the capabilities of a heart that has a regurgitant mitral lesion, treatment for congestive heart failure should be carried out in a routine manner.

*Mitral Valve Prolapse*

This syndrome is common enough to warrant mention, but it is not clear that the occasional problems associated with prolapse (endocarditis, arrhythmia, cerebral emboli, mitral regurgitation) are more likely to occur during pregnancy. The only treatment recommended is the use of *antibiotics* at the time of labor and delivery.

*Aortic Stenosis*

Aortic stenosis is uncommon in pregnant women, but when present it can cause congestive heart failure. However, it is *hypovolemia* that puts these patients at greatest risk. Maternal mortality rates of up to 17 percent with aortic stenosis have been reported. Severe aortic stenosis should be corrected prior to pregnancy. If a pregnant woman with aortic stenosis develops symptoms, one should limit her activity; if that is unsuccessful, she should be treated in standard medical fashion. If symptoms are progressive and cannot be controlled, aortic valvuloplasty or valve surgery should be performed.

*Aortic Regurgitation*

Like the other volume-overload lesions, aortic regurgitation is generally well tolerated during pregnancy. If aortic regurgitation results in, or is caused by, endocarditis, and if the infection is not rapidly controlled or hemodynamic deterioration occurs, early surgery should be considered despite the pregnancy.

*Pulmonary and Tricuspid Valve Disease*

Significant pulmonary valve disease is uncommon in pregnancy. Regurgitant lesions appear to be well tolerated. Pulmonary stenosis is also well tolerated, unless the woman has been symptomatic prior to the pregnancy. Tricuspid valve lesions—particularly tricuspid regurgitation—also are uncommon and seem to be well tolerated during pregnancy.

## Congenital Heart Disease

Increasing numbers of women with congenital heart disease are reaching childbearing age; most have had complete or partial surgical correction, and many are capable of conception. The normal hemodynamic changes of pregnancy are poorly tolerated by some women, and maternal heart disease can adversely affect fetal development. Further, live-born children of such mothers are more likely to have congenital heart defects (see Table 26-3).

*Congenital Heart Lesions Without Associated Cyanosis*

**Left-to-Right Shunts** Although left-to-right shunting increases the chances of pulmonary hypertension, ventricular arrhythmias, thromboembolism, and congestive heart failure, it is not clear that any of these are made more likely by pregnancy. With atrial and ventricular septal defects and with a patent ductus arteriosus, the degree of shunting is affected by the relative resistances in the systemic and pulmonary vascular circuits; both fall during pregnancy. Normally the changes are similar, so that there is no significant alteration in the degree of shunting during pregnancy.

**Obstructive Lesions** Obstruction to outflow from the *left* side of the heart is due to the previously described aortic-valve stenosis, as well as supra- and sub-aortic valvular stenosis. In symptomatic women, surgical correction prior to pregnancy is preferable; it increases the safety of the mother and the fetus. Two conditions warrant some discussion: One is *coarctation of the aorta.* Although more common in males, this lesion may occur in women. The risk of aortic dissection, or of cerebral hemorrhage due to rupture of associated intracranial aneurysms, is increased during pregnancy. The overall maternal mortality rate is approximately 3 percent. Surgical correction should be undertaken prior to pregnancy; if

TABLE 26-3 Congenital Heart Disease in the Offspring of a Parent with
Congenital Heart Disease

| Congenital heart defect in a parent | Risk of congenital heart disease in offspring if one parent is affected,*† % |
|---|---|
| Intracardiac shunts | |
| ASD | 3–11 |
| VSD | 4–22 |
| PDA | 4–11 |
| Obstruction to flow | |
| Left-sided obstruction‡ | 3–26 |
| Right-sided obstruction | 3–22 |
| Complex abnormalities | |
| Tetralogy of Fallot | 4–15 |
| Ebstein's anomaly | Uncertain |
| Transposition of the great arteries | Uncertain |

*The high numbers in these ranges all come from the same large series. The incidence of congenital heart disease in the offspring tends to be closer to the *low* numbers in most other reported series.

†The risk in obstructive lesions is decreased by corrective surgery prior to pregnancy.

‡Includes coarctation, aortic stenosis, discrete subaortic stenosis, supravalvular stenosis. It does not include IHSS; with this the child has a 50-percent chance of having IHSS.

pregnancy occurs in a woman with coarctation, treatment of hypertension is required, and care should be taken to avoid major swings in blood pressure. The other condition that is noteworthy here is *hypertrophic obstructive cardiomyopathy.* Affected women have an increase in both the number and the severity of symptoms. Only one maternal death has been reported. Management of these patients should include avoidance of hypovolemia. The use of prophylactic beta-adrenergic blocking agents at the time of labor and delivery is controversial.

Obstruction to *right* ventricular outflow is also preferably corrected prior to pregnancy. If pregnancy does occur, treatment should be directed at avoiding intravascular volume depletion. The dangers of right ventricular obstruction due to increased pulmonary vascular resistance have been emphasized under "Pulmonary Hypertension," above.

*Cyanotic Congenital Heart Disease*

Congenital cardiac lesions resulting in cyanosis are frequently complex. Women with these syndromes may carry to term, but they and their fetuses are at increased risk of morbidity and mortality. *The risk warrants avoidance of pregnancy;* if such a patient becomes pregnant, interruption is recommended. If interruption is not accepted, treatment should be directed toward minimizng hypovolemia and preventing a fall in systemic vascular resistance. Surgical correction prior to pregnancy has resulted in excellent long-term results and safe pregnancies. This is particularly true for tetralogy of Fallot.

*Marfan Syndrome*   The risk of death to the mother from aortic rupture or dissection is higher during pregnancy than at other times. This may be particularly true if the aortic root is enlarged (>40 mm, by echocardiogram, has been used as one criterion). If the diagnosis of Marfan syndrome is definite, we advise avoidance of pregnancy—and interruption if pregnancy has begun. Should the patient choose to continue with the pregnancy, her activity should be restricted, hypertension prevented, and a beta$_1$-selective blocking agent given on a prophylactic basis.

### Congestive (Dilated) Cardiomyopathies

Because pregnancy is likely to aggravate symptoms—and, more important, is associated with a maternal mortality rate of up to 10 percent—the presence of *symptomatic* dilated cardiomyopathy is a reason to advise avoidance of pregnancy. If pregnancy does occur, interruption is recommended. The maternal risk in women with *asymptomatic* dilated cardiomyopathy is less well defined. We advise avoidance of pregnancy.

Cardiomyopathy can occur in association with pregnancy during the peripartum period. This "peripartum cardiomyopathy" is more common in multiparas, as well as in women who are older, are pregnant with twins, have associated hypertension, or are black. If cardiomegaly persists after pregnancy, the prognosis is poor and repeat pregnancy is inadvisable.

### Coronary Artery Disease

Myocardial infarction and angina pectoris, though rare, have been reported during pregnancy. The etiology is less likely to be atherosclerotic and more likely to be thromboembolic or related to vascular dissection or coronary spasm. *Medical treatment* should be used, with resort to mechanical approaches only when symptoms cannot be controlled.

### Cardiac Arrhythmias

It is not clear that arrhythmias are more likely to occur during pregnancy then at other times, but they are not uncommon. When necessary, standard medical treatment should be used. Cardioversion, if necessary, is tolerated by mother and fetus.

Bradyarrhythmias may also occur during pregnancy. They do not require treatment unless they result in symptoms or in clear maternal compromise. Temporary or permanent pacemakers can be placed if necessary.

## Pregnancy and Cardiac Surgery

Any patient who has undergone valve surgery or surgery for congenital heart disease has some residual deformity. For such patients, *antibiotic prophylaxis against endocarditis* is advised at the time of labor and delivery.

The risks of pregnancy in patients with congenital lesions depend on the residual shunts, the pulmonary vascular resistance, and ventricular function.

Pregnancy in patients with *prosthetic valves* is associated with increased risks. All patients with mechanical prosthetic valves require full anticoagulation. Because of the risk to the fetus from the warfarin derivatives, women with mechanical prostheses should be instructed in the use of heparin when contemplating pregnancy or when pregnant. It is an advantage for young valve-replacement candidates planning pregnancy to receive natural-tissue valves, and to go without anticoagulants throughout pregnancy; but if this approach is taken, it must be acknowledged that there will be a high rate of need for early valve replacement due to subsequent valve degeneration.

At time of writing, there are five reported cases of successful pregnancy following cardiac transplantation. No problems have been mentioned.

## Use of Cardiovascular Drugs During Pregnancy

It is best to avoid medications during pregnancy whenever possible; but if the cardiovascular function of the mother indicates a need, drugs should not be withheld.

### Diuretics

Diuretics should be reserved for women with congestive heart failure not controlled by sodium restriction, and for those with hypertension. They should *not* be used for isolated pedal edema. The relative advantages and risks of the available preparations are not altered by pregnancy.

### Inotropic Agents

Indications for the use of *digitalis* are not changed by pregnancy. Both digoxin and digitoxin cross the placental barrier; fetal serum levels of these drugs approximate those in the mother. The same dose of digoxin will, in general, yield lower maternal serum levels during pregnancy than in the nonpregnant state. Intravenous inotropic or vasopressor agents may be used when required, but the fetus is jeopardized—all of the available preparations cause decreased uterine blood flow.

### Adrenergic Receptor Blocking Agents

There are concerns about increased fetal and maternal side effects from beta-blocking drugs during pregnancy; but large experience, particularly with the beta$_1$-selective agents, suggests that they can be used with reasonable safety for treatment of hypertension or tachyarrhythmias. If they are used, then the heart rate, blood sugar, and respiratory status of the newborn infant should be monitored.

### Antiarrhythmic Agents

These drugs cross the placenta. Information on their fetal effects is sparse. Quinidine has been used most often and has no clear adverse effects on the fetus. Potential risks of the other, unevaluated, drugs must be weighed against their hoped-for benefits.

### Calcium Antagonists

Nifedipine, verapamil, and diltiazem, though each can lower uterine blood flow, have not been demonstrated to affect pregnancy adversely. Each, if used in pregnancy, will cross the placenta and will be found in breast milk.

### Vasodilator Agents

Preload- and afterload-reducing agents may have adverse effects on uterine perfusion. Hydralazine and the nitrate preparations have been most frequently used, with good fetal tolerance. There is little information available on the effects of the angiotensin-converting enzyme (ACE) inhibitors. Nitroprusside may cause fetal accumulation of cyanide, but its use is justified in life-threatening situations.

### Anticoagulants

Warfarin is contraindicated throughout pregnancy. The word "throughout" is controversial here. Warfarin crosses the placenta, and fetal exposure during the first 2 months results in a 15- to 25-percent incidence of malformations from the so-called warfarin embryopathy syndrome (facial abnormalities, epitracheal deformity, digital abnormalities, epithelial changes, and mental impairment). Because organogenesis is reasonably complete by the end of the first trimester, some physicians say that warfarin can be used after that time. Still, because wafarin has been associated with continued fetal and maternal bleeding problems in the second and third trimesters, women requiring anticoagulation should be instructed in the use of 3-times-per-day administration of subcutaneous heparin (total daily dose of 15,000 to 36,000 units) throughout pregnancy.

## SUGGESTED READING

Elkayam U, Gleicher N (eds): *Cardiac Problems in Pregnancy: Diagnosis and Management of Maternal and Fetal Disease*. New York, Alan R Liss, Inc, 1982.

McAnulty JH, Metcalfe J, Ueland K: The heart and certain physiological conditions, in Hurst JW et al (eds): *The Heart,* 7th ed. New York, McGraw-Hill, Chap 74, pp 1465–1478, 1990.

Metcalfe J, McAnulty JH, Ueland K: *Heart Disease and Pregnancy: Physiology and Management,* 2d ed. Boston, Little, Brown and Company, 1986.

Sullivan JM, Ramanathan KB: Management of medical problems in pregnancy—severe cardiac disease. *N Engl J Med* 313:304–309, 1985.

Whittemore R, Hobbins JC, Engle MA: Pregnancy and its outcome in women with and without surgical treatment of congenital heart disease. *Am J Cardiol* 50:641–651, 1982.

*27* Exercise and the Heart

*Peter M. Buttrick, M.D.*
*James Scheuer, M.D.*

This chapter reviews the physiological responses that accompany acute exercise, and the chronic cardiovascular adaptations that occur as a result of physical conditioning. In addition, the clinical features of the athlete's heart and the risks and benefits of conditioning will be described.

## ACUTE HEMODYNAMICS

In general, exercise is divided into two distinct types: *isotonic* (or dynamic) and *isometric* (or static). These differ in the physiological responses they evoke and in the demands they place on the heart—which, in turn, define the chronic adaptations that develop in conditioned athletes.

The earliest hemodynamic response to dynamic exercise is a fall in systemic vascular resistance, which reflects vasodilatation of the resistance vessels in the exercising muscle. This is marked even at mild exercise intensity. Afterload falls and cardiac output is redistributed, so that during maximal effort more than 80 percent of the cardiac output may be directed to working muscle, versus only 18 percent at rest. Since the aerobic capacity of skeletal muscle is far greater than that of the splanchnic and renal tissues (and since local factors may actually increase the capacity of skeletal muscle to extract oxygen), the net result of this redistribution of flow is an increase in systemic oxygen consumption. The primary cardiac response to dynamic exercise is an increased heart rate. However, heart rate alone does account for the increased cardiac output seen during exercise. There is an increase in venous return, probably mediated by vasoconstriction of the large veins as well as the mechanical effects of muscular contraction, which results in increased end-diastolic volume and augmented stroke volume (by the Frank-Starling mechanism). There is also an increase in neurohumoral sympathetic drive that augments cardiac contractility.

During isometric exercise, a discrete muscle group is enlisted and no external work is performed. The oxygen requirements necessary to sustain isometric exercise are proportional to the muscle mass involved and are generally modest. However, these demands cannot be met by an increase in blood flow, as local vasodilatation is limited by mechanical compression of the resistance vessels. Flow to the exercising muscle may actually decrease. Muscle perfusion tends to be maintained via a rise in arterial pressure that is initiated by a reflex arc emanating from the contracting muscle, which results in increased systemic vascular resistance even in the face of only modest exertion. In concert with this, stroke volume may actually fall, and the heart rate response to isometric exercise is exaggerated. Thus, in contrast to isotonic exercise, isometric exercise imposes a significant systolic, or pressure, load on the heart.

## CHRONIC ADAPTATIONS

With conditioning induced by chronic bouts of dynamic exercise, a series of cardiovascular adaptations develop which are reflected by a significant increase in maximal oxygen consumption. In addition to increasing maximal exercise capacity, these allow sustained submaximal work with economy of effort. The adaptations that develop affect both skeletal muscle and the heart. In skeletal muscle, capillary density increases, as does the number of mitochondria and the respiratory capacity of the muscle. Oxygen extraction by a conditioned skeletal muscle is increased at any given blood flow. The primary cardiac adaptations are a decrease in heart rate, both at rest and at any submaximal level of exercise, and an increase in heart size, manifested mainly by greater right and left ventricular end-diastolic chamber dimensions. This is a result both of the lower heart rate and greater diastolic filling and of cardiac hypertrophy, which results in greater ventricular circumferences. These changes allow an increase in stroke volume. In addition, the mechanical properties of the conditioned heart are altered so that increased rates of systolic contraction and diastolic relaxation occur. Capillary density and coronary collaterals are also increased, but the clinical significance of these changes remains unclear.

## THE ATHLETE'S HEART

Characteristic features in the clinical assessment of an athlete include a resting bradycardia, a slightly lateralized PMI, and both an $S_3$ and an $S_4$ (heard in up to 50 percent of athletes). Short ejection murmurs are usual. ECG abnormalities are common and include sinus arrhythmias with pauses of up to 2.5 s. First-degree and Mobitz I second-degree AV blocks occur frequently, largely reflecting increased vagal tone. An increase both in the P wave and in the QRS voltages, associated with lateral T-wave inversions, may also be seen. QRS prolongation, axis deviations, and supraventricular and ventricular tachycardias are not characteristic and may warrant further workup. Echocardiographic findings in a dynamically trained athlete include a slight symmetric increase in left ventricular wall thickness associated with an increase in end-diastolic dimension, and a normal (or even slightly diminished) end-systolic dimension. Concentric left ventricular hypertrophy may be seen in the isometrically conditioned athlete. Asymmetric septal hypertrophy is unusual.

## EXERCISE AND SUDDEN DEATH

Cardiovascular death during exercise is extremely rare. Autopsy data overwhelmingly suggests that it is associated with recognized or occult cardiac diseases. In persons under 35, common causes of sudden death during exercise include coronary anomalies and hypertrophic obstructive cardiomyopathy, and, less commonly, coronary artery disease, mitral valve prolapse, aortic rupture, and myocarditis. In persons over 35, coronary artery disease is the predominant risk factor, though other entities, such as valvular heart disease and cardiomyopathies, are also seen.

A related question is whether exercise conditioning can prevent cardiovascular death. Several large longitudinal studies suggest that it can. These include studies of Harvard alumni, San Francisco longshoremen, and British civil servants, all of which showed that increased physical activity, independent of known coronary risk factors, was associated with a delay in the onset of symptomatic coronary disease and a reduction in cardiovascular risk.

## SUGGESTED READING

Asmussen E: Similarities and dissimilarities between static and dynamic exercise. *Circ Res* 48(Suppl 2):13–110, 1981.

Buttrick PM, Scheuer J: Exercise and the heart, in Hurst JW (ed): *The Heart*, 7th ed. New York, McGraw Hill, Chap 75, pp 1479–1488, 1990.

Hanson P (ed): Exercise and the heart. *Cardiol Clin* 5:147–348, 1987.

Huston TP, Puffer JC, Rodney WM: The athletic heart syndrome. *N Engl J Med* 313:24–32, 1985.

Maron BJ: Structural features of the athlete's heart as defined by echocardiography. *J Am Coll Cardiol* 7:190–203, 1986.

Paffenbarger RS, Hyde RT, Wing AL, et al: Physical activity, all-cause mortality and longevity in college alumni. *N Engl J Med* 314:605–613, 1986.

Schaible TF, Scheuer J: Cardiac adaptations to chronic exercise. *Prog Cardiovasc Dis* 27:297–324, 1985.

Scheuer J: Effects of physical training on myocardial vascularity and perfusion. *Circulation* 66:491–495, 1982.

## 28 | Cardiovascular Aging and Adaptation to Disease

*Robert C. Schlant, M.D.*

### INTRODUCTION

Aging is associated with selective changes in the cardiovascular system. The overall function of the left ventricle at rest remains relatively normal evidenced by the maintained ability of the aged cardiac muscle to develop tension and to respond to inotropic stimulation with calcium or with post-extrasystolic potentiation. On the other hand, there is a significant decrease in the inotropic response to beta-sympathetic stimulation, manifest by a decreased response to catecholamines, and to digitalis. In addition, there is a decreased heart rate response to sympathetic stimulation and a decreased arterial vasodilatation during exercise. In aged animals there is usually only a small decrease in the velocity of shortening in cardiac muscle, but a very striking prolongation of the duration both of contraction and of relaxation. Some of the age-associated prolongation of contraction may be related to deconditioning and to the mild left ventricle hypertrophy that occurs with aging.

While there are no major changes in left ventricular function in healthy aged human subjects at rest, the elderly heart does respond to exercise or stress in a different manner than the young heart. The prolonged diastolic relaxation of the aged myocardium can more easily limit blood flow to the subendocardium of the left ventricle, which receives almost all of its blood flow during diastole. Subendocardial ischemia is even more likely to occur when the ventricle is hypertrophied or when the ventricular end-diastolic pressure is elevated. Tachycardia, which produces a shorter period of diastole per minute, may also contribute to an increase in left ventricular diastolic pressure.

Additional cardiovascular changes with aging include an increase in stiffness of both the left ventricle and the peripheral blood vessels. Because of the increase in stiffness of the aorta and large vessels, there is increased impedance to left ventricular ejection. This, in turn, results in some degree of left ventricular hypertrophy. Furthermore, during exercise the aged peripheral vasculature fails to dilate normally and to decrease peripheral resistance. Aging is associated with a significant decrease in the maximum heart rate response to exercise or to beta-sympathetic stimulation. It is

**237**

interesting that exercise conditioning in the aged can, to some slight degree, increase the maximum heart rate response.

## CARDIOVASCULAR RESPONSE TO EXERCISE IN THE AGED

The aged human being has an age-associated decrease in the maximum rate of oxygen consumption during exercise, in association with a decreased capacity for maximum exercise. The healthy aged individual responds differently to exercise than a young individual. First, the aged individual has a significant decrease in the maximum heart rate response to exercise. Second, he or she has a less-than-normal decrease in left ventricular afterload during exercise. This is produced by both a decreased arterial vasodilator response and an increase in the end-systolic volume which does not decrease with exercise as in younger subjects. Third, there is a significant increase in the end-diastolic left ventricular volume and in the left ventricular stroke volume during exercise. Accordingly, the elderly use the Frank-Starling mechanism to increase stroke volume during exercise much more than young individuals. In most healthy elderly individuals, the left ventricular ejection fraction during exercise decreases only mildly in the absence of disease.

## HYPERTENSION IN THE AGED (See Chap. 13)

The diastolic blood pressure may normally increase slightly during early adulthood. In general, however, a diastolic pressure consistently above 90 mmHg is thought to indicate the presence of disease. Abnormal systolic blood pressure in an aged patient may be partially related to increased stiffness of the aorta and great vessels. Epidemiologically, the development of coronary artery disease or heart failure is more strongly related to systolic than to diastolic blood pressure. Many elderly patients with hypertension respond well to therapy with angiotensin-converting enzyme (ACE) inhibitors or calcium antagonists.

## CORONARY ARTERY DISEASE IN THE AGED

Age is a major risk factor for the development of coronary artery disease. In addition, the prognosis with angina pectoris or acute myocardial infarction or coronary bypass graft surgery is poorer for aged patients than for younger patients. Coronary artery disease may more likely be "silent" in the elderly than in the young. Thus, aged patients may have more episodes of "silent" acute myocardial infarction and more episodes of silent or asymptomatic angina. At times coronary artery disease is manifest by "angina equivalents," which may include dyspnea on exertion, chronic fatigue, or arrhythmias.

## CONGESTIVE HEART FAILURE IN THE AGED
(See Chap. 1)

The decreased responsiveness and reserve capacity of the elderly cardiovascular system and of the kidneys in the aged is not thought to produce congestive heart failure. On the other hand, the cardiovascular system of the aged is less able to tolerate tachycardia, a sudden load of intravenous fluid, or other acute stress. Coronary artery disease and hypertensive heart disease are the most common causes of heart failure in the aged. Amyloid heart disease may also occur. (See Chap. 18.)

## CARDIAC ELECTROPHYSIOLOGY IN THE AGED
(See Chaps. 3 and 4)

Elderly patients may have dysfunction of the sinus node, the atrioventricular node, the His-Purkinje system, and the bundle branches. In addition, the elderly have an increase in supraventricular and ventricular arrhythmias.

## VALVULAR HEART DISEASE IN THE AGED
(See Chaps. 8 and 9)

The most common type of valvular heart disease in the elderly is calcific aortic stenosis, which is usually due to a congenital bicuspid aortic valve in patients under the age of 70 years and to idiopathic fibrocalcific changes in a tricuspid aortic valve (Mönckeberg's stenosis) in older patients. These changes can also produce aortic regurgitation. Calcification of the mitral anulus may also occur in the elderly. Mitral regurgitation may occur, due to coronary artery disease and papillary muscle dysfunction or to myxomatous changes in the mitral valve. Rheumatic mitral stenosis or regurgitation also may occur. Balloon valvuloplasty may be useful for highly selected elderly patients with aortic or mitral stenosis who are not candidates for surgery.

## SUGGESTED READING

Messerli FH (ed): *Cardiovascular Disease in the Elderly.* Boston, Martinus Nijhoff, pp 1–347, 1984.

Weisfeldt ML, Gerstenblith G: Cardiovascular aging and adaptation to disease, in Hurst JW et al (eds): *The Heart,* 7th ed. New York, McGraw-Hill, Chap 76, pp 1488–1496, 1990.

Weisfeldt ML (ed): *The Aging Heart: Its Function and Response to Stress.* New York, Raven Press, pp 1–323, 1980.

Wenger NK, Furberg CL, Pitt E (eds): *Coronary Heart Disease in the Elderly.* New York, Elsevier, pp 1–412, 1986.

*Frederick S. Fein, M.S.*
*Edmund H. Sonnenblick, M.D.*

## ACROMEGALY

Cardiomegaly is characteristic. In many patients the extent of cardiomegaly is proportional to the enlargement seen in other viscera. The heart may be disproportionately enlarged, especially if there is concomitant hypertension or congestive heart failure (cardiomyopathy).

## HYPERTHYROIDISM

### Typical Cardiovascular Manifestations

Patients frequently complain of palpitations and exertional dyspnea. They usually have sinus tachycardia, systolic hypertension, low diastolic blood pressure, increased stroke volume, and decreased systemic vascular resistance. Pulses are brisk. The cardiac impulse is prominent, with increased $S_1$ and $P_2$ sounds; frequently there are $S_3$ gallops and systolic flow murmurs. Cardiovascular signs and symptoms may predominate in patients with apathetic hyperthyroidism.

### Congestive Heart Failure

This is most common in the setting of underlying valvular, myocardial, or coronary artery disease. For example, if mitral stenosis is present, pulmonary hypertension and pulmonary vascular congestion will be worsened by the tachycardia and increased cardiac output.

### Arrhythmias

Atrial arrhythmias are common, including PACs, paroxysmal atrial tachycardia, atrial flutter, and atrial fibrillation. The latter predisposes to systemic embolization.

### Angina

Patients with obstructive coronary artery disease frequently develop worsening symptoms of ischemia with the development of thyrotoxicosis.

## Mitral Valve Prolapse

The incidence of this disorder is increased, primarily in patients with Graves' disease.

## Treatment

Beta blockers, such as intravenous or oral propranolol, have often been used to treat the cardiovascular manifestations of hyperthyroidism while other modalities are used to render the patient euthyroid. If there is doubt about the adequacy of left ventricular systolic function, a trial of intravenous esmolol may be considered. Beta blockers do not influence the increased oxygen consumption that is characteristic of hyperthyroidism. Higher-than-normal doses of digitalis may be needed to control the heart rate during atrial arrhythmias. Anticoagulation is recommended for atrial fibrillation (especially if it lasts for 3 days or more); it should be continued for 4 weeks after conversion to sinus rhythm and reestablishment of the euthyroid state.

## HYPOTHYROIDISM

### Typical Cardiovascular Manifestations

Generally there is sinus bradycardia, mild hypertension (especially in the elderly), decreased pulse pressure, decreased stroke volume, and increased systemic vascular resistance. The ECG frequently shows low voltage, and sometimes prolonged QT intervals and conduction disturbances.

### Congestive Heart Failure

Uncomplicated hypothyroidism generally does not cause sufficient myocardial dysfunction to bring about overt congestive heart failure. However, treatment of hypothyroidism may precipitate congestive heart failure in patients with underlying valvular, myocardial, or coronary artery disease. Digitalis should be used with caution in hypothyroid patients with congestive heart failure.

### Pericardial Effusion

High-protein-content effusions are common and may be massive at times, even resulting in cardiac tamponade. Low voltage on the ECG and an enlarged cardiac silhouette often occur. Echocardiography is an extremely valuable diagnostic tool. The effusion resolves with thyroid hormone replacement, but this may take several months.

### Coronary Artery Disease

Signs of coronary artery disease may be masked by hypothyroidism. Extreme caution in thyroid hormone replacement is necessary in patients with known coronary artery disease.

## HYPERPARATHYROIDISM

Hypercalcemia is responsible for the basic cardiovascular abnormalities in hyperparathyroidism, including shortened QT interval, increased sensitivity to digitalis (and increased tendency to digitalis toxicity), and occasional conduction disturbances. The frequency of hypertension is increased.

## HYPOPARATHYROIDISM

Prolonged QT interval is common. Congestive heart failure has been described rarely.

## CUSHING'S SYNDROME

The major cardiac manifestations reflect hypertension and hypokalemia.

## ADDISON'S DISEASE

The major cardiac manifestation is hypotension, with decreased pulse pressure and low cardiac output. The cardiac silhouette is small. The hypotension of glucocorticoid deficiency alone is not related to volume deficiency; it responds poorly to all therapies except glucocorticoids. In Addison's disease, however, there is deficiency of both cortisol and aldosterone; lack of aldosterone leads to volume depletion and contributes to hypotension. ECG signs of hyperkalemia may also occur.

## DIABETES MELLITUS

### Coronary Artery Disease

The incidence and severity of coronary artery disease are increased in type I and type II diabetics. Silent infarction and silent ischemia are also more frequent. The short- and long-term mortality rates following myocardial infarction are greater in diabetics than in nondiabetics. The effects of tight metabolic control on short-term mortality are uncertain. Long-term beta blockade has similar cardiovascular benefits in diabetics and diabetics following myocardial infarction, but the use of these drugs requires caution, especially in type I diabetics.

## Autonomic Neuropathy

Decreased heart rate variation during respiration and standing are markers for increased cardiac mortality in diabetics. Some of this mortality represents sudden death, which may be related to the high incidence of QT prolongation in this population.

## Cardiomyopathy

Patients have been described with features of either restrictive or congestive cardiomyopathy in the absence of coronary atherosclerosis. Hypertension is an important risk factor for this complication of diabetes. Congestive heart failure in diabetics may also be the consequence of coronary artery disease. The cardiovascular response to captopril or enalapril in diabetics with congestive heart failure is at least as beneficial as that in nondiabetics. Attention to renal function and serum potassium levels is important.

## SUGGESTED READING

Fein FS, Sonnenblick EH: Diabetic cardiomyopathy. *Prog C Vasc Dis* 27:255–270, 1985.

Fleischer N, Fein FS, Sonnenblick EH: The heart and endocrine diseases, in Hurst JW et al (eds): *The Heart*, 7th ed. New York, McGraw Hill, Chap 77, pp 1497–1513, 1990.

Jaffe AS, Spadaro JJ, Schechtman K, et al: Increased congestive heart failure after myocardial infarction of modest extent in patients with diabetes mellitus. *Am Heart J* 108:31–37, 1984.

Skelton CL: The heart and hyperthyroidism. *N Engl J Med* 307:1206–1208, 1982.

Ulvenstam G, Aberg A, Bergstrand R, et al: Long-term prognosis after myocardial infarction in men with diabetes. *Diabetes* 34:787–792, 1985.

Zimmerman J, Yahalom J, Bar-On H: Clinical spectrum of pericardial effusion as the presenting feature of hypothyroidism. *Am Heart J* 106:770–771, 1983.

## 30

The Heart and Connective Tissue
Disease

*Robert C. Schlant, M.D.*

The connective tissue, or collagen vascular, diseases are systemic disorders of unknown origin characterized by inflammatory lesions of many organs, including the joints, muscles, blood vessels, pleurae, and pericardium. The prognosis is often related to involvement of the kidney, brain, or heart. The cardiac manifestations of five common connective tissue diseases are shown in Table 30-1.

## SYSTEMIC LUPUS ERYTHEMATOSUS (SLE)

### Clinical Manifestations

SLE occurs most often in the second and third decades of life, and affects women more frequently than men. Frequent early signs include fever, arthralgias, arthritis, skin rash, myalgias, and pleuritis.

SLE can produce a *pancarditis* with involvement of the heart valves, endocardium, myocardium, coronary arteries, and pericardium. Pericardial involvement is most frequent; *pericarditis* can be the first manifestation of SLE. Pericardial involvement is usually manifested by effusion or by pericarditis with fibrofibrinous fluid. Rarely, purulent pericarditis, cardiac tamponade, and pericardial constriction may occur. Uremic pericarditis may occur in patients with severe renal failure.

*SLE endocarditis and valvulitis* is produced by fibrofibrinous sterile vegetations that may occur on any of the heart valves, especially the mitral and aortic. "Atypical verrucous endocarditis" was first described by Libman and Sacks. The lesions are usually clinically silent, but they can produce murmurs from either stenosis or regurgitation and, rarely, can produce severe valve dysfunction and require valve replacement. The lesions also predispose to infective endocarditis.

*SLE myocarditis* is uncommon clinically. A severe form can occur, however, with ventricular arrhythmias, conduction disturbances, and congestive heart failure.

SLE may involve the small intramyocardial arteries and produce fibrinoid necrosis and thromboembolic occlusions. Involvement of the vessels to the SA and AV nodes may produce disturbances of rhythm and conduction, including complete heart block. Systemic

TABLE 30-1 Primary Cardiac Manifestations in Connective Tissue Diseases

| Disease | Pericardium | Myocardium | Endocardium | Coronary arteries |
|---------|-------------|------------|-------------|-------------------|
| SLE | + + | + | + + | +/− |
| PAN | +/− | + | 0 | + + |
| RA | + + | + | + | 0 |
| AS | 0 | +/− | + + | 0 |
| PSS | + | + + | 0 | + + |

+ + = Major site of involvement; + = may be involved, but less frequently; +/− = rarely involved; 0 = not involved.

*Source:* Adapted from Healy BP: The heart and connective tissue disease, in Hurst JW, Schlant RC, Rackley CE, Sonnenblick EH, Wenger NK (eds): *The Heart,* 7th ed. New York, McGraw-Hill, Chap 78, pp 1513–1522, 1990.

hypertension is frequently associated with renal involvement and may result in heart failure. Coronary atherosclerosis may be accelerated by the hypertension, renal failure, and steroid therapy.

### Special Diagnostic Tests

Serum gamma globulin and cryoproteins are frequently elevated, while serum complement is usually decreased. Lupus-erythematous (LE) cell preparations are characteristic. Antinuclear antibody (ANA), anticytoplasmic, and rheumatoid factors are frequently positive, but are nonspecific.

### Natural History and Prognosis

Survival is greater than 80 percent over a 10-year period; most deaths are related to infection, renal failure, or cerebritis.

### Differential Diagnosis

This includes rheumatic heart disease, infective endocarditis, myocarditis, acute purulent or tuberculous pericarditis, dilated cardiomyopathy, glomerulonephritis, sickle-cell disease, and other connective tissue diseases.

### Therapy

Therapy for SLE includes nonsteroidal anti-inflammatory drugs, corticosteroids, and cytotoxic agents. Systemic hypertension, congestive heart failure, and arrhythmias are managed in the usual ways. Pericardial effusions can produce tamponade and can require pericardiocentesis. SLE valvulitis can require valve replacement.

## POLYARTERITIS NODOSA (PAN)

PAN produces segmental necrotizing arteritis of the medium-sized or small arteries throughout the body, especially in the skin, kidneys, gastrointestinal tract, spleen, lymph nodes, central nervous system, skeletal muscles, and heart.

### Diagnosis

The diagnosis is based on the clinical evidence of multisystem involvement and on biopsy evidence of arteritis. The sedimentation rate and serum gamma globulins are frequently elevated, and rheumatoid factor and antinuclear antibodies may be present.

### Natural History and Prognosis

PAN may produce focal myocardial infarction or conduction system abnormalities. Involvement of the renal arteries often leads to renal failure and hypertension, which can produce congestive heart failure. In general, the prognosis of PAN is poor.

### Differential Diagnosis

This includes giant-cell arteritis, hypersensitivity angitis, temporal arteritis, Takayasu's arteritis, and arteritis from other connective tissue disorders.

### Therapy

Corticosteroids and other anti-inflammatory drugs are used to treat PAN. Hypertension, heart failure, and conduction system abnormalities are treated in the usual ways.

## RHEUMATOID ARTHRITIS (RA)

### Clinical Manifestations

RA is the most common connective tissue disease. It usually affects the joints, with arthralgia and arthritis, fever, anemia, weight loss, subcutaneous nodules, and lymphadenopathy. Pleuritis and necrotizing vasculitis occur less often. Pericarditis may occur in up to 30 percent of patients, but is usually overshadowed by other symptoms. Large pericardial effusions can require pericardiocentesis; pericardial constriction can require pericardiectomy. Rheumatoid nodules can involve the myocardium and the heart valves, where they can produce mild-to-severe valvular regurgitation. Very rarely, extensive rheumatoid nodules and myocarditis can produce arrhythmias, conduction disturbances, and congestive heart failure.

## Therapy

Arrhythmias, conduction disturbances, heart failure, and acute pericarditis are treated in the usual ways. Therapy for RA usually consists of corticosteroids and nonsteroidal anti-inflammatory agents.

## ANKYLOSING SPONDYLITIS (AS)

### Clinical Manifestations

Ankylosing spondylitis, or rheumatoid spondylitis, usually affects young men, with inflammation of the spinal joints and, eventually (over 20 or 30 years), immobilization of the spine due to fusion of the costovertebral and sacroiliac joints. Most patients have the HLA-B27 histocompatibility antigen, as do patients with Reiter's syndrome and juvenile arthritis.

The aorta of a patient with ankylosing spondylitis may have an inflammatory sclerosis, just above and below the aortic valve, that produces aortic regurgitation. Extension to the mitral valve can produce mitral regurgitation; extension into the ventricular septum can produce conduction defects. Reiter's syndrome and psoriatic arthritis can each produce a similar inflammatory sclerosis of the aortic root, and aortic regurgitation.

### Therapy

Conduction disturbances and heart failure are treated in the usual ways. Aortic regurgitation can require valve replacement.

## PROGRESSIVE SYSTEMIC SCLEROSIS (PSS)

### Clinical Manifestations

PSS (formerly called *scleroderma*) is associated with fibrous thickening of the skin and fibrous and degenerative changes and diffuse vascular lesions in the fingers, esophagus, small and large bowels, kidneys, heart, and lungs. Systemic hypertension due to renal involvement is common. Most patients have Raynaud's disease of the fingers. A similar phenomenon also occurs in the vasculature of involved internal organs.

The clinical course varies from short and severe to long and benign. A variant of PSS is the *CREST syndrome* (*c*alcinosis, *R*aynaud's phenomenon, *e*sophageal abnormality, *s*clerodactylia, *t*elangiectasia), in which symptoms of lung disease and pulmonary hypertension may predominate.

PSS may produce patchy myocardial necrosis and fibrosis, possibly due to Raynaud's vasospastic phenomenon of the small coronary vessels. This can result in angina pectoris, myocardial infarction, sudden cardiac death, arrhythmias, and biventricular congestive heart failure. Pericarditis may occur due to PSS or, more often, to chronic renal failure. Very rarely, constrictive pericarditis can occur. PSS can involve the pulmonary vasculature and produce severe pulmonary vascular disease, with lesions similar to those of primary pulmonary hypertension (see Chap. 14) and with a similar clinical picture, including possible sudden cardiac death.

### Therapy

Arrhythmias and congestive heart failure are treated as usual. Calcium channel blockers, such as nifedipine, may help patients with Raynaud's phenomenon involving the myocardium as well as the fingers, but the benefit of such therapy is not proven. Corticosteroids and D-penicillamine are also of unproven efficacy.

## SUGGESTED READING

Alexander EL, Firestein GS, Weiss JL: Reversible cold-induced abnormalities in myocardial perfusion and function in systemic sclerosis. *Ann Intern Med* 105:661–668, 1986.

Alpert MA, Goldberg SH, Singsen BH, et al: Cardiovascular manifestations of mixed connective tissue disease in adults. *Circulation* 68:1182–1193, 1983.

Ellis WW, Baer AN, Robertson RM, et al: Left ventricle dysfunction induced by cold exposure in patients with systemic sclerosis. *Am J Med* 80:385–392, 1986.

Healy BP: The heart and connective tissue disease, in Hurst JW et al (eds): *The Heart*, 7th ed. New York, McGraw-Hill, Chap 78, pp 1513–1522, 1990.

Kahan A, Devaux JY, Amor B, et al: Nifedipine and thallium-201 myocardial perfusion in progressive systemic sclerosis, *N Engl J Med* 314:1397–1402, 1986.

## 31

# The Heart, Alcoholism, and Nutritional Disease

*Timothy J. Regan, M.D.*

## ALCOHOLIC CARDIOMYOPATHY

Cardiomyopathy related to long-term alcohol abuse has gained renewed recognition in recent years. Alcoholism has been reported to be the most common identifiable etiologic factor in congestive cardiomyopathy, accounting for up to one-third of cases.

As with other causes of primary myocardial disease, a diffuse abnormality of the myocardium is present, unrelated to coronary atherosclerosis, arterial hypertension, valvular disease, or congenital heart disease. Though symptoms of congestive heart failure may be the most common presentation in primary myocardial disease of multiple etiologies, congestive heart failure may be found on initial examination in fewer than half of patients. In a significant proportion of patients, arrhythmias without congestive heart failure may be the first evident abnormality. Chest pain is not uncommon; occasionally, classic angina pectoris is the only symptom despite normal coronary arteriograms.

### Etiology

The evidence that ethanol and/or its metabolites are the etiologic basis for alcoholic cardiomyopathy is circumstantial. The major supportive feature for this idea is the history of ethanol ingestion in intoxicating amounts for many years, frequently marked by periods of spree drinking. The reduced mortality rate in patients who become abstinent further supports the view that ethanol is the major factor in the development of the disease.

In an epidemiological survey of a working population the risk of cardiovascular death was increased when chronic alcohol consumption exceeded six drinks a day. As a variable that may contribute to the development of cardiomyopathy, cigarette use is common. In contrast to alcoholic cirrhosis, clinically evident malnutrition usually is not present in the cardiac patient. In females, the disease is rare before the age of menopause.

### Diagnosis

Clinical reports of cardiomyopathy have emphasized the problem of denial in attempting to elicit a history of alcoholism. There is male predominance. Suggestive diagnostic aspects include a family history of chronic alcoholism, social disruption, and accident-proneness. The major positive diagnostic feature is the history of ethanol ingestion in intoxicating amounts for many years, frequently marked by periods of spree drinking. Often this information can be obtained only through persistent questioning in multiple visits with the patient or by communication with relatives. Altered blood composition may support the suspicion of addiction. The mean corpuscular red cell volume may be enhanced, serum albumin and transferrin reduced. Platelet adenyl cyclase responses to appropriate stimulation may be reduced; this condition may persist for months to years after the individual becomes abstinent.

## Heart Failure

Almost 50 percent of individuals addicted to ethanol show subclinical abnormalities of left ventricular function on noninvasive testing. In those in whom cardiac dysfunction progresses to low-cardiac-output heart failure, exertional or nocturnal dyspnea is present. Patients may also complain of weakness and fatigue, presumably because of the reduction in cardiac output. The physical signs of cardiac decompensation seen in these individuals are similar to those observed with other forms of congestive cardiomyopathy—i.e., early and late diastolic gallop and cardiomegaly. The murmur of mitral regurgitation is usually well differentiated from that related to rheumatic valvular disease. This murmur is characteristically confined to a portion of systole, is only rarely holosystolic, and, as a rule, changes as cardiac compensation is restored. A holosystolic murmur due to tricuspid regurgitation may be heard in the third and fourth intercostal spaces along the sternal border. It is also diminished with the amelioration of heart failure.

Since the addicted person may frequently delay seeking medical assistance for weeks to months, evidence of right-sided heart failure is not uncommon, with distended jugular veins; also common is an enlarged, tender liver, as well as edema of the dependent portions of the body.

A common complication of cardiomyopathy is the development of pulmonary or peripheral arterial emboli. Systemic emboli can originate from mural thrombi in the left ventricle and left atrium. Pulmonary emboli are often associated with thrombi in the dilated right heart and with thrombophlebitis in the venous system.

### ECG

The electrocardiogram at this time may be relatively normal or show nonspecific changes. Poor progression of the R wave across the precordium is fairly common, particularly as the disease advances. This is thought to be due to progression of the ventricular disease and conduction delay. Evidence of left ventricular and atrial enlargement is common, but left anterior hemiblock occurs in a minority of patients, while left or right bundle branch block appears in approximately 10 percent. A variety of arrhythmias may be present, including atrial or ventricular ectopic beats and atrial fibrillation. Usually these are secondary to heart failure.

### Hemodynamics

The hemodynamic characteristics of the left ventricle in patients who are compensated from heart failure show a qualitative similarity to those found in patients in the subclinical state. Presentation with noncoronary chest pain rather than heart failure can be associated with a significant increase of end-diastolic pressure but a slight reduction of end-diastolic volume consistent with diminished compliance. Moreover, indices of contractility are frequently diminished in this state. When shortness of breath appears, there is an increase in end-diastolic volume and a further reduction of systolic function as measured by ejection fraction.

### Precipitating Factors

Usually there are no evident factors other than ethanol that can be readily associated with the episode of heart failure. However, occasional, small, isolated outbreaks appear to be associated with the combination of ethanol abuse and the trace metals lead, cobalt, and/or arsenic. Several other factors have to be considered potentially important. Clinically evident malnutrition usually is not present in the cardiac patient, though it is commonly associated with liver disease. In females, the disease is rare before menopause.

### Natural History and Prognosis

The course of alcoholic cardiomyopathy is variable, depending largely on the extent of cardiac involvement. The outlook is relatively poor in persons who continue to ingest ethanol in substantial amounts. In one study a series of 64 alcoholic patients with cardiomyopathy was followed over a 4-year period. One-third remained abstinent, and the mortality rate in this group was 9 percent, though only a minority exhibited clinical improvement paralleling the response in hepatic cirrhosis. Of those who remained actively alcoholic, more than one-half succumbed. Presumably, at certain stages of the disease the pathogenic mechanisms may continue unabated despite traditional pharmacological management and abstinence from alcohol.

### Management

Pharmacological therapy for cardiac decompensation depends on the state of cardiac disease when the patient is first encountered.

During the first episode of heart failure, if the patient has had symptoms for a relatively short time with only modest cardiomegaly and pulmonary congestion then he or she may be managed initially by diuretics to diminish volume overload. As the disease progresses, there is a role for preload- and afterload-reducing agents. Presumably the latter may provide long-term efficacy as reported for other causes of heart failure. Digitalis can contribute to the management of congestive failure in the advanced stages of the disease and is most useful in the control of atrial fibrillation or sinus tachycardia, assuming the patient's compliance.

### Arrhythmias

The patient may present with an arrhythmia as the initial manifestation of disease. Supraventricular arrhythmias predominate; atrial fibrillation is the most common arrhythmia. Cardioversion or pharmacological intervention is frequently required, but sinus rhythm is restored spontaneously in some patients. Plasma electrolytes on admission are usually normal. During a subsequent recurrence the same arrhythmia may be present as during the original episode.

This entity has been called the *holiday heart syndrome* because of frequent presentation over holidays or weekends. In this syndrome the acute cardiac rhythm disturbance occurs in association with heavy ethanol consumption in a person who has chronically abused ethanol without other clinical evidence of heart disease. Under unusual circumstances, such as a prolonged period of sleeplessness, the arrhythmia may be induced acutely without chronic abuse.

Sudden unexpected death in alcoholics has been reported from several countries. This phenomenon has been attributed to cardiac arrest; this conclusion is supported by the observation of a reduced ventricular fibrillation threshold in an animal model of chronic alcoholism. In one series, young and middle-aged persons without coronary disease made up 8 percent of all sudden deaths. A subsequent investigation in the Soviet Union revealed an incidence of 17 percent in the apparent absence of other toxins. Frequently there was no evidence of cardiac hypertrophy; the liver involvement was often in the form of fatty liver rather than hepatic cirrhosis.

### Pathology

In examinations of biopsy specimens from living patients and of autopsy tissue preparations, no distinctive features have been revealed in the patients with alcoholic heart disease as compared to those with congestive cardiomyopathy of other causes. Quite early in the prefailure stage there seems to be dilitation of the sarcoplasmic reticulum and the undifferentiated portion of the intercalated disk, but these changes are apparently obscured at later stages of disease, when considerable myocytolysis may be seen. An increase of fibrous tissue is a usual finding; it may take the form of an increase in the interstitial collagen component or replacement of myocardial fibers. Intramural vessels are usually normal, but in the areas of fibrous-tissue accumulation they may show wall thickening.

## ALCOHOL AND HYPERTENSION

Diagnosis of alcoholic cardiomyopathy is often obscurred when the patient presents with elevated arterial blood pressure. When seen with other causes of heart failure, this phenomenon is usually considered to be secondary to compensatory peripheral vasoconstriction during cardiac decompensation. Hypertensive episodes may be more frequent in the alcoholic, particularly if measurements are made shortly after a period of ethanol intake. During the late intoxication–early withdrawal period this response has been reported in up to one-half of noncardiac alcoholics observed in an outpatient setting, usually without the development of classic withdrawal illness. Other evidence of hypertension, such as retinopathy, usually is absent.

Arterial pressure may be moderately elevated for several days, with spontaneous decline to normal thereafter. Substantial elevations may require up to a week for spontaneous normalization. After a short period of abstinence arterial pressures are normalized in all but 10 percent of noncardiac alcoholics, which represents the incidence of hypertension in a control group.

## SELECTED VITAMIN AND MINERAL DEFICIENCIES

### Thiamine

Beriberi is a high-cardiac-output state associated with arteriolar vasodilatation. Although it has been the classic view that right ventricular failure is dominant when symptoms develop, several studies have documented a significant elevation of left ventricular end-diastolic and pulmonary capillary wedge pressure that is reversible with thiamine therapy.

### Vitamin C

Scurvy can be associated with sudden death. Human volunteers on a vitamin C–deficient diet have reported dyspnea and chest pain associated with PR prolongation and ST-segment abnormalities. These symptoms may be reversible with the administration of vitamin C.

### Vitamin E and Selenium

Selenium deficiency has been associated with a cardiomyopathy in children. The disease has a regional distribution in agricultural areas where the selenium content of the staple grains and soil is reduced. Supplementation of the diet with selenium has been found to be preventive. Although isolated selenium deficiency that produces cardiomyopathy has not been described in animal models, combined deprivation of selenium and vitamin E has been shown experimentally to produce patchy necrosis of the myocardium.

### Cachexia

Severe weight loss in individuals who have relatively normal initial body weight may have important cardiovascular consequences, particularly in infants and children, where primary congestive heart failure resulting from either marasmus or kwashiorkor may occur. In adults the nutritional deficiency that characterizes protein-calorie undernutrition is marked by a significant reduction of heart rate, stroke volume, and cardiac output associated with a diminished left ventricular end-diastolic diameter and mass. The ECG is generally unremarkable, but some patients exhibit ST-T wave changes. The QT interval is usually normal. Patients who recover from anorexia show improvement in heart rate, posterior wall dimension, systolic wall stress, and left ventricular internal dimension. A potential for arrhythmias and sudden death has been postulated.

### Hyperalimentation

Therapeutic feeding by the enteric or parenteral route has assumed increasing importance in the management of a variety of acute illnesses. Adults with chronic undernutrition without underlying heart disease may develop heart failure during hyperalimentation: a state resembling congestive heart failure may develop, characterized by hypermetabolism, ventricular gallop, augmented cardiac output, and normal ejection fraction. Rapid resolution follows diuretic therapy, slowing of the rate of hyperalimentation, and a reduction in the daily intake of sodium.

### SUGGESTED READING

Dyer AR, Stamler J, Paul O, et al: Alcohol consumption and 17-year mortality in the Chicago Western Electric Company Study. *Prev Med* 9:78–90, 1980.

Ettinger PO, Wu CF, DeLa Cruz C Jr, et al: Arrhythmias and the 'holiday heart'. *J Am Coll Cardiol* 1:816–818, 1983.

Klatsky AL, Freidman GD, Siegelaub AB: Alcohol use and cardiovascular disease: The Kaiser-Permanente experience. *Circulation* 64(suppl III):32, 1981.

Regan TJ: The heart, alcoholism, and nutritional disease, in Hurst, JW et al (eds): *The Heart,* 7th ed. New York, McGraw-Hill, Chap 81, pp 1533–1538, 1990.

Rosengren A, Wilhelmsen L, Wedel H: Separate and combined effects of smoking and alcohol abuse in middle-aged men. *Acta Med Scand* 223:111–118, 1988.

Urbano-Marquez A, Estruch R, Navarro-Lopez F, et al: The effects of alcoholism on skeletal and cardiac muscle. *N Engl J Med* 320:409–415, 1989.

Vikhert AM, Tsiplenkova VG, Cherpachenko NM: Alcoholic cardiomyopathy and sudden cardiac death. *J Am Coll Cardiol* 8:3A–11A, 1986.

## 32 | Obesity and the Cardiovascular System

*James K. Alexander, M.D.*

### HYPERTENSION

Although there is a well-established association of obesity and hypertension, blood pressure elevation does not correlate well with increase in relative weight, and most overweight subjects are normotensive. However, where obesity and hypertension coexist, the initial approach to therapy should include weight reduction and dietary sodium restriction, measures which reduce blood pressure in most cases.

### ATHEROSCLEROTIC CORONARY ARTERY DISEASE

While epidemiological data suggest that the markedly overweight individual is at increased risk for coronary events, a large body of anatomic and arteriographic evidence indicates no correlation of adiposity with coronary disease. The link, if any, between obesity and coronary disease has proved elusive. The association of obesity with hypertension appears to play some role. Except for morbid obesity and/or sleep apnea, adiposity is not a risk factor for sudden death. In diabetic women experiencing acute myocardial infarction, obesity predisposes to the development of congestive heart failure. A reduction in weight of more than 20 percent may be required for amelioration of symptoms in obese men with angina pectoris.

### SLEEP APNEA

More than half of individuals with sleep apnea are obese. Apneic episodes may be associated with hypoxemia and hypercapnia, as well as systemic and pulmonary hypertension. In persons with underlying coronary disease, arrhythmias are common, including sinus arrest, AV block, ventricular tachycardia, and asystole. Predisposition to daytime somnolence may be an important diagnostic clue. When this syndrome is identified by sleep study, tracheostomy and weight reduction are useful measures.

### CARDIOMYOPATHY

Virtually all morbidly obese people develop eccentric left ventricular hypertrophy, in some cases associated with a chronic circulatory congestive state. Clinical manifestations of pulmonary and systemic congestion are associated with increased blood volume and high cardiac output, elevated left ventricular filling pressure, pulmonary hypertension at rest or during exercise, and, in 50 to 60 percent of cases, modest-to-moderate systemic hypertension. Echocardiographic findings include increased left ventricular wall thickness and left ventricular mass, modest increase in left ventricular cavity dimension, and enlargement of the left atrium. In some cases left ventricular ejection fraction is depressed, but in others systolic function may be well preserved despite repeated bouts of severe circulatory congestion over a period of many years. Thus, left ventricular systolic function must be assessed by echocardiographic, angiographic, or radionuclide techniques, and cannot be predicted on bedside examination. Left ventricular diastolic dysfunction associated with hypertrophy and diminished chamber compliance is regularly present. It is thought that chronic volume overload, with or without systemic hypertension, results in eccentric left ventricular hypertrophy. In patients with preserved left ventricular systolic function, wall stress, as indicated by wall thickness–to–cavity radius ratio, remains normal, suggesting "adequate" hypertrophy. In those with depressed systolic function, wall thickness–to–cavity radius ratio is reduced, reflecting increased wall stress and "inadequate" hypertrophy. About 5 percent of extremely obese persons develop marked hypoventilation associated with a syndrome of somnolence, hypoxemia and cyanosis, respiratory acidosis, and polycythemia. Sleep apnea appears to initiate this syndrome in many, but not all, of these patients. In this setting, pulmonary vasoconstriction secondary to hypoxemia and acidosis results in an additional component of pulmonary hypertension and a transpulmonary diastolic pressure gradient superimposed upon underlying left ventricular hypertrophy and elevated filling pressure. Biventricular hypertrophy supervenes, and occasionally right-sided involvement may predominate.

Frequent electrocardiographic findings in very obese subjects are left axis deviation and low voltage in the standard leads. Despite marked anatomical involvement, electrocardiographic evidences of left ventricular hypertrophy are usually absent. In those subjects with hypoventilation, right axis deviation and P pulmonale may be seen. Recurrent bouts of congestion predispose to the development of atrial fibrillation or flutter. Also sudden death frequently occurs.

## THERAPEUTIC CONSIDERATIONS

- Diuretic therapy is well tolerated, and together with dietary sodium restriction is usually the most effective measure for symptomatic relief.

- Digitalis and vasodilator therapy have proved useful in some cases involving systolic left ventricular dysfunction. Digitalis dosage should *not* be based on body weight—this might lead to toxicity.
- Antihypertensive therapy is indicated when blood pressure is high. Angiotensin-converting enzyme inhibitors, calcium channel blockers, or other agents known to result in regression of myocardial hypertrophy are probably preferable.
- Low-dose subcutaneous heparin should be considered for patients who present in an acute congestive state, as prophylaxis against venous thrombosis and pulmonary embolism.
- With relief of acute symptoms, a program to achieve weight reduction is indicated. Hemodynamic alterations and left ventricular hypertrophy are reversible with weight reduction.

## SUGGESTED READING

Alexander JK: The heart and obesity, in Hurst JW et al (eds): *The Heart*, 7th ed. New York, McGraw-Hill, Chap 81, pp 1533–1537, 1990.

Barrett-Connor EL: Obesity, atherosclerosis, and coronary artery disease. *Ann Intern Med* 103:1010–1019, 1985.

Bray GA: Complications of obesity. *Ann Intern Med* 103:1052–1062, 1985.

Bray GA: Obesity and the heart. *Mod Concepts Cardiovasc Dis* 56:67–71, 1987.

## The Interrelationship of Heart Disease and Kidney Disease

*Vera Delaney, M.D., Ph.D.*
*Edmund Bourke, M.D.*

### RENAL CONSEQUENCES OF HEART FAILURE

The kidney plays a central role in the pathogenesis and management of congestive heart failure. Its major response to failure of the heart is progressive retention of salt and water. The afferent and efferent mechanisms through which this is mediated are not completely understood. Diuretics are the cornerstone of management. The benefits of other counterregulatory drugs acting on the kidney are not yet established.

In early heart failure, the accompanying decreased renal blood flow is associated with a greater constriction of the efferent than of the afferent arteriole, with a rise in the filtration fraction and preservation of glomerular filtration rate (GFR). In advanced cases, constriction of the afferent arteriole results in a fall in GFR and, ultimately, in prerenal azotemia. There is a greater rise in blood urea nitrogen (BUN) than in serum creatinine, exceeding the 10:1 ratio generally seen. A serum creatinine level above 3 mg/dl, when attributable to cardiac failure alone, is a poor prognostic sign. Iatrogenic causes must, however, be excluded, in particular the misuse of diuretics. Attempts to improve cardiac function, including afterload reduction, are indicated.

Prerenal azotemia is invariable in cardiogenic shock. Here, recovery of renal function is determined by the underlying cardiac lesion. Acute tubular necrosis in this setting is a grave sign, usually heralding cardiac death.

### CARDIAC CONSEQUENCES OF RENAL FAILURE

Altered cardiovascular physiology in renal failure is attributable to:

- *Factors primarily affecting preload or afterload.* These include renal anemia, shunting from vascular access, nephrogenic pericardial disease, salt and water overload, and hypertension.
- *Factors primarily affecting myocardial contractility.* These are most often attributable to the electrolyte abnormalities seen in renal failure, including hyperkalemia and severe metabolic acidosis. No specific "uremic cardiomyopathy" has yet been established.

A primary cardiac disease—especially coronary artery disease—may coexist with renal insufficiency. There is also an increased incidence of aortic sclerosis and of infective endocarditis in dialysis patients.

The use of cardiac drugs requires cognizance of their half-life and dialyzability. Digitalis toxicity is the most common culprit. Its potential interaction with alterations in plasma electrolytes requires attention.

## NEPHROGENIC PERICARDIAL DISEASE

Uremic pericarditis is less common than it used to be, except where patients, by virtue of poor compliance or other socioeconomic factors, present at the later stages of renal failure. It is an ominous sign, a harbinger of hemorrhagic tamponade. It constitutes an indication for emergency dialysis and generally responds to it.

About 15 percent of apparently adequately dialyzed patients develop "dialysis pericarditis," implying a separate entity. It often precipitates atrial flutter or fibrillation. It is a source of morbidity and mortality. About 50 percent of patients respond to short-term intensification of dialysis, the initial treatment of choice. Administration of low-dose heparin during dialysis is prudent. The role of nonsteroidal anti-inflammatory agents and oral or intrapericardial steroids is not yet established. Except in cases of mortal danger, pericardiocentesis should be performed only in the cardiac catheterization laboratory, following echocardiographic confirmation. There is no general agreement on the relative indications for pericardiectomy or a pleuropericardial window.

## INFECTIVE ENDOCARDITIS AND ENDOVASCULITIS

Manifestations of renal involvement, including advanced renal failure, may be the presenting features of endocarditis in patients with previously normal renal function.

The dialysis population is at increased risk of endocarditis. The vascular access is the portal of entry. The aortic valve is the valve most frequently involved. *Staphylococcus aureus* and *S. epidermidis* are the most common infecting organisms.

Endovasculitis of the access site is accompanied by signs of inflammation; failure of resolution on administration of appropriate antibiotics requires surgical removal of the access graft.

## ATHEROSCLEROSIS AND CORONARY ARTERY DISEASE IN CHRONIC RENAL FAILURE

When allowance is made for such major atherogenic risk factors as hypertension and diabetes, there is no conclusive evidence for accelerated atherosclerosis in chronic renal failure *per se*, either before or after the institution of maintenance dialysis. The very high incidence of cardiovascular death (52 percent) in dialyzed patients is attributable to coexisting morbid conditions. Surprising is the recently reported low incidence of deaths due to myocardial infarction (12.5 percent). Most of these cardiovascular deaths are "sudden cardiac deaths of unknown cause."

The hyperlipidemia generally seen does not correlate significantly with the degree of atherosclerosis in this population; therapeutic intervention is not warranted.

## ATHEROEMBOLIC DISEASE OF THE KIDNEYS

Embolization of cholesterol crystals, from eroded atherosclerotic plaques, frequently affects the microvessels of the kidney. Predominantly a disease of older males, it may follow surgery on atherosclerotic aortas, or angiography, or may occur *de novo*. Progressive renal failure frequently ensues. Clues include episodic hypertension, livedo reticularis, focal ischemia of toes, elevated sedimentation rate, eosinophilia, and eosinophiluria. There is no effective therapy. Anticoagulants are contraindicated, since they prevent fibrin formation on eroded plaques.

In contrast to these microemboli, thromboembolic disease of the major renal vessels is most often due to cardiac valvular vegetations or mural thrombi. Flank pain and/or hematuria are classic presenting features. Timely consideration is required for possible renal angiography, anticoagulants, streptokinase, or possible early surgical intervention.

## DISEASES THAT AFFECT THE HEART AND THE KIDNEY

While enumeration of these diseases is outside the scope of this summary, they should be considered before renal malfunction is definitively attributed to a primary cardiac lesion (or vice versa).

### Cardiac Surgery in Renal-Failure Patients

Cardiac surgery in patients with chronic renal failure, including those on maintenance dialysis, is frequently an acceptable risk when adequate nephrologic backup is available.

In patients being considered for renal transplantation, if coronary artery bypass or valve replacement is warranted, it is generally carried out prior to the renal transplantation.

### Hemofiltration and Peritoneal Dialysis in the Management of Refractory Congestive Heart Failure

Short-term subjective and objective improvements have been reported in some cases of intractable congestive failure.

## Cardiac Transplant Recipients and Renal Function

The absence of intrinsic renal disease and a creatinine clearance above 50 ml/min are renal requirements for cardiac transplantation.

Cyclosporine-A nephrotoxicity is an important, albeit not insurmountable, complication of cardiac transplantation.

## CARDIAC DRUGS IN PATIENTS WITH RENAL FAILURE

Possible modifications of dosage or intervals of administration require consultation of appropriate reference sources.

Drugs requiring decreased dosage in renal failure include digoxin, procainamide, disopyramide, and nitroprusside. Those not requiring decreased dosage include diuretics, digitoxin, lidocaine, most beta blockers, antihypertensives, calcium channel blockers, and phenytoin. Quinidine increases plasma digoxin levels.

Removal by dialysis is insufficient to require dose adjustments for digoxin, digitoxin, phenytoin, propranolol, and verapamil. Substantial dialysis of procainamide, N-acetylprocainamide, methyldopa, and nitroprusside does occur.

## SUGGESTED READING

Berlyne GM, Giovaretti S (eds): Contributions to nephrology, the heart in end state renal failure, vol 52. Basel, Karger, 1986.

Brenner BM, Stein JH (eds): Contemporary issues in nephrology, in O'Rourke RA (guest ed): *The Heart and Renal Disease.* New York, Churchill Livingstone, 1984.

Delaney V, Bourke E: The interrelationship of heart disease and kidney disease, in Hurst JW et al (eds): *The Heart,* 7th ed. New York, McGraw-Hill, Chap 83, pp 1543–1556, 1990.

Seyffart G: Drugs in renal failure: Dosing guidlines for frequently used drugs in end stage renal disease and dialysis patients. *Blood Purif* 3:140–154, 1985.

## 34 | Electrolytes and the Heart

*David P. Rardon, M.D.    Charles Fisch, M.D.*

## INTRODUCTION

Potassium ($K^+$), sodium ($Na^+$), and calcium ($Ca^{2+}$) are the major ions responsible for normal electrical activity of the heart. $Ca^{2+}$ is also the messenger that initiates excitation-contraction coupling, and, along with magnesium ($Mg^{2+}$) and phosphorus (P), is involved in myocardial contraction. These ions are responsible for the resting and action potentials of cardiac cells and for diastolic depolarization of pacemaker cells. Abnormally high or low concentrations of $K^+$, $Ca^{2+}$, and $Mg^{2+}$ may alter the surface electrocardiogram or result in cardiac arrhythmias.

## POTASSIUM

The normal range of $K^+$ is 3.5 to 5.0 meq/liter. Common causes for deviation above and below this range are listed below.

### Causes of Hyperkalemia

- Increased intake
  - Salt substitutes
  - Potassium penicillin
- Increased input
  - Rhabdomyolysis
  - Hemolysis
- Decreased excretion
  - Acute renal failure
  - Chronic renal failure
  - Addison's disease
  - Hyporeninemic hypoaldosteronism
- Other
  - Acidosis
  - Pseudohyperkalemia

### Causes of Hypokalemia

- Poor dietary intake
- Gastrointestinal loss
  - Vomiting
  - Diarrhea

- Urinary loss
  - Diuretic therapy
- Renal tubular acidosis
- Chronic interstitial nephritis
- Excessive mineralocorticoid effect
  - Hyperaldosteronism
  - Excessive glucocorticoid hormones (Cushing's syndrome)

## Potassium and the Electrocardiogram

The electrocardiographic manifestations of high and low $K^+$ and the corresponding $K^+$ concentrations required to produce these effects are listed below and illustrated in Fig. 34-1.

*Hyperkalemia*

|  | $K^+$, *meq/liter* |
|---|---|
| Peaked or tented T waves | 5.5–6.5 |
| Low-amplitude P waves | 7.0–8.0 |
| QRS widening | 9.0–11.0 |

*Hypokalemia*

| Increased U-wave amplitude | <3.0 |
|---|---|
| Decreased T-wave amplitude | <2.7–3.0 |

## Hyperkalemia and Arrhythmias

The effect of hyperkalemia on cardiac rhythm is complex; virtually any arrhythmia, including sinus bradycardia or arrest, AV block, idioventricular rhythm, or asystole, may be seen. At $K^+$ levels >12 meq/liter, ventricular fibrillation is common.

## Treatment of Hyperkalemia

The treatment of hyperkalemia depends not only on the level of $K^+$, but upon the neuromuscular and electrocardiographic effects of this elevation. Treatment may include one or more of the following:

*Elimination of Cause*

Stopping $K^+$-sparing diuretic, treatment of acidosis, etc.; when level of $K^+$ is <6.5 meq/liter and accompanied only by tented T waves.

*Calcium Gluconate*

10 to 30 ml of 10% solution IV over 1–5 min; used only for $K^+$ levels >6.5 meq/liter with ECG or neuromuscular changes.

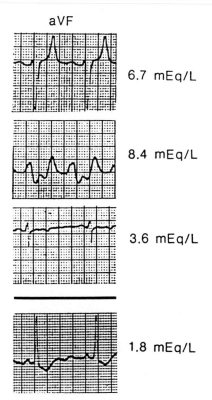

aVF

6.7 mEq/L

8.4 mEq/L

3.6 mEq/L

1.8 mEq/L

FIG. 34-1 Electrocardiographic manifestations of altered K$^+$. The top three panels are lead aV$_F$ recorded in the same patient at different K$^+$ levels. K$^+$ 6.7 meq/liter, "tented" T waves; K$^+$ 8.4 meq/liter, widened QRS; K$^+$ 3.6 meq/liter, nonspecific T-wave changes. The lower panel is lead aV$_F$ from a patient with K$^+$ of 1.8 meq/liter. The T waves are flattened and the U waves increased in amplitude.

*NaHCO₃*

50 meq IV over 5 min.

*D50W*

50-ml ampule, plus 10 units regular insulin IV over 5 min.

*Sodium Polystyrene Sulfonate (Kayexalate)*

20 to 50 g in 100 to 200 ml sorbitol PO, which can be repeated every 3–4 h up to 5 doses per day.

## Hypokalemia and Arrhythmias

Hypokalemia <3.5 meq/liter promotes the appearance of both supraventricular and ventricular ectopic rhythms.

## Treatment of Hypokalemia

*Oral*

KCl elixer or capsules; 10 to 30 meq every 1–2 h.

*IV*

Do not exceed 20 meq/h, and do not use a concentration greater than 50 meq/liter.

*Ca and Mg*

These may need to be replaced concurrently in patients with these deficits.

## Hypokalemia and Digitalis

Characteristic arrhythmias in digitalis-intoxicated patients include nonparoxysmal junctional tachycardias, atrial tachycardia with block, and increased ventricular ectopy. Hypokalemia exacerbates arrhythmias secondary to digitalis intoxication. When $K^+$ is low, the administration of K is safe and effective in suppressing these arrhythmias.

## CALCIUM

The normal range of $Ca^{2+}$ is 8.5 to 10.5 mg/dl. Common causes of high and low $Ca^{2+}$ are listed below. The electrocardiographic effects of altered serum $Ca^{2+}$ are illustrated in Fig. 34-2.

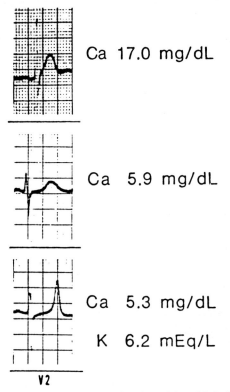

V2

FIG. 34-2  Electrocardiographic manifestations of altered $Ca^{2+}$. The top panel ($Ca^{2+}$ 17 mg/dl) shows a QT interval shortened primarily by reduction of the ST-segment duration. The middle panel ($Ca^{2+}$ 5.9 mg/dl) shows a QT interval lengthened primarily by prolongation of the ST segment. The bottom panel ($Ca^{2+}$ 5.3 mg/dl; $K^+$ 6.2 meq/liter) shows a prolonged QT interval with "tented" T waves. This pattern is commonly seen with chronic renal failure.

### Causes of Hypercalcemia

- Hyperparathyroidism
- Malignancy
- Thiazides
- Hypervitaminosis D
- Sarcoidosis
- Multiple endocrine adenomatosis

### Causes of Hypocalcemia

- Hypoparathyroidism
- Chronic renal failure
- Pancreatitis
- Malabsorption
- Malnutrition
- Hyperphosphatemia
- Hypomagnesemia

### Calcium and the Electrocardiogram

Hypercalcemia shortens the QT interval, primarily by reducing the duration of the ST interval. Hypocalcemia prolongs the QT interval secondary to an increase in the duration of the ST segment. Clinically, abnormalities of serum $Ca^{2+}$ rarely produce arrhythmias.

### Treatment of Hypercalcemia

*Normal Saline Solution*

4 to 5 liters/day IV plus furosemide 80 to 120 mg every 4–6 h IV.

*Mithramycin*

25 to 50 μg/kg IV may lower $Ca^{2+}$ to normal within several days.

### Treatment of Hypocalcemia

*IV*

10 ml 10% Ca gluconate (90 mg Ca) or 10 ml 10% Ca chloride (360 mg Ca) over 5 min.

*Oral*

- Ca carbonate 500 mg four times a day.
- Vitamin D: ergocalciferol 1.25 to 3.75 mg/day or dihydrotachysterol 0.25 to 1.0 mg/day.

- Phosphate binders 30 ml three times a day if hyperphosphatemia is present.
- Associated hypomagnesemia may also need to be corrected.

## MAGNESIUM

The normal range of $Mg^{2+}$ is 1.4 to 2.0 meq/liter. Common causes of high and low magnesium are listed below.

### Causes of Hypermagnesemia

- Acute renal failure
- Adrenocortical insufficiency

### Causes of Hypomagnesemia

- Diabetic ketoacidosis
- Chronic alcoholism
- Furosemide
- Malabsorption syndromes
- Acute tubular necrosis
- Primary aldosteronism
- Acute pancreatitis

### Magnesium and the Electrocardiogram

$Mg^{2+}$ is an important metalloenzyme for many enzyme reactions, including Na-K ATPase. Intracellular $Mg^{2+}$ deficiency may be associated with increases in intracellular $Na^+$ and $Ca^{2+}$ and a loss of $K^+$. The interdependence of $Mg^{2+}$, $Ca^{2+}$, $Na^+$, and $K^+$ makes the ECG recognition of $Mg^{2+}$ alterations difficult. In early $Mg^{2+}$ deficiency the QRS complex narrows and the T wave may be peaked. With more severe deficiency the ECG resembles that in hypokalemia, with a wider QRS complex, ST-segment depression and low-amplitude T waves.

### Magnesium and Arrhythmias

Hypomagnesemia may potentiate digitalis-induced arrhythmias. Hypermagnesemia may produce SA and AV block at the level of 15 meq/liter, and cardiac arrest at levels of 15 to 22 meq/liter. Neuromuscular and respiratory paralysis usually precede cardiac arrest.

Even in patients with normal serum $Mg^{2+}$, Mg has been reported to be useful in either automatic or reentrant arrhythmias secondary to low $K^+$, including atrial flutter, atrial fibrillation, or ventricular ectopic beats. Mg may be useful as an initial treatment of patients with a prolonged QT interval and torsade de pointes.

### Treatment of Hypomagnesemia

*IV (50% MgSO₄, 8.13 meq Mg/gm)*

- Emergency treatment of torsade de pointes
  - 16.2 meq IV over 5–10 min.
- Replacement therapy
  - Initially 12 ml (49 meq Mg) in 1000 ml D5W over 3h, followed by 10 ml (40 meq Mg) in each of two 1-liter solutions to be administered throughout the day, followed by 12 ml (49 meq Mg) distributed in total daily IV fluids over the next 24 h.

### SUGGESTED READING

Lauber DP: A symposium: Magnesium deficiency—pathogenesis, prevalence, and strategies for repletion. *Am J Cardiol* 63:1G–46G, 1989.

Rardon DP, Fisch C: Electrolytes and the Heart, in Hurst JW et al (eds): *The Heart,* 7th ed. New York, McGraw-Hill, Chap 84, pp 1557–1570, 1990.

Seelig MS: Electrocardiographic patterns of magnesium depletion in alcoholic heart disease. *Ann NY Acad Sci* 162:906–917, 1969.

## 35 | Evaluation and Management of Patients with Heart Disease who Undergo Noncardiac Surgery

*Peter C. Gazes, M.D.*

Hunter and his associates have reported that, preoperatively, 38 percent of 141 randomly selected surgical patients aged 35 years or older had historic or physical evidence of heart disease, hypertension, or diabetes mellitus. Forty-nine percent had abnormal preoperative electrocardiograms. Patients with cardiac disease may have limited ability to respond to the hemodynamic and metabolic stresses of surgery and anesthetic agents.

## PREOPERATIVE EVALUATION

### History

The history should include the symptoms of heart disease and a meticulous review of all current medications. An increasing number of drugs have been found to alter cardiac hemodynamics during and after surgery.

### Cardiovascular Drugs

Many cardiovascular medications can interact with anesthetics, because both groups of agents can alter the peripheral and central sympathetic and parasympathetic tone, depolarize the membranes of the heart, and alter contractility and peripheral vascular resistance directly or indirectly.

Digitalis may be continued parenterally during or after surgery. Antiarrhythmic drugs should be continued up to the time of surgery or discontinued earlier, during electrocardiographic monitoring, if they are being taken for no clear reason. Most supraventricular arrhythmias and ventricular arrhythmias should be treated for several days prior to elective surgery. If they exist just prior to emergency surgery, the supraventricular types can be controlled by digitalis, propranolol, verapamil, or a combination of these; the ventricular type can be controlled by lidocaine.

Nitrates, beta blockers, calcium channel blockers, and afterload-reducing agents such as hydralazine and ACE inhibitors should be continued to the day of surgery.

### Antihypertensive Agents

Most physicians agree that patients with hypertension who are maintained on antihypertensive drugs with good control of blood pressure have less pressure fluctuation during anesthesia than those who are untreated. In fact, abrupt cessation of some drugs, such as beta blockers and clonidine, may initiate rebound hypertension, tachyarrhythmia, worsening of angina, and even myocardial infarction in patients with coronary disease; this may occur either during or after surgery.

Diuretic agents may deplete body potassium, sodium, chloride, and total body water, and may decrease peripheral vascular resistance. Metabolic alkalosis predisposes the patient to cardiopulmonary arrest. Thus, before the operation, the blood volume should be restored and any electrolyte imbalance corrected.

### Antiplatelet Drugs

The average life span of blood platelets is about 9 days. For at least 5 days prior to elective surgery the patient should avoid all medications that adversely affect platelet function and so might enhance bleeding (e.g., aspirin and other nonsteroidal anti-inflammatory agents).

### Anticoagulants

Oral anticoagulants should be omitted from the regimen prior to surgery. These drugs pose a problem primarily in patients who have prosthetic valves—especially mitral—or conditions that place them at high risk for thromboembolism (e.g., prior history of emboli). Generally, in such patients, warfarin should be discontinued at least 3 days before surgery (prothrombin time should be restored to within 20 percent of normal), and constant intravenous heparin should be begun (maintaining partial thromboplastin times at about twice control values). The effect of heparin should be reversed just before surgery by intravenous administration of protamine sulfate. After surgery, when there is no evidence of bleeding, heparin and warfarin should be restarted; only oral warfarin should be continued once the prothrombin time has become therapeutic. However, in one study of 159 patients with prosthetic valves undergoing noncardiac surgical procedures, no thromboembolic complications were noted when the anticoagulant was discontinued an average of 2.9 days preoperatively (allowing prothrombin time to return to within 20 percent of the normal range) and restarted 2.7 days postoperatively.

## Corticosteroids

Adrenal insufficiency may follow withdrawal of corticosteroid therapy, because of inhibition of adrenal corticotropin releasing factor, or adrenal atrophy, or both. Patients who are receiving, or at any time during the past year have received, high-dose and long-term corticosteroid therapy require therapy to be supplemented or reinstituted.

## Hypoglycemic Agents

The management of the insulin-dependent diabetic patient prior to elective surgery depends on the patient's insulin program and the fluid and electrolyte requirements of the surgical procedure. In addition, major surgery can render the patient glucose-intolerant and insulin-resistant. Therefore, no arbitrary insulin program to control blood glucose during surgery should be used; it would not achieve the intended goals. Each case should be individualized to maintain the blood glucose in a range of 80 to 120 mg/dl.

## Physical Examination and Other Studies

The consultant should begin by taking a history and performing a complete physical examination. Recommended studies include urinalysis, routine blood determinations (complete blood count, hematocrit, blood urea nitrogen, blood sugar, and electrolytes), a chest x-ray, and an electrocardiogram. The results of these tests may prompt further studies to determine the possible presence of other abnormalities. It seems appropriate to obtain a preoperative ECG for any patient aged 40 years or more, and a stress test (thallium for women and for any patient whose resting ECG is abnormal) in any patient whose history suggests ischemic heart disease. Abnormalities such as nonspecific ST-T wave changes, bundle branch block, and arrhythmias may be found in patients with no other evidence of heart disease. This information is very valuable in following patients—especially the knowledge that these changes have not developed during or after surgery. Echocardiography and Doppler and radionuclide studies may be indicated; in some instances, pulmonary function studies and cardiac catheterization may be necessary. The consultant should determine if the patient is a poor risk and needs Swan-Ganz catheter monitoring.

Some other factors to be considered by the consultant before advising noncardiac surgery in a cardiac patient are the type and severity of the patient's heart disease; the length, magnitude, and stresses of the operation; the patient's age; the anesthesia to be administered; and the patient's prior experiences with anesthetic agents and reactions to drugs. A herniorrhaphy or transurethral resection poses much less surgical risk than intrathoracic surgery, gastric resection, cholecystectomy, or other intraperitoneal surgery.

After the preoperative evaluation, the consultant should be able to give some indication of the patient's surgical risk. For many years the New York Heart Association functional classification was used. It is still popular today, especially since it has been revised into "Cardiac Status and Prognosis".

Goldman and his associates have proposed a multifactorial index of cardiac risks (Table 35-1). Based on total points, patients are separated into four classes of risk. Patients in Class 1 (0 to 5 points) and Class 2 (6 to 12 points) have significantly fewer

TABLE 35-1  Computation of the Cardiac Risk Index

| Criteria | Points |
|---|---|
| History | |
| age >70 years | 5 |
| MI in previous 6 months | 10 |
| Physical examination | |
| S₃ gallop or JVD | 11 |
| Important valvular aortic stenosis | 3 |
| Electrocardiogram | |
| Rhythm other than sinus, or PACs on last preoperative ECG | 7 |
| >5 PVCs/min at any time before operation | 7 |
| General status | |
| P_O2 <60 or P_CO2 >50 mmHg, K <3.0 or HCO₃ <20 meq/liter, BUN >50 or Cr >3.0 mg/dl, abnormal SGOT, signs of chronic liver disease, or patient bedridden from noncardiac causes | 3 |
| Operation | |
| Intraperitoneal, intrathoracic, or aortic operation | 3 |
| Emergency operation | 4 |
| Total possible | 53 |

MI = Myocardial infarction; JVD = Jugular-vein distension; PACs = premature atrial contractions; PVCs = premature ventricular contractions; $P_{O2}$ = partial pressure of oxygen; $P_{CO2}$ = partial pressure of carbon dioxide; K = Potassium; HCO₃ = Bicarbonate; BUN = Blood urea nitrogen; Cr = creatinine; SGOT = serum glutamic oxalacetic transaminase.

Source: Reprinted by permission of Goldman L et al and the New England Journal of Medicine. (From the New England Journal of Medicine 297:845, 1977.

complications than do those in Class 3 (13 to 25 points) and Class 4 (26 points or more). The progression from Class 1 to Class 4 shows an increase in the proportion of patients with life-threatening, but nonfatal, complications. Class 4 patients also account for over half of cardiac deaths. Since 28 of the 53 points represent potentially controllable or reversible situations, surgery should be delayed, if possible, in order to lower the risk with therapy. This multifactorial index is useful, but some subgroups need additional testing (e.g., ECG or radionuclide stress testing or cardiac catheterization).

The life expectancy of the patient should be considered before elective surgery, because to operate on a patient who cannot live to enjoy the benefits is foolish. Elective surgery should be postponed until the patient is stable and has no such problems as fever, heart failure, electrolytic imbalance, anemia, unstable angina, recent infarction, or other organ system conditions.

## PREOPERATIVE AND OPERATIVE MANAGEMENT OF SPECIFIC PROBLEMS

### Coronary Artery Disease

Coronary artery disease is the most common type of heart disease and accounts for most of the operative mortality. In noncardiac surgery, patients with chronic stable angina (NYHA Class II) usually tolerate anesthesia and surgery with appropriate monitoring for ischemia. Often, however, it is best to delineate the coronary anatomy by coronary arteriography—especially prior to major noncardiac surgery procedures. Patients with unstable angina tolerate surgery poorly, and should be considered for myocardial revascularization (bypass surgery or angioplasty) prior to elective surgery.

The results of noncardiac surgery after acute myocardial infarction depend on the myocardial reserve and the time that has passed since the infarction occurred. Since 1962, several studies have shown that the sooner noncardiac surgery is performed after infarction the greater are the morbidity and mortality. In a recent study the incidence of reinfarction within 3 months after infarction was 5.7 percent; between 4 and 6 months, 2.3 percent. In the past, the incidence of reinfarction was much greater; invasive hemodynamic monitoring and new cardiac drugs probably account for the decrease. Elective surgery should be postponed, therefore, until at least 6 months after an infarction—unless a life-threatening emergency develops, in which case invasive hemodynamic monitoring should be done.

Nitroglycerin, in ointment or patches, can be applied before surgery to an area away from the surgical site where it will not be wiped off or removed. Intravenous nitroglycerin should be available in the operating room.

Sudden withdrawal of beta blockers has been known to produce a rebound syndrome with symptoms of exacerbated hypertension, increase in frequency and severity of angina, acute myocardial infarction, and arrhythmias. Thus propranolol (or any other beta blocker) should be kept in the regimen up to the morning of surgery and resumed postoperatively.

Verapamil should be used with special caution in the presence of left ventricular dysfunction, because most anesthetic agents also reduce myocardial contractility.

Several studies suggest that coronary bypass grafting can alter the mortality and morbidity of patients having noncardiac surgery. The Coronary Artery Surgery Study (CASS), in particular, documented that coronary artery bypass grafting in patients with severe coronary artery disease reduced mortality in noncardiac surgery.

### Hypertension

Controlled hypertension usually does not increase the risks of general anesthesia or major surgery. Patients maintained on antihypertensive agents up to the time of surgery, with good control of blood pressure, suffer the fewest episodes of hypotension and hypertension during anesthesia.

### Valvular Heart Disease

The lesions and their hemodynamic significance, as well as endocarditis prophylaxis, anticoagulants, and arrhythmias, should be evaluated. Patients with valvular heart disease whose cardiac status is NYHA Class I or II usually tolerate surgery as well as patients without cardiac disease. Patients whose cardiac status is Class III or IV, especially those with critical aortic or mitral stenosis, often suffer surgical complications. They have the worst prognosis. Patients with significant symptomatic valvular disease should have corrective surgery before undergoing elective noncardiac operations. In some cases it may be feasible to have aortic or mitral balloon valvuloplasty for stenotic lesions.

Patients with valvular disease (including calcified mitral anulus) or prosthetic valves (a very high-risk group for endocarditis) who are undergoing dental or surgical procedures should receive prophylactic antibiotic therapy in order to prevent bacterial endocarditis (see Table 35-2). Those with midsystolic clicks (which indicate mitral prolapse) or ejection sounds (which may indicate aortic or pulmonic valvular stenosis), with or without an associated murmur, also should receive prophylaxis. However, some physicians give antibiotic prophylaxis only if these extra sounds are associated

TABLE 35-2 Prophylaxis Against Bacterial Endocarditis (Adults)

| Procedure | Medications | |
| --- | --- | --- |
| | Before procedure | After procedure |
| Dental and upper respiratory tract | 2.0 g penicillin V orally 1 h prior to procedure | 1.0 g 6 h later |
| | *or* | |
| | 2 million units aqueous penicillin G, IV or IM, 30–60 min prior to procedure | 1 million units 6 h later |
| | *Allergic to penicillin* | |
| | Erythromycin 1.0 g orally 1 h prior to procedure | 500 mg 6 h after initial dose |
| | *Prosthetic valves and other higher risks* | |
| | Ampicillin 1.0–2.0 g plus gentamicin 1.5 mg/kg IM or IV, both given 30 min before procedure | Penicillin V 1.0 g orally 6 h later |
| | Vancomycin 1 g IV over 60 min, begun 60 min before procedure | No repeat dose necessary |
| Gastrointestinal and genitourinary tract surgery and instrumentation | *Most patients* | |
| | Ampicillin 2.0 g IM or IV, plus gentamicin 1.5 mg/kg IM or IV, both 30 min before procedure | One follow-up dose 8 h later |
| | *Allergic to penicillin* | |
| | Vancomycin 1.0 g IV given over 60 min, plus 1.5 mg/kg gentamicin IM or IV, both 1 h before procedure | Dose repeated once 8–12 h later |
| | *Minor or repetitive procedures in low-risk patients* | |
| | Amoxicillin 3.0 g orally 1 h before procedure | 1.5 g 6 h after initial dose |

*Source:* Adapted from Shulman ST et al: Prevention of bacterial endocarditis. American Heart Association Committee Report, *Circulation* 70:1123A, 1984.

with murmurs or the valves appear thickened on echocardiography, which may ignore the fact that a murmur may be intermittent. See also Chapter 15 and Table 15-6.

## Congenital Heart Disease

Patients with noncyanotic congenital heart lesions who do not have evidence of heart failure generally tolerate surgery with very few complications. However, cyanotic patients pose greater risks, especially regarding problems of postoperative hemorrhage, hypotension, and vascular thrombosis.

Patients with congenital heart disease should receive antibiotic prophylaxis in the same manner as for valvular heart disease.

## Pulmonary Heart Disease

In addition to having routine preoperative studies, cardiac patients with lung disease should be evaluated by pulmonary function studies and arterial blood gas measurements.

Problems with anesthetics and intra- and postoperative complications (such as hypoxia, hypercapnia, atelectasis, and infection) occur more often in cardiac patients with lung disease as compared to those without lung disease. These patients should be prepared preoperatively by the use of bronchodilators, expectorants, and aerosols, with intermittent positive pressure; and by cessation of smoking. Use of opiates should be avoided, and antibiotics should be given empirically.

### Tachyarrhythmias

Premature atrial or junctional beats occurring rarely do not require therapy. If they are frequent, preoperative digitalization should be considered.

When premature ventricular beats are of the complex type (more than five per minute, multifocal, in runs or pairs, or R-on-T phenomenon), lidocaine should be begun preoperatively in patients with cardiac disease—especially in those with ischemic heart disease. This regimen should be continued during the operation. Patients with supraventricular tachyarrhythmias should be digitalized and, in some cases, cardioverted. Beta blockers or verapamil have also been used.

### Bradyarrhythmias

Patients with SA pause or block, second- or third-degree AV block, or clear histories of Stokes-Adams attacks should have temporary pacers and, in some cases, permanent pacemakers. However, the need for temporary pacing in patients with bifascicular block (left or right bundle branch block with left anterior or posterior fascicular block) has been controversial. Most physicians now agree that patients with such asymptomatic bifascicular blocks do not require prophylactic pacemaker insertion before surgery. However, a noninvasive pacemaker or a pacing catheter should be available in the operating room.

## Congestive Heart Failure

Patients with evidence of systolic dysfunction and congestive heart failure should receive digitalis, diuretics, and vasodilator therapy, as indicated, both preoperatively and postoperatively. Nonemergency surgical procedures should be delayed until compensation is restored.

Patients with heart failure and normal ejection fraction often have primarily left ventricular diastolic dysfunction. Only disease states such as hypertrophic and restrictive cardiomyopathy used to be placed in this category. However, diastolic dysfunction may occur with such common conditions as hypertension or ischemic heart disease with a normal ejection fraction. The standard treatment for congestive heart failure often may be harmful in such conditions. Some patients respond best to calcium antagonists and beta blockers.

There is controversy about routine preoperative digitalization in the absence of signs of overt systolic dysfunction and heart failure, or atrial fibrillation or flutter. Many physicians prefer not to give prophylactic digitalization. In some cases, however, findings of myocardial dysfunction may be present without such congestive-failure phenomena as rales, edema, or hepatomegaly. Such patients may have moderate or severe cardiomegaly, abnormal height of the deep jugular venous pulsations, an $S_3$ gallop, pulsus alternans, or x-ray evidence of interstitial edema. The author prefers to digitalize such patients preoperatively, and those who are undergoing lobectomy or pneumonectomy (in whom there is a 15-percent incidence of supraventricular arrhythmias).

## GENERAL OPERATIVE MANAGEMENT

During major surgery, patients with significant heart disease should have intraarterial pressure monitoring, continuous electrocardiographic monitoring, and, in poor-risk cases, pressure and cardiac output monitoring with a Swan-Ganz catheter. With less severe cardiac disease, patients may require only electrocardiographic monitoring, blood pressure measurement by cuff, and application of a chest stethoscope.

Cardiac arrest associated with anesthesia is not very common today, because anesthesiologists do not allow hypoxia or hypercapnia to develop. Cardiac arrest during surgery should be managed similarly to arrest occurring from other causes.

When cardiac arrhythmias appear during surgery, the anesthesiologist must determine whether they are produced by the anesthesia, poor oxygenation, carbon dioxide retention, hypotension, or reflex cardiac stimulation due to surgical maneuvers. If these causes can be eliminated and the arrhythmias persist, specific antiarrhythmic therapy should be instituted.

The concurrent replacement of fluid or blood loss is essential during an operation, especially a long, difficult procedure.

Fluid overload, anesthetic-induced myocardial depression, myocardial ischemia, and hypertension are some factors that may precipitate pulmonary edema. Pulmonary edema may be treated by elevation of the chest, administration of intravenous morphine, positive-pressure oxygen delivery, and furosemide given intravenously. Preload reducing agents, such as nitroglycerin and nitroprusside, are also often very effective. When the patient has not been digitalized, digitalis should also be given intravenously. However, digitalis and arterial vasodilators should not be used if there is predominantly diastolic dysfunction.

The inhibition of demand pacemakers by their inappropriate sensing of extrinsic electric sources has been recognized for several years. Electromagnetic forces of the electrocautery may be sensed and so cause temporary suppression of the pacemaker, despite electrical shielding and the introduction of filters. During surgery, the electrosurgical tip and the ground plate should be as far from the pacemaker as possible, and electrosurgery should be limited to intermittent 2- to 3-s periods if any pacemaker suppression is produced.

## POSTOPERATIVE COMPLICATIONS AND MANAGEMENT

The stress of surgery can result in increases in antidiuretic hormone, ACTH, cortisol, and catecholamines, and changes in the acid-base and electrolyte balances. These, plus other factors, may contribute to such postoperative problems as electrolyte disturbances, hypo- or hypervolemia, hypotension, oliguria, respiratory depression (hypoxia and hypercapnia), arrhythmia, congestive heart failure, fever, and thrombophlebitis and pulmonary embolism.

Electrolyte disturbances should be corrected, for these (e.g., hypokalemia) can produce arrhythmias, especially in digitalized patients. Hypovolemia may be due to fluid or blood loss and electrolyte disturbance.

Myocardial infarction, arrhythmias, or catecholamine depletion due to drugs may cause hypotension. The signs and findings of postoperative myocardial infarction often are atypical.

The prolonged effects of anesthesia or the indiscriminate use of opiates can cause respiratory depression and suppression of the cough reflex. Hypercarbia is the primary indication for mechanical support in the postoperative period. Early pulmonary failure should be suspected if the pulse and respirations are rapid and the patient appears restless and anxious. The chest x-ray may not be helpful, but blood gas studies (arterial oxygen, arterial carbon dioxide, and pH) are diagnostic. The use of oxygen is most important in treating ventilatory failure. It may be necessary to use an endotracheal tube connected to a mechanical ventilator. If artificial ventilation is required for several days, then a tracheostomy may be required.

Arrhythmias or congestive heart failure after surgery should be managed as when they occur before or during surgery.

Postoperative fever in the cardiac patient may be due to lung infection (especially secondary to atelectasis), urinary tract infection, bacterial endocarditis, pulmonary emboli, or wound infection. Gram-negative sepsis may produce shock; thus, when infections are noted, every attempt should be made to isolate the microorganisms and give appropriate antibiotic therapy. Sometimes antibiotics must be administered empirically.

Postoperative thrombophlebitis and pulmonary embolism may be prevented by frequent movement of the patient, use of elastic stockings, and early ambulation. Prophylactic administration of low-dose heparin (5000 units subcutaneously every 12 h) postoperatively appears to diminish the risk in patients aged 40 or older who have had major general, urologic, orthopedic, or gynecologic surgery.

## SUGGESTED READING

Foster ED, Davis KB, Carpenter JA, et al: Risk of noncardiac operation in patients with defined coronary disease: The Coronary Artery Surgery Study (CASS) Registry experience. *Ann Thorac Surg* 41:42–50, 1986.

Gazes PC: Noncardiac surgery in the cardiac patient, in Hurst JW et al (eds): *The Heart*, 7th ed. New York, McGraw-Hill, Chap 87, pp 1602–1613, 1990.

Goldman L, Caldera DL, Nussbaum SR, et al: Multifactorial index of cardiac risk in noncardiac surgery procedures. *N Engl J Med* 297:845–850, 1977.

Hunter PR, Endrey-Walder P, Bauer GE, et al: Myocardial infarction following surgical operations. *Br Med J* 4:725–728, 1968.

Rao TLK, Jacobs KH, El-Etr AA: Reinfarction following anesthesia in patients with myocardial infarction. *Anesthesiology* 59:499–505, 1983.

Salem DN, Chuttani K, Isner JM: Assessment and management of cardiac disease in the surgical patient. *Curr Prob Cardiol* 14:171–224, 1989.

Shulman ST, Amren DP, Bisno AL, et al: Prevention of bacterial endocarditis. A statement for health professionals by the Committee on Rheumatic Fever and Infective Endocarditis of the Council on Cardiovascular Disease in the Young. *Circulation* 70:1123A–1127A, 1984.

Tinker JH, Noback CR, Vlietstra RE, et al: Management of patients with heart disease for noncardiac surgery. *JAMA* 246:1348–1350, 1981.

*36* | Drugs Used to Control Vascular
Resistance and Capacitance

*Subodh K. Agrawal, M.D.*
*Robert C. Schlant, M.D.*

Vasoactive drugs that alter vascular resistance and capacitance are used to support or control systemic arterial blood pressure, to maximize cardiac output in both acute and chronic congestive heart failure, and to reduce myocardial oxygen consumption in myocardial ischemic syndromes. It is important to understand the effects of these drugs on left ventricular performance and regional circulation, and on the interactions between the right and left ventricles. Some of these agents are listed in Table 36-1. The antihypertensive drugs are discussed in Chap. 13; calcium antagonists in Chap. 39; and nonglycosidic cardiotonic agents in Chap. 41.

## HEMODYNAMIC EFFECTS OF VASODILATORS

Vasodilators, which cause arteriolar and/or venular dilatation, can affect cardiac performance by altering preload, afterload, and/or blood volume.

### Role of Preload Changes in Cardiac Performance

Right ventricular preload (end-diastolic fiber length) is influenced by systemic venous capacitance and intravascular volume. Left ventricular preload is influenced by the capacitance of the pulmonary vascular bed and right ventricular output. According to classic Frank-Starling curves, end-diastolic myocardial fiber length (preload) is a major factor in determining ventricular stroke volume. Frank-Starling curves indicate that, up to a certain limit, increased initial fiber length influences the strength of myocardial contraction. The following should be borne in mind in considering the effects of pre-load on cardiac performance:

- When the left ventricle is markedly dilated, it may lose much of its responsiveness to preload; if this happens, stroke volume no longer increases significantly with an increase in preload.
- Marked dilatation of the left ventricle is due to slippage of myocardial fibers, and to an increase in fiber length.
- Changes in left ventricular compliance may significantly alter the relationship between diastolic pressure and diastolic volume.

- Left ventricular dilatation increases wall tension, which results in increased oxygen consumption. If the dilated ventricle is operating on a flattened Frank-Starling curve, the increase in oxygen consumption may not be associated with an increase in stroke volume.

## Role of Afterload Changes in Cardiac Performance

Arterial vasodilators may improve cardiac performance by reducing afterload. The following should be borne in mind in considering the effects of afterload on cardiac performance:

- Although the normal left ventricle is able to maintain its performance in the face of fairly wide changes in afterload, the damaged myocardium loses this ability, and ventricular performance may decrease significantly with an increase in afterload.
- Changes in vascular resistance and compliance produced by vasodilator drugs can counteract some of the neurohormonal changes produced by the sympathetic nervous system and the renin-angiotensin system in heart failure.
- Cardiac output may respond to changes in total left ventricular afterload, but the effect on flow to a specific vascular bed is controlled by local vascular changes.

## DIRECT-ACTING VASODILATOR DRUGS

### Arterial and Venous Vasodilator Drugs

*Nitroglycerin* and various nitrate preparations activate soluble guanylate cyclase and increase cyclic guanosine monophosphate in vascular smooth muscle. They dilate veins, large muscular arteries, collateral coronary vascular channels, and pulmonary arterioles; they increase venous capacitance, decrease systemic resistance, decrease pulmonary resistance, lower right and left ventricular filling pressures, reduce blood pressure, and reduce cardiac work load. They are used in patients with angina pectoris, acute myocardial infarction, congestive heart failure, and acute pulmonary edema. When these agents are employed chronically, many patients need a drug-free interval of 8 to 12 h to avoid the development of tolerance.

*Sodium nitroprusside* produces a dose-dependent reduction of arterial pressure in patients with hypertension, and a dose-dependent decrease of left ventricular impedance in patients with congestive heart failure. Continuous blood pressure monitoring is necessary during infusion. This drug is used to control blood pressure in hypertensive crises or aortic dissection, and to augment left ventricular performance in selected patients with acute myo-

TABLE 36-1 Vasodilators

| Drugs | Route of administration | Routes and doses |
|---|---|---|
| Agents acting at adrenergic receptors | | |
| Prazosin (Minipres) | Oral | 1 mg—1st dose 2–10 mg bid |
| Labetalol (Normodyne, Trandate) | Oral Intravenous | PO: 100–400 mg bid IV: 1–2 mg/kg/min |
| Clonidine (Catapres) | Oral Transdermal | PO: 0.1–0.3 mg bid Transdermal: 0.1–0.3 mg per week |
| ACE inhibitors | | |
| Captopril (Capoten) | Oral | 6.25 mg—1st dose, 12.5–50 mg bid or tid (1 h before meals) |
| Enalapril (Vasotec) (Enalaprit) | Oral Intravenous | PO: 2.5 mg—1st dose 5 to 20 mg q d IV: 1.25 mg over 5 min q 6 h |
| Lisinopril (Zestril) | Oral | 5 mg—1st dose, 10–40 mg q d |
| Direct vasodilators* | | |
| Sodium nitroprusside (Nipride) | Intravenous | 0.5–10 µg/kg/min |
| Nitroglycerin (Tridil, Nitro-Bid) | Intravenous | 5–200 µg/min |
| Nitroglycerin (Nitrostat) | Sublingual | 0.15–0.6 mg prn |
| Nitroglycerin (Nitro-Bid) | Oral | 2.5–9.0 mg bid or tid |
| Nitroglycerin (Nitrol ointment 2%, Nitro-Dur, Transderm-Nitro, Nitrodisc, Deponit) | Transdermal | 1.25–5.0 cm q 8–24 h 2.5–15 mg patch/day |
| Nitrolingual spray | Oral spray | 0.4 mg/spray dose prn |
| Isosorbide dinitrate (Isordil, Sorbitrate, Dilatrate-SR) | Sublingual or oral | S.L.: 2.5–20 mg q 6 h PO: 5–80 mg q 8–12 h |
| Hydralazine (Apresoline) | Oral, IV, or IM | PO: 10–75 mg q 6 h IV: 5–20 mg q 6 h IM: 5–40 mg q 6 h |
| Diazoxide (Hyperstat) | Intravenous | 1–3 mg/kg q 10–15 min |
| Minoxidil (Loniten) | Oral | 5–40 mg q d in single or divided doses |

* Chronic nitrate therapy should include a daily 8- to 12-h period without nitrate administration to prevent the development of tolerance.

| Onset of effect | Side effects |
| --- | --- |
| 30 min | 1st-dose hypotension, dizziness, syncope, edema, tolerance |
| 30 min Immediate | Hypotension, dizziness, may exacerbate congestive heart failure |
| 1 h 2–3 days | Withdrawal hypertension, dry mouth |
| 15 min | Renal insufficiency, neutropenia, hypotension, rash, cough, dysgeusia |
| 1–2 h 15 min | Renal insufficiency, rash, hypotension, angioedema, headache, dizziness |
| 1 h | Renal insufficiency, hypotension, dizziness, headache, fatigue, cough |
| Immediate | Hypotension, metabolic acidosis, accumulation of thiocyanate |
| Immediate | Headache, hypotension, withdrawal symptoms, methemoglobinemia, tolerance |
| 30 s | Headache, hypotension, tolerance |
| 1 h | Headache, hypotension, tolerance |
| 1 h | As above |
| 30 s | As above |
| 5–30 min | As above |
| 30 min Few min 15 min | Headache, tachycardia, autoimmune lupus-like reaction, increased toxicity in slow acetylators, angina, edema, tolerance |
| Immediate | Hyperglycemia, hypotension, tachycardia, hyperuricemia |
| 30 min | Tachycardia, water retention, pericardial effusion, hirsutism |

cardial infarction or severe congestive heart failure. (See Chap. 13.)

## Arterial Vasodilator Drugs

*Diazoxide, hydralazine,* and *minoxidil* act independently of the calcium channel to lower systemic vascular resistance in patients with hypertension, and to reduce impedance to left ventricular ejection in patients with heart failure. Reflex tachycardia and fluid retention are possible side effects. (See Chap. 13.) The combination of hydralazine and isosorbide dinitrate, which reduces systemic vascular resistance and raises venous capacitance, has been used in combination with digoxin and diuretics to treat chronic congestive heart failure.

## NEUROHORMONAL ANTAGONISTS

### Central Adrenergic Inhibitors

*Clonidine* and *guanabenz* stimulate central alpha$_2$ receptors and thereby decrease sympathetic outflow, which results in arterial and venous dilatation, decreased heart rate, and decreased myocardial contractility. These agents are used mainly to treat patients with systemic hypertension. Their negative inotropic effects limit their usefulness as vasodilator agents for the treatment of heart failure. The effects of *methyldopa* and *reserpine* are related, at least in part, to central inhibition. (See Chap. 13.)

### Sympathetic Vasoconstrictor Inhibitors

Vascular smooth-muscle tone in arteries, arterioles, and veins depends, in part, on sympathetic vasoconstrictor activity mediated largely through alpha-adrenoreceptor stimulation. Inhibition of this sympathetic vasoconstriction results in reduction of systemic vascular resistance, redistribution of peripheral blood flow, and/or increase in venous capacitance. Sympathetic blockade, which tends to produce orthostatic hypotension, may occur at numerous sites in the sympathetic vasoconstrictor apparatus. Sympathetic ganglionic blocking drugs effectively inhibit sympathetic vasoconstriction, but are unacceptable to most patients because of such side effects as constipation, urinary retention, and uncontrollable orthostatic hypotension.

*Guanethidine, guanadrel, bethanidine,* and *bretylium* all inhibit postganglionic release of norepinephrine and are effective in controlling hypertension. Because of such side effects as orthostatic hypotension and diarrhea, these agents are usually reserved for patients in whom more tolerable agents have proved ineffective. *Labetalol* is an antihypertensive, nonspecific beta-adrenoreceptor antagonist that also has alpha-adrenoreceptor blocking activity. Orthostatic hypotension is a possible side effect. (See Chap. 13.)

Alpha-adrenoreceptor blockers like *phentolamine* and *Dibenzyline* exert their action nonselectively on both presynaptic and postsynaptic alpha receptors. Intravenous phentolamine is useful acutely to control systemic blood pressure. These agents can cause significant orthostatic hypotension and reflex tachycardia. *Prazosin* is mainly a postsynaptic alpha-receptor blocker and has a decreased incidence of reflex tachycardia. Prazosin should be given as a last dose of 1 mg orally at bedtime, to avoid first-dose-induced severe orthostasis. Some patients develop tolerance to prazosin-induced hemodynamic changes. (See Chap. 13.)

## CONVERTING-ENZYME INHIBITORS

The converting-enzyme inhibitors block *angiotensin-converting enzymes* (ACE) at relatively low doses. In general, higher doses prolong the duration of inhibition rather than increase its peak effect. These agents (captopril, enalapril, lisinopril) are very useful in the treatment of hypertension and congestive heart failure. (See Chap. 13.)

## SUGGESTED READING

Chatterjee K, DeMarco T, Rouleau J: Vasodilator therapy in chronic congestive heart failure. *J Am Coll Cardiol* 62:46A–54A, 1988.

Cohn JN: Drugs used to control vascular resistance and capacitance, in Hurst JW et al (eds): *The Heart*, 7th ed. New York, McGraw-Hill, Chap 94, pp 1673–1681, 1990.

Cohn JN, Archibald DG, Ziesche S, et al: Effect of vasodilator therapy on mortality in chronic congestive heart failure. *N Engl J Med* 314:1547–1552, 1986.

The CONSENSUS Trial Group: Effects of enalapril on mortality in severe heart failure: Results of the Cooperative North Scandinavian Enalapril Survival Study, CONSENSUS. *N Engl J Med* 316:1429–1435, 1987.

Opie LH, Chatterjee K, Harrison DC: Vasodilating drugs, in Opie LH (ed): *Drugs for the Heart*, 2d ed. Boston, Grune & Stratton, pp 131–147, 1987.

| Drugs Used to Treat Cardiac Arrhythmias

*Raymond L. Woosley, M.D., Ph.D.*

## INTRODUCTION

The antiarrhythmic drugs are some of the most controversial drugs in cardiology. They have the greatest potential for harm and are among the least studied for possible benefit. Controversy abounds in the literature, with conflicting results on the value of, for example, prophylactic lidocaine in acute myocardial infarction, or chronic therapy to suppress asymptomatic ventricular arrhythmias. Because of their toxicity, these drugs should be prescribed only when benefit is likely. The reader should carefully review the indications for use of these drugs before prescribing any of them.

Table 37-1 lists the classes of *antiarrhythmic actions* of drugs as proposed by Vaughan-Williams. This table is printed here only because of its general usefulness and its value as a shorthand for discussing drug action. Many physicians use it, erroneously, as a classification of *drugs;* such use is not recommended. (The reader should refer to Chapter 95 of Hurst JW et al [eds], *The Heart* [7th ed, New York, McGraw-Hill, 1990], for a full explanation of the limitations of the classification.) Suffice it to say that there are few examples of clinical utility for the classification and many examples where it is misleading.

## QUINIDINE

Quinidine is one of the oldest antiarrhythmic agents, but there is still much to be learned about its actions. It is effective for both ventricular and supraventricular arrhythmias and is one of the most effective drugs for preventing recurrence of atrial fibrillation or flutter. Because it enhances AV nodal conduction, patients in atrial fibrillation or flutter should be given digoxin prior to starting quinidine. As with other antiarrhythmic agents with class I action, it has only limited efficacy in preventing recurrence of ventricular tachycardia. Approximately 20 to 25 percent of patients respond when programmed ventricular stimulation is used to guide therapy. The use of lower doses in combination with mexiletine is often necessary to increase effectiveness and reduce the incidence of side effects. Because of quinidine's effects to slow conduction and increase refractoriness in accessory pathways, it may be effective in preventing rapid ventricular response during atrial fibrillation

TABLE 37-1 Classification of Antiarrhythmic Actions

| Class | Action | Effect on ECG | Drugs with predominant action |
|-------|--------|---------------|-------------------------------|
| I | Sodium channel block | ↑ QRS | |
| IA | Sodium channel w/some K+ channel block | ↑ QRS & QT | quinidine; procainamide; disopyramide |
| IB | Sodium channel block (weak) | None | lidocaine; mexiletine; tocainide; phenytoin |
| IC | Potent sodium channel block | ↑ ↑ QRS | flecainide; encainide; propafenone |
| II | Antagonism of sympathetic nervous system | ↓ heart rate | beta blockers |
| III | Increased refractoriness | ↑ QT | bretylium; amiodarone; sotalol |
| IV | Blockade of slow inward calcium current | ↓ heart rate | verapamil; diltiazem |

in patients with the Wolff-Parkinson-White (WPW) syndrome. Digoxin may be deleterious in this setting, as it may counteract a beneficial effect in the bypass tract tissue.

Quinidine is very poorly tolerated because of side effects which characteristically occur both early and late. The most common early side effect is diarrhea, which has been reported in 10 to 40 percent of patients during the first 4 weeks of therapy. During chronic therapy, rash, fever, photosensitivity of the skin, and thrombocytopenia are occasionally seen. Excessive dosages lead to a classic toxicity called *cinchonism* (tinnitus, blurred vision, and headache). Another classic toxicity of serious concern is the syndrome of torsade de pointes; it has been estimated to occur in 1 to 4 percent of patients and is usually self-limiting, but can be lethal if unrecognized. It generally occurs in one of three settings during quinidine therapy: (1) within the first few days of therapy at usual dosages; (2) later, during stable therapy, when a patient becomes hypokalemic; and (3) at high dosages. It is facilitated by any factors that prolong repolarization, slow heart rate, or reduce potassium levels. Examples are diuretic therapy, congenital long-QT syndrome, hypothyroidism, sick sinus syndrome, and diarrhea. It is preceded by marked prolongation of the QT interval, usually with plasma quinidine concentrations that are in the low or subtherapeutic range. It is treated best by (1) increasing the heart rate (pacing or isoproterenol infusion), (2) administration of sodium (bicarbonate or lactate injection), and (3) normalizing the potassium and magnesium levels. If these fail, trials of intravenous magnesium sulfate (2–3 g over 5–10 min) have been reported to be effective. The use of other antiarrhythmic drugs can be dangerous in this setting and has led to death in some patients.

The usual initial dose of quinidine sulfate is 200 mg every 6 h. The elimination half-life ranges from 4 to 20 h, so steady state is reached in 1 to 4 days. Since the metabolites are active, it is best to wait 2 to 3 days between dose escalations when possible. The QT interval and QRS duration should be monitored regularly; continuous ECG monitoring is advisable. Many cardiologists recommend hospitalization and ECG monitoring during initiation of any antiarrhythmic drug, especially quinidine. Measurement of trough levels is helpful, concentrations between 2 and 5 µg/ml are usually required. Side effects may occur at any concentration; the measurement of peak levels is of no value. Many patients require dosages of quinidine sulfate of 300 or 400 mg every 6 h. Patients who are receiving drugs that induce hepatic metabolism may require 400 to 600 mg every 6 h to achieve a therapeutic plasma concentration.

The sustained-release forms of quinidine have slower absorption and often have trough levels below the usual therapeutic range. The quinidine gluconate formulation is said to be better tolerated, but this is probably due to the fact that it contains less quinidine base—60 percent, versus 80 percent for quinidine sulfate. The gluconate salt is also available for intravenous infusion, but should be given at rates ≤20 mg/min to prevent serious hypotension. Because quinidine is an alpha blocker and reduces afterload, it only rarely worsens heart failure. However, it may produce excessive orthostatic hypotension if the patient is taking vasodilators, especially nitrates or dipyridamole. Digoxin or digitoxin dosages should be reduced, and/or plasma concentrations monitored, to prevent accumulation to toxic levels when they are used with quinidine. Quinidine blocks the metabolism of many drugs; interactions should be watched for with metoprolol, timolol, encainide, flecainide, propafenone, and many of the tricyclic antidepressants.

## PROCAINAMIDE

Procainamide is widely thought to be similar to quinidine. However, they are very different drugs with few similarities. Procainamide has similar potency for preventing recurrence of ventricular tachycardia (about 20 percent of patients), but it may be effective in patients refractory to quinidine—and vice versa. It is said to be effective in preventing recurrence of atrial fibrillation, but no controlled studies are available to prove this and it is generally considered less effective than quinidine. In general, it is not a good drug for chronic oral therapy because of a very high incidence of side effects (see below). Intravenous therapy is often effective for ventricular arrhythmias, but requires approximately 20 to 30 min to reach effective levels safely. Rapid infusion ($>50$ mg/min) can lead to hypotension because of ganglionic blocking actions seen at high levels and/or negative inotropic actions. A relatively safe regimen is 20 mg/min for 30 to 40 min. This yields concentrations in the effective range ($4–8$ $\mu$g/ml) in most patients with little effect on blood pressure or intraventricular conduction. Some patients may require a total loading dose of 1 to 2 g, but this produces levels that are usually not tolerated during chronic therapy. Blood pressure and the QRS interval should be monitored during the infusion. If the patient has recently been given other cardioactive drugs, lower initial dosages of procainamide should be used. Response to intravenous procainamide does not predict response to oral therapy, because of the varied production of procainamide's potentially active metabolite, N-acetylprocainamide (NAPA). Because NAPA has mainly class III antiarrhythmic action and little, if any, potency as a sodium channel blocker, it is very difficult to predict clinical response to oral therapy. Plasma level monitoring is of limited value, and there is no validity in the often-recommended practice of using the sum of the procainamide and NAPA concentrations to monitor therapy. This is due to their different electrophysiological actions and from the nonconcordance of clinical responses to the two agents when given as single agents.

During chronic oral therapy approximately 50 percent of patients withdraw because of intolerable side effects. Nausea and vomiting are common early problems. Rash and drug fever occur sporadically during therapy, and approximately 20 percent of patients per year develop a lupus-like syndrome. Antinuclear antibodies (ANA) are seen in almost all patients after 9 to 12 months, but only those with high or rapidly rising titers develop symptoms, which include a malar rash, arthralgias, and fever. If this lupus-like syndrome goes undiagnosed and the drug is continued, the syndrome can progress to a more generalized rash, arthritis, and/or pleuritis. Several cases of pericarditis have been described; some have progressed to tamponade and death. The symptoms usually resolve with a time course similar to that of their onset. However, ANA may remain intermittently positive for years. The current estimates are that 1 patient out of 500 will develop agranulocytosis due to procainamide. Regular monitoring of WBC is recommended by the manufacturers every 2 weeks for the first 3 months.

Oral dosages are variable and highly influenced by renal function. Because of its short half-life, the usual starting dose (500 mg) is administered every 3 to 4 h. The slow release formulations allow dosing every 6 to 8 h. Because NAPA accumulates more slowly and reaches greater levels than procainamide in rapid acetylators (55 percent of Caucasians and 90 percent of Orientals), one should wait at least 2 days to allow achievement of steady state (>4 days in renal failure). Many patients require total daily dosages of 6–8 g/day (750 mg every 3 h or, for the sustained-release formulation, 1.5–2.0 g every 6 h).

## DISOPYRAMIDE

Disopyramide is of limited use for patients with ventricular arrhythmias, because of its negative inotropic actions; but it is useful in patients with preserved left ventricular function or with supraventricular arrhythmias and WPW syndrome. Dose-related anticholinergic side effects limit therapy in many patients by causing urinary retention, dry mouth, and blurred vision. The usual dosage is 150 mg every 6 h. Some patients require dosages of 200 to 250 mg every 8 h. The sustained-release form allows dosing every 12 h, and is usually initiated at 200 mg every 12 h.

Plasma concentration monitoring is of little value because of variable and saturable binding of the drug to plasma proteins. A doubling of total concentration in blood may actually be a sixfold increase in the *free* drug level, potentially causing toxicity. For this reason, loading doses or rapid increases in dosage are very dangerous and not recommended. There is no organ toxicity associated with chronic therapy; if the drug is initially tolerated, chronic therapy is usually without problems. Disopyramide is metabolized by the liver. Agents that induce hepatic metabolism (phenytoin, rifampin, and barbiturates) can cause levels to fall, with loss of clinical benefit.

## TOCAINIDE

Tocainide is an orally active lidocaine congener that should be used only for life-threatening ventricular arrhythmias that have failed to respond to other agents, including mexiletine. Only 10 to 15 percent of patients evaluated respond to therapy. Approximately 1 patient in 500 develops agranulocytosis or pulmonary fibrosis, making tocainide a dangerous agent for chronic therapy. Troublesome side effects, such as tremor, lightheadedness, pruritis, and nausea, occur in 30 to 40 percent of patients, limiting therapy. Because tocainide is cleared mainly by the kidneys, patients with renal disease require much lower dosages. Usual doses are from 400–600 mg q 8 h. Lower doses must be used in renal patients.

## MEXILETINE

Mexiletine is another lidocaine congener, similar to tocainide in many ways. It has no serious organ toxicity and therefore need not always be reserved for refractory patients. However, only 10 to 15 percent of patients with ventricular tachycardia respond, and it is best used in combination with quinidine to increase efficacy and reduce side effects.

The most common side effects are seen early in therapy; 30 to 35 percent of patients may develop nausea, vomiting, tremor, blurred vision, or pruritus. A rare case of hepatitis has been described. Most side effects are dose-related and may be controlled by lowering the size of each dose and/or giving it with food or aluminum antacids. Monitoring of plasma concentrations is of little value. Dosage usually begins with 150 mg orally every 8 h, and may be increased every 2 to 3 days to 200 mg q 8, 250 mg q 8, or 250 mg q 6 h.

## ENCAINIDE AND FLECAINIDE

Encainide and flecainide (see below) are potent drugs that prolong the QRS and PR intervals at dosages usually required to suppress arrhythmias. They have been found to increase mortality in patients with prior myocardial infarction and asymptomatic ventricular arrhythmias, and are therefore recommended only for patients with life-threatening ventricular tachycardia or fibrillation in whom other agents have failed. Unfortunately, it is this population that has a low response rate (about 20 percent) and a very high incidence of aggravation of the arrhythmia (10 to 25 percent). Obviously, therapy should be initiated under monitored conditions by physicians experienced in the care of such patients. Patients with supraventricular arrhythmias, particularly those with WPW syndrome, have been reported to respond to these two agents. However, their very restrictive labeling requires that they be used in highly symptomatic patients.

## LIDOCAINE

Lidocaine is one of the most effective, and most often misused, drugs in cardiology. There is controversy over its prophylactic use in patients with presumed myocardial infarction. However, it is rapidly effective in suppressing ventricular arrhythmias in the setting of acute ischemia. If reversible causes have been excluded, it should be given as a series of loading and maintenance infusions. In patients *without* heart failure, the initial injection of 1 mg/kg should be given over 2 min, and a maintenance infusion of 2 mg/

min started as soon as possible. After 8, 16, and 24 min, additional 0.5-mg/kg loading injections should be given. If the patient develops side effects at any time during the loading, subsequent loading infusions should not be given. If serious side effects, such as heart block or hypotension, are seen, the drug should be discontinued entirely and, if necessary, pacing or volume expanders given to correct the side effects. Most side effects are transient and require nothing more than observation. The sizes of the initial injection and the three serial loading injections should be halved in patients with heart failure. For those with severe heart failure or liver disease the maintenance infusion, too, should be halved. Plasma concentration monitoring is essential to adjust dosage to prevent excessive accumulation or subtherapeutic levels.

## VERAPAMIL

Verapamil is a very effective agent for converting paroxysmal supraventricular tachycardia. Diagnosis of the arrhythmia is essential, because inadvertent administration to patients in ventricular tachycardia almost uniformly produces hemodynamic decompensation, shock, or even death. Verapamil is contraindicated in patients with WPW syndrome and atrial fibrillation, who have occasionally been reported to develop acceleration of ventricular rhythm after administration of verapamil. In contrast, patients with WPW syndrome and narrow-complex supraventricular tachycardia respond well to verapamil. It is usually given as an infusion of 5–10 mg over 2–5 min. Oral therapy is in the range of 80–160 mg q 8 h.

## PROPRANOLOL

Propranolol, like many of the other beta blockers, is an effective antiarrhythmic. By slowing conduction in the AV node, it can convert or suppress supraventricular arrhythmias, and when used with digoxin it can be used to slow ventricular response in atrial fibrillation. Patients with exercise-induced tachyarrhythmias can often be controlled with oral therapy. Propranolol is often effective for acute termination of supraventricular tachycardia, and occasionally effective for ventricular tachycardia. However, severe hypotension is frequently seen after intravenous administration to patients in ventricular tachycardia.

Intravenous dosages of 0.1 mg/kg at a rate of 1 mg/min can be administered for acute therapy of arrhythmias. A maintenance infusion of 0.1 mg/min will maintain an effective level of propranolol in patients with relatively normal hepatic and cardiac function. Oral therapy requires titration from a usual starting dose of 40 mg q 6–8 h. The dosage can be increased every 1 to 2 days.

There is little benefit above 120 mg q 6 h. Neither propranolol nor any other beta blocker is generally effective as a single agent for prevention of recurrent sustained ventricular tachycardia, unless the tachycardia is reproducibly induced by exercise. Propranolol is often used in combination with the local-anesthetic class of drugs (e.g., quinidine).

## ESMOLOL

Esmolol is an effective cardioselective beta blocker for intravenous use that was specifically developed to be ultra-short-acting. It can be useful for any arrhythmias responsive to beta blockers, and has the advantage of short duration of action in case adverse effects occur. Therapy should be initiated with a loading infusion of 500 μg/kg over 1 min, followed by 50 μg/kg/min. If inadequate efficacy is obtained, additional loading doses of 500 μg/kg should be given and the maintenance dose increased by 50 μg/kg/min. The usually effective maintenance dose is 100 μg/kg/min; few patients require over 200 μg/kg/min. Hypotension is a frequent complication.

## BRETYLIUM

Bretylium is a very effective antiarrhythmic drug for malignant ventricular arrhythmias, available only for intravenous use. Because of its complex pharmacological actions, it is usually reserved for patients who have failed to respond to lidocaine and, in some cases, procainamide. For patients with recurrent ventricular fibrillation or sustained ventricular tachycardia, it should be given as a rapid intravenous injection into a central line. If the patient is awake, rapid injection will often cause nausea and vomiting; the drug should be given at a rate of 8–10 mg/min in such cases.

Bretylium is cleared entirely by the kidneys. The dosage should be reduced in patients with renal insufficiency. The usual initial dose is 5 mg/kg as a rapid injection, or slow infusion of 8–10 mg/min. A second dose of 5–10 mg/kg is usually given if the patient fails to respond to the first loading dose. A maximum loading dose of 20 mg/kg is recommended, though no dose-related toxicity other than nausea has been described. Maintenance doses of 1–2 mg/min are usually recommended. Very low doses of bretylium block adrenergic neuronal function, and blood pressure is not reduced further by high dosages. Supine blood pressure should be regulated by volume expansion to maintain CNS perfusion and urine production.

## AMIODARONE

Amiodarone is available for oral therapy of life-threatening ventricular tachycardia or fibrillation, but because of severe and sometimes lethal toxicity it should be reserved for patients in whom all other drugs available have failed. The toxic effects are generally dose-related, but have been seen in some patients with low dosages within 2 to 3 months of beginning therapy. During initial therapy, loading doses of 300–600 mg b.i.d. are given for 10–14 days. Variable regimens have been used in the past; there are no studies allowing comparison of different methods. Abrupt changes in dosage can lead to recurrence of the arrhythmia, so tapering of the dose in the first few weeks to the lowest effective dosage is essential. Most patients require 400 mg/day as a single dose, but a few can be controlled on 200 mg/day. Some require 600 mg/day.

During the loading period, the patient should be observed for evidence of amiodarone's effects on conduction (heart block, bundle branch block, severe bradycardia). Worsening of the arrhythmia, including torsade de pointes, has been reported, but is unusual and may simply reflect inadequate therapy in some cases. Before or soon after the beginning of therapy, baseline tests to screen for toxicity should be obtained. These tests include chest x-ray, pulmonary function tests (including CO diffusion capacity), thyroid function, serum chemistry (including liver function tests), and an ophthalmologic exam. These should be repeated whenever toxicity is suspected; the chest x-ray and serum chemistry should be repeated every 3 months. Approximately 30 percent of patients develop elevated serum transaminases that usually resolve with dosage reduction. The most serious side effect is pulmonary toxicity, which can occur acutely or develop slowly and insidiously. It is estimated to occur in 5 to 10 percent of patients each year; 10 percent of cases are lethal. Other serious toxic effects include hypo- and hyperthyroidism, peripheral neuropathy, and incapacitating nausea and vomiting. There are many other side effects and drug interactions. (See Chap. 95 of *The Heart.*)

## SUGGESTED READING

CAST investigators: Preliminary report: Effect of encainide and flecainide on mortality in a randomized trial of arrhythmia suppression after myocardial infarction. *N Engl J Med* 321:406–412, 1989.

Katzung BG: New Concepts in antiarrhythmic drug action, in Yu PN, Goodwin JF (eds): *Progress in Cardiology,* vol 15. Philadelphia, Lea and Febiger, pp 5–18, 1987.

Kudenchuk PJ, Pierson DJ, Greene HL, et al: Prospective evaluation of amiodarone pulmonary toxicity. *Chest* 86:541–548, 1984.

Lie KI, Wellens HJ, van Capelle FJ, et al: Lidocaine in the prevention of primary ventricular fibrillation. A double-blind, randomized study of 212 consecutive patients. *N Engl J Med* 291:1324–1326, 1974.

Stewart RB, Bardy GH, Greene HL: Wide complex tachycardia: Misdiagnosis and outcome after emergent therapy. *Ann Intern Med* 104(6):766–771, 1986.

Vaughn-Williams EM: A classification of antiarrhythmic actions reassessed after a decade of new drugs. *J Clin Pharmacol* 24:129, 1984.

Wellens HJJ, Brugada P, Penn OC: The management of preexcitation syndromes. *JAMA* 257:2325–2333, 1987.

Woosley RL: Antiarrhythmic agents, in Hurst JW et al (eds): *The Heart*, 7th ed. New York, McGraw-Hill, Chap 95, pp 1682–1711, 1990.

Woosley RL, Funck-Brentano C: Overview of the clinical pharmacology of antiarrhythmic drugs. *Am J Cardiol* 61:61A–69A, 1988.

## 38 | Beta-Adrenergic Blocking Drugs

*William H. Frishman, M.D.*
*Eliot J. Lazar, M.D.*

The beta-adrenergic blocking drugs (beta blockers) were used originally for the treatment of angina pectoris and arrhythmias. They have gained widespread acceptance for treatment of many other conditions, both cardiac and noncardiac, including hypertrophic cardiomyopathy, systemic hypertension, dissecting aneurysm, mitral valve prolapse, migraine, glaucoma, and essential tremor. The drugs are also indicated, in oral and parenteral forms, for reducing the risk of death and nonfatal reinfarction in survivors of acute myocardial infarction.

### BASIC PHARMACOLOGICAL DIFFERENCES

Thirteen beta blockers are currently approved for use in the United States (Table 38-1): propranolol, atenolol, nadolol, timolol, carteolol, metoprolol, penbutolol, pindolol, acebutolol, esmolol, labetalol, betaxolol, and oxprenolol. Others are in clinical trials or are about to be approved. These include bisoprolol, carvedilol, celiprolol, dilevalol, and flestolol.

Most marketed beta blockers are racemic mixtures of optical isomers (D, L). More beta-blocking activity is found in the L, or levorotatory, form. This difference between the activities of the two types of isomer allows differentiation of the pharmacological properties of membrane-stabilizing activity and beta blockade.

#### Membrane-Stabilizing Activity

In high concentrations, some beta blockers have a quinidine-like effect on the cardiac action potential. This is unrelated to beta blockade, and is exhibited equally by the two stereoisomers of each drug.

#### Beta₁ Selectivity

Beta blockers can be classified as selective or nonselective, according to their ability to block the action of endogenous catecholamines in some tissues at lower drug concentrations than are required in other tissues. In relatively low therapeutic doses, selective agents, such as atenolol, betaxolol, metoprolol, acebutolol, and esmolol, block cardiac beta₁ receptors more than they do the beta₂ receptors found in bronchial or vascular smooth muscle. In higher doses, selective agents block both types of beta receptors; thus they should not be used in patients with absolute contraindications to beta blockade (e.g., bronchospasm).

### Intrinsic Sympathomimetic Activity

Some beta blockers exhibit intrinsic sympathomimetic activity or partial agonist activity (PAA) at the beta receptor. These agents cause less slowing of the heart rate than beta blockers without this property; exercise-induced elevations in heart rate are similarly blunted. Agents with either nonselective (pindolol) or beta$_2$-selective (dilevalol) PAA reduce peripheral vascular resistance and, theoretically, might be better tolerated in patients with peripheral vascular disease. These agents may also have less effect on serum lipids than nonselective beta blockers without PAA.

### Alpha-Adrenergic Blocking Ability

Several beta blockers, such as labetalol, have the additional property of alpha-adrenergic blockade. Labetalol has been shown to be 4 to 16 times less potent at alpha receptors than at beta receptors. Theoretically the property of alpha blockade should produce a decrease in peripheral vascular resistance, which in turn should act to preserve cardiac output. Whether this is clinically significant is unclear. One advantage of these agents is their efficacy in certain populations in which conventional beta blockers are less effective (e.g., blacks). Labetalol is available in parenteral form for treatment of hypertensive emergencies and urgencies. Labetalol also has a neutral effect on plasma lipids.

### CLINICAL EFFECTS AND THERAPEUTIC APPLICATIONS (Table 38-2)

#### Hypertension

Beta blockers have been shown to be effective in reducing blood pressure in patients with systemic hypertension. The mechanism by which they reduce blood pressure is not entirely clear; it is likely that a number of drug actions account for this, including negative chronotropic and inotropic effects, and effects to lower peripheral vascular resistance (beta blockers with PAA and alpha$_1$ antagonism) and plasma renin.

#### Angina Pectoris

Beta blockers act primarily on the demand side of the myocardial oxygen supply/demand equation. The three main factors contrib-

TABLE 38-1 Pharmacodynamic Properties and Cardiac Effects of β-Adrenoceptor Blockers

| Drug | Relative β₁ selectivity* | Partial agonist activity | Membrane-stabilizing activity | Resting heart rate | Exercise heart rate | Resting myocardial contractility | Resting blood pressure | Exercise blood pressure | Resting atrioventricular conduction | Antiarrhythmic effect |
|---|---|---|---|---|---|---|---|---|---|---|
| Acebutolol | + | + | + | ↕→ | → | → | → | → | → | + |
| Atenolol | ++ | 0 | 0 | → | → | → | → | → | → | + |
| Betaxolol | ++ | 0 | + | → | → | → | → | → | → | + |
| Bevantolol | ++ | 0 | 0 | → | → | → | → | → | → | + |
| Carteolol | 0 | + | 0 | ↕↓ | → | ↕↓ | → | → | ↕↓ | + |
| Carvediol** | 0 | + | 0 | ↕↓ | → | ↕↓ | → | → | ↕↓ | + |
| Celiprolol† | + | + | 0 | ↕↓ | → | ↕↓ | → | → | ↕↓ | + |
| Dilevalol‡ | 0 | + | 0 | ↕ | → | ↕↓ | → | →↑ | ↕ | + |
| Esmolol | ++ | 0 | 0 | → | → | → | → | → | → | + |
| Labetalol§ | 0 | 0 | 0 | ↕↓ | → | ↕↓ | → | → | ↕↓ | + |
| Meloprolol | ++ | 0 | + | ↕↓ | → | ↕↓ | → | → | ↕↓ | + |
| Nadolol | 0 | 0 | 0 | → | → | → | → | → | → | + |
| Oxprenolol | 0 | + | + | → | → | → | → | → | → | + |
| Penbutolol | 0 | + | 0 | → | → | → | → | → | → | + |
| Pindolol | 0 | ++ | + | ↕↓ | → | ↕↓ | → | → | ↕↓ | + |
| Propranolol | 0 | 0 | ++ | → | → | → | → | → | → | + |
| Solalol | 0 | 0 | 0 | → | → | → | → | → | → | + |
| Timolol | 0 | 0 | 0 | ↕ | ↕ | ↕ | ↕ | ↕ | ↕ | + |
| Isomer: D-propranolol | 0 | 0 | ++ | ↕→↓ | | →↓ | | | →↓ | +‾ |

300

* $\beta_1$ selectivity is seen only with low therapeutic drug concentrations. With higher concentrations, $\beta_1$ selectivity is not seen.

** Carvedilol has additional $\alpha_1$-adrenergic blocking activity without $\beta_2$ agonism.

† Celiprolol has peripheral $\beta_2$ agonism and may have additional $\alpha_2$-adrenergic blocking activity at high doses.

‡ Dilevalol is an isomer of labetalol with peripheral $\beta_2$ agonism but no $\alpha_1$-blocking activity.

§ Labetalol has additional $\alpha_1$-adrenergic blocking properties and direct $\beta_2$-adrenergic vasodilator activity.

¶ Effects of D-propranolol with doses in human beings well above the therapeutic level. The isomer also lacks $\beta$-blocking activity.

Two pluses indicate a strong effect; one plus, modest effect; zero, absent effect; upward-pointing arrow = elevation; downward-pointing arrow = reduction; double-headed horizontal arrow = no change.

*Source:* Frishman WH: *Clinical Pharmacology of the β-Adrenoreceptor Blocking Drugs, 2d ed* Norwalk, Appleton-Century-Crofts, p 32, 1984; adapted and reproduced with permission. Also from Frishman WH: *Int J Cardiol* 2:167, 1982; adapted and reproduced with permission. Also from Frishman WH: Beta-adrenergic blockers, *Med Clin North Am* 72:52, 1988, reproduced with the permission of the publisher and author.

TABLE 38-2 Reported Cardiovascular Indications for β-Adrenoreceptor Blocking Drugs

| |
|---|
| Hypertension* |
| Angina pectoris* |
| "Silent" myocardial ischemia |
| Supraventricular arrhythmias* (including those seen with thyrotoxicosis) |
| Ventricular arrhythmias* |
| Reducing the risk of mortality and reinfarction in survivors of acute myocardial infarction* |
| Hyperacute phase of myocardial infarction* |
| Dissection of the aorta |
| Hypertrophic cardiomyopathy* |
| Reversing left ventricular hypertrophy |
| Digitalis intoxication |
| Mitral valve prolapse |
| QT-interval prolongation syndrome |
| Tetralogy of Fallot |
| Mitral stenosis |
| Congestive cardiomyopathy |
| Fetal tachycardia |
| Neurocirculatory asthenia |

*Indications formally approved by FDA.

uting to myocardial oxygen demand are heart rate, systolic blood pressure, and left ventricular wall tension. The first two appear to be most important. Beta blockers slow the resting heart rate. This has two favorable effects: blood pressure is decreased, and the longer diastolic filling time that accompanies a slower heart rate may also allow an increased coronary perfusion time. Beta blockade also decreases the increments in heart rate and blood pressure that accompany exercise. Most available beta blockers cause an increase in work capacity in patients with stable angina pectoris. Beta blockers have also been shown to decrease nitroglycerin consumption and the frequency of chest pain. They have been used successfully in combination with nitrates, and with some of the calcium antagonists. (In the latter case, one must watch for negative inotropic effects and impairment of cardiac conduction).

### Arrhythmias

Beta blockers function as antiarrhythmic drugs predominantly by competitive inhibition of adrenergic stimulation. This reduces the slope of Phase 4 depolarization as well as the spontaneous firing rate of sinus or ectopic pacemakers. Some of these agents also may have membrane-stabilizing activity—the "quinidine-like," or "local anesthetic," effect. These drugs have been used to treat various supraventricular and ventricular tachyarrhythmias.

## Survivors of Acute Myocardial Infarction

Several studies have demonstrated the efficacy of beta blockers in reducing mortality and nonfatal reinfarction in survivors of acute myocardial infarction. Propranolol and timolol have been approved for reducing the risk of mortality in infarct survivors when initiated 5 to 28 days after myocardial infarction. Metoprolol and atenolol are similarly approved, and can also be given intravenously during the initial stages of an infarction, with and without thrombolysis.

## Other Cardiovascular Applications

Beta blockers are used to treat patients with hypertrophic cardiomyopathy. Propranolol, for example, controls the symptoms of dyspnea and chest pain seen with this condition, and may lower the intraventricular pressure gradient. Beta blockers have also been used to treat asymptomatic myocardial ischemia, with reductions in the amount and degree of ST-segment depression on ECG, as determined by 24-h ambulatory Holter recording. In patients with mitral valve prolapse, these drugs also relieve chest pain and palpitations. In the initial management of dissecting aortic aneurysm, they have been used in combination with arterial vasodilators. Other clinical conditions in which these agents have been used include tetralogy of Fallot, QT-prolongation syndrome, and thyrotoxicosis. For more detailed discussion of these subjects, we refer the reader to "Suggested Reading," at the end of the chapter.

## Other Non-Cardiovascular Uses

Some beta blockers are now approved in topical form for reducing intraocular pressure in patients with open-angle glaucoma, and in oral form for treating benign essential tremor and for prophylaxis against migraine headache syndrome.

## ADVERSE EFFECTS

The adverse effects of beta blockers fall into two categories: those related to beta-adrenergic blockade, and those related to other reactions. The former group includes asthma, heart failure, bradycardia and heart block, intermittent claudication, Raynaud's phenomenon, glycemic changes, and central nervous system effects. There may be some variation in the frequencies of these side effects, depending on the particular agent used. It is important to remember that the property of $beta_1$ specificity is relative; thus, in patients with absolute contraindications to $beta_2$ blockade, the use of a "$beta_1$-selective" agent may still be unacceptable (e.g., bronchospasm).

TABLE 38-3 Clinical Situations That Would Influence the Choice of a β-Blocking Drug

| Condition | Choice of β blocker |
|---|---|
| Asthma, chronic bronchitis with bronchospasm | Avoid all β blockers if possible, but small doses of $\beta_1$-selective blockers (acebutolol, atenolol, metoprolol) can be used; $\beta_1$ selectivity is lost with higher doses; drugs with partial agonist activity (pindolol, oxprenolol) and labetalol with α-adrenergic blocking properties can also be used. |
| Congestive heart failure | Drugs with partial agonist activity and labetalol may have an advantage, though β blockers are usually contraindicated. |
| Angina | In patients with angina at low heart rates, drugs with partial agonist activity are probably contraindicated; patients who have angina at high heart rates but who have resting bradycardia may benefit from a drug with partial agonist activity; in vasospastic angina, labetalol may be useful; other β blockers should be used with caution. |
| Atrioventricular conduction defects | β blockers generally contraindicated, but drugs with partial agonist activity and labetalol can be tried with caution. |
| Bradycardia | β blockers with partial agonist activity and labetalol have less pulse-slowing effect and are preferable. |
| Raynaud's phenomenon, intermittent claudication, cold extremities | $\beta_1$-Selective blocking agents, labetalol, and agents with partial agonist activity may have an advantage. |
| Depression | Avoid propranolol; substitute a β blocker with partial agonist activity. |
| Diabetes mellitus | $\beta_1$-Selective agents and partial agonist drugs are preferable. |
| Thyrotoxicosis | All agents will control symptoms, but agents without partial agonist activity are preferred. |
| Pheochromocytoma | Avoid all β blockers unless an α blocker is given; labetalol may be used as a treatment of choice. |

| | |
|---|---|
| Renal failure | Use reduced doses of compounds largely eliminated by renal mechanisms (nadolol, sotalol, atenolol) and drugs whose bioavailability is increased in uremia (propranolol, alprenolol); also consider possible accumulation of active metabolites (propranolol). |
| Insulin and sulfonylurea use | Danger of hypoglycemia; possibly less using drugs with $\beta_1$ selectivity. |
| Clonidine | Avoid sotalol (and other nonselective $\beta$ blockers); severe rebound effect with clonidine withdrawal. |
| Oculomucocutaneous syndrome | Stop drug; substitute any $\beta$ blocker. |
| Hyperlipidemia | Avoid nonselective $\beta$ blockers; use agents with partial agonism or $\beta_1$ selectivity, or labetalol. |

*Source:* Frishman WH: *Clinical Pharmacology of the β-Adrenoceptor Blocking Drugs,* 2d ed. Norwalk, Appleton-Century-Crofts, p. 162, 1984; reproduced with permission from the publisher and author. Also from Frishman WH: The beta–adrenoceptor blocking drugs. *Int J Cardiol* 2:173, 1982; reproduced with permission from the publisher and author.

*Source:* Frishman WH: *Clinical Pharmacology of the β-Adrenoceptor Blocking Drugs,* 2d ed. Norwalk, Appleton-Century-Crofts, p 162, 1984; reproduced with permission from the publisher and author.

A number of rare side effects unrelated to beta blockade have been reported. These include uveitis and sclerosing peritonitis, purpura, and agranulocytosis.

### Overdosage

Deliberate and accidental over-ingestions of beta blockers have been reported. The competitive pharmacological properties of these drugs permit antidotal treatment with parenteral infusions of beta agonists such as isoproterenol or dobutamine. Glucagon and amrinone have also been used for this purpose. Close monitoring of cardiopulmonary status is especially important in patients with known or suspected beta-blocker overdosage.

### Beta-Blocker Withdrawal

Exacerbation of angina pectoris, myocardial infarction, and arrhythmias—and, in some instances, death—have been reported in patients in whom beta-blocker therapy was abruptly halted. Recently, exacerbation of silent myocardial ischemia has been observed after abrupt cessation of beta-blocker therapy. Double-

TABLE 38-4 Drug Interactions That May Occur With β-Blocking Drugs

| Drug | Possible effects | Precautions |
|------|------------------|-------------|
| Aluminum hydroxide gel | Decreases β-blocker absorption and therapeutic effect | Avoid β blocker–aluminum hydroxide combination |
| Aminophylline | Mutual inhibition | Observe patient's response |
| Amiodarone | Cardiac arrest | Combination should be used with caution |
| Antidiabetic agents | Enhanced hypoglycemia; hypertension | Monitor for altered diabetic response |
| Calcium channel inhibitors (e.g., verapamil, diltiazem) | Potentiation of bradycardia, myocardial depression, and hypotension | Avoid use, although few patients show ill effects |
| Cimetidine | Prolongs half-life of propranolol | Combination should be used with caution |
| Clonidine | Hypertension during clonidine withdrawal | Monitor for hypertensive response; withdraw β-blocker before withdrawing clonidine |
| Digitalis glycosides | Potentiation of bradycardia | Observe patient's response; interactions may benefit angina patients with abnormal ventricular function |
| Epinephrine | Hypertension; bradycardia | Administer epinephrine cautiously; cardioselective β blocker may be safer |
| Ergot alkaloids | Excessive vasoconstriction | Observe patient's response; few patients show ill effects |
| Glucagon | Inhibition of hyperglycemic effect | Monitor for reduced response |
| Halofenate | Reduced β-blocking activity; production of propranolol withdrawal rebound syndrome | Observe for impaired response to β blockade |
| Indomethacin | Inhibition of antihypertensive response to β blockade | Observe patient's response |

| | | |
|---|---|---|
| Isoproterenol | Mutual inhibition | Avoid concurrent use or choose cardioselective β blocker |
| Levodopa | Antagonism of levodopa's hypotensive and positive inotropic effects | Monitor for altered response; interaction may have favorable results |
| Lidocaine | Propranolol pre-treatment increases lidocaine blood levels and potential toxicity | Combination should be used with caution; use lower doses of lidocaine |
| Methyldopa | Hypertension during stress | Monitor for hypertensive episodes |
| Monamine oxidase inhibitors | Uncertain, theoretical | Manufacturer of propranolol considers concurrent use contraindicated |
| Phenothiazines | Additive hypotensive effects | Monitor for altered response especially with high doses of phenothiazine |
| Phenylpro-pranolamine | Severe hypertensive reaction | Avoid use, especially in hypertension controlled by both methyldopa and β blockers |
| Phenytoin | Additive cardiac depressant effects | Administer IV phenytoin with great caution |
| Quinidine | Additive cardiac depressant effects | Observe patient's response; few patients show ill effects |
| Reserpine | Excessive sympathetic blockade | Observe patient's response |
| Tricyclic antidepressants | Inhibits negative inotropic and chronotropic effects of β blockers | Observe patient's response |
| Tubocurarine | Enhanced neuromuscular blockade | Observe response in surgical patients, especially after high doses of propranolol |

blind controlled trials have also confirmed the existence of a true beta-blocker withdrawal reaction. Thus, patients on chronic beta-blocker therapy should be tapered off of this therapy slowly and observed closely.

## CLINICAL USE AND DRUG INTERACTIONS

Situations in which particular beta blockers or beta-blocker subclasses should be used are shown in Table 38-3. The common drug interactions with beta-blockers are shown in Table 38-4.

## SUGGESTED READING

Frishman WH: β-Adrenergic blockade in the treatment of coronary artery disease, in Hurst JW (ed): *Clinical Essays on the Heart,* vol. II. New York, McGraw-Hill, pp 25–63, 1984.

Frishman WH: *Clinical Pharmacology of the Beta-Adrenoceptor Blocking Drugs,* 2d ed. New York, Appleton-Century-Crofts, 1984.

Frishman WH: β-Adrenergic blockers. *Med Clin North Am* 72(1):37–81, 1988.

Frishman WH, Skolnick AE, Lazar EJ, et al: β-Adrenergic blockade and calcium-channel blockade in myocardial infarction. *Med Clin North Am* 73(2):409–36, 1989.

Frishman WH, Sonnenblick EH: Beta-adrenergic blocking drugs, in Hurst JW et al (eds): *The Heart,* 7th ed. New York, McGraw-Hill, Chap 96, pp 1712–1730, 1990.

*39* | Calcium Antagonists

*William H. Frishman, M.D.*
*Eliot J. Lazar, M.D.*

## INTRODUCTION

There are three main classes of calcium antagonists available today. *Nifedipine* and *nicardipine* represent the dihydropyridines, *diltiazem* the benzothiazepines, and *verapamil* the papaverine-like agents. Unlike the beta-adrenergic blocking drugs, calcium antagonists differ from one another in structure. The predominant effect of these agents is on the slow channels of the cell membrane; their exact mechanisms of action vary considerably. In addition to their membrane effects calcium channel blockers can inhibit the availability of calcium ions for excitation coupling at intracellular sites.

## CARDIOVASCULAR EFFECTS (Tables 39-1, 39-2)

Calcium antagonists inhibit contraction of vascular smooth muscle and, to a lesser extent, of cardiac and skeletal muscle. This differential effect is due to the greater reliance of vascular smooth muscle on external calcium entry. Cardiac and skeletal muscle tissues rely on recirculating internal calcium stores. This allows for dilatation of arterial smooth muscle with less effect on myocardial contractility and virtually no effect on skeletal muscle. The calcium antagonists are less active on venous smooth muscle, and at therapeutic doses are ineffective for decreasing venous capacitance.

All calcium antagonists exert some degree of negative inotropic effect, which appears to be dose-dependent. Since the excitation-contraction coupling in smooth muscle is 3 to 10 times more sensitive to the action of calcium antagonists than that in myocardial fibers, the usual therapeutic doses may not produce significant negative inotropic effects. Additionally, the negative inotropic effect may be attenuated by the reflex augmentation of beta-adrenergic tone that accompanies arterial vasodilatation. However, this mechanism is unlikely to help patients with significantly impaired left ventricular function in whom the baroreceptor reflex is markedly attenuated.

## ELECTROPHYSIOLOGICAL EFFECTS

The three classes of calcium antagonists differ somewhat in their effects on the cardiac conduction system. Verapamil and diltiazem

**309**

**TABLE 39-1 Pharmacological Effects of the Calcium Antagonists**

| | Heart rate | | Conduction | | Myocardial contractility | Peripheral vasodilator | Cardiac output | Coronary blood flow | Myocardial O₂ demand |
|---|---|---|---|---|---|---|---|---|---|
| | Acute | Chronic | SA node | AV node | | | | | |
| Diltiazem | ↑ | ↑ | ↓ | ↓ | ↓ | ↑↑ | V | ↑ | ↓ |
| Verapamil | ↑ | ↑ | ↓ | ↓ | ↓↓ | ↑↑ | V | ↑ | ↓ |
| Amlodipine | ↑ | — | — | — | ↑ | ↑↑ | ↓ | ↑ | ↓ |
| Isradipine | ↑ | ↑ | — | — | — | ↑↑ | ↓ | ↑ | ↓ |
| Nifedipine | ↑ | ↓ | — | ↑ | ↓ | ↑↑ | ↓ | ↑ | ↓ |
| Nicardipine | ↑ | ↓ | — | ↑ | — | ↑↑ | ↓ | ↑ | ↓ |
| Nitrendipine | ↑ | — | — | ↑ | — | ↑↑ | ↓ | ↑ | ↓ |

*Note:* ↑ = increase; ↓ = decrease; — = no change; V = variable; SA = sinatrial; AV = atrioventricular.
*Source:* Frishman WH et al. Calcium-channel blockers in systemic hypertension. *Med Clin North Am* 72:454, 1988. Reproduced with permission from the publisher and authors.

prolong conduction and refractoriness in the atrioventricular (AV) and sinoatrial (SA) node. Sinus node discharge rates are depressed by all calcium antagonists. However, clinically this effect may be compensated for by baroreceptor reflexes, particularly with short-acting dihydropyridines.

## CLINICAL APPLICATIONS (Table 39-3)

Currently there are four calcium antagonists available in the United States. A host of others have been submitted for approval or are undergoing clinical trials.

The antianginal action of these agents appears to be multifactorial. These drugs exert vasodilator effects on the coronary and peripheral vessels, in addition to their mild effects on contractility. They are particularly effective in coronary spasm. Calcium antagonists seem to be as effective as beta blockers in controlling chronic stable angina pectoris and combined angina pectoris/hypertension, when used as monotherapy. However, there may be some limitations when short-acting dihydropyridines are used, because of the reflex tachycardia that sometimes occurs. Combination therapy with nitrates and/or beta blockers may be more efficacious than monotherapy. Because adverse effects can occur with combination therapy, patients must be carefully selected and monitored.

Verapamil has been widely used for atrial fibrillation and flutter, and for paroxysmal supraventricular tachycardia. In atrial fibrillation the predominant effect is reduction of ventricular response, rather than conversion to normal sinus rhythm. Diltiazem has been studied recently in these settings, but is not yet approved as routine therapy. One caution should be remembered in dealing with wide-complex tachyarrhythmias: *If there is any question about the origin of the rhythm, it should be treated as ventricular in origin.* A number of adverse outcomes have been reported when verapamil was used for presumed supraventricular tachycardia with aberrancy that turned out, in fact, to be ventricular tachycardia.

Calcium antagonists are effective in treating systemic hypertension and are now considered a first-line drug option along with diuretics, beta blockers, and ACE inhibitors. Calcium antagonists are effective in reducing both systolic and diastolic blood pressures, and have been found to be effective in blacks and in the elderly. They have also been shown to cause regression of left ventricular hypertrophy.

Other conditions in which calcium antagonists have been used include hypertensive emergencies, silent myocardial ischemia, and hypertrophic cardiomyopathy, although FDA approval has not been granted for these indications. Calcium antagonists have also

TABLE 39-2 Clinical Use of Calcium Antagonists

| | Dosage | | Onset of action | | Therapeutic plasma concentration | Site of metabolism | Active metabolites | Excretion, % |
|---|---|---|---|---|---|---|---|---|
| | Oral | IV | Oral | IV | | | | |
| Diltiazem | 30–90 mg q 6–8 h | 75–150 μg/kg (10–20 mg) | <30 min | <10 min | 50–200 ng/ml | Deacetylation N-demethylation O-demethylation Major hepatic first-pass effect | No | 60 fecal |
| Diltiazem SR | 60–80 mg q 12 h | | | | | | No | |
| Verapamil | 80–120 mg q 6–12 h | 150 μg/kg (10–20 mg) | <30 min | <5 min | >100 ng/ml | N-dealkylation N-demethylation Major hepatic first-pass effect | Yes | 15 fecal 70 renal |
| Verapamil SR | 240–280 mg q 12 or 24 h | | <30 min | | >50 ng/ml | | Yes | 15 fecal 70 renal |
| Amlodipine | 5–10 mg | | <30 min | | | Oxidation Major hepatic first-pass effect | No | 60 renal |

| | | | | | | | |
|---|---|---|---|---|---|---|---|
| Isradipine | 2.5–20 mg q 12 h | | <20 min | 1–10 ng/ml | Oxidation Major hepatic first-pass effect | No | 65 renal 35 fecal |
| Nifedipine | 10–40 mg q 6–8 h | 5–15 µg/kg | <20 min — (3 min sl) | 25–100 ng/ml | A hydroxycarboxylic acid and a lactone with no known activity; major hepatic first-pass effect | No | 20–40 fecal 50–80 renal |
| Nifedipine-GITS | 30–120 mg q 24 h | | | | | No | |
| Nicardipine | 10–20 mg tid | 1.15 mg/h | <20 min <5 min | 28–50 ng/ml | Major hepatic first-pass effect | No | 35 fecal 60 renal |
| Nitrendipine | 20–40 mg (once or twice daily) | | <60 min | 12–16 ng/ml | Major hepatic first-pass effect | No | 15 renal 77 fecal |

*Note:* tid = three times daily; sl = sublingual.
*Source:* Frishman WH et al: Calcium-channel blockers in systemic hypertension. *Med Clin North Am* 72:487, 1988. Reproduced with permission from the publisher and authors.

TABLE 39-3 Cardiovascular Uses of Calcium Antagonists

| |
|---|
| Angina pectoris* |
|   Effort angina |
|   "Rest" angina |
|   Prinzmetal's variant |
| Arrhythmia treatment and prophylaxis* (acute and chronic)— verapamil |
| Systemic hypertension*—verapamil, diltiazem SR, nifedipine GITS |
| Hypertensive emergencies*—nicardipine |
| Hypertrophic cardiomyopathy—verapamil, nicardipine, diltiazem |
| Congestive heart failure—nifedipine |
| Myocardial infarction (containing size of infarct) |
| Myocardial infarction (prevention Q-wave infarcts in non-Q-wave infarctions)—diltiazem |
| Primary pulmonary hypertension—nifedipine |
| Peripheral vascular disease |
|   Raynaud's phenomenon |
|   Intermittent claudication |
|   Cerebral arterial spasm* (subarachnoid hemorrhage)— nimodipine |
|   Stroke—nimodipine |
|   Mesenteric insufficiency |
|   Migraine headache prophylaxis—nimodipine |
| Deacceleration of atherosclerosis |
| Prevention of cardiomyopathy |

\* Use approved by the Food and Drug Administration.

been studied in use against congestive heart failure and primary pulmonary hypertension; however, current data suggest that they should not be used as routine therapy in these conditions.

## ADVERSE EFFECTS (Table 39-4)

Besides their expected effects on the cardiovascular system, these drugs have a wide array of side effects. Nifedipine has a fairly high incidence of minor side effects; major side effects are far less common. The most frequent side effects reported with nifedipine include headache, pedal edema, flushing, parasthesias, and dizziness. More serious side effects include exacerbation of ischemic symptoms and hypotension. These effects appear to be less common with the new long-acting form of nifedipine (nifedipine GITS). Diltiazem and verapamil can potentiate conduction system dysfunction. The most common adverse effect with verapamil is constipation, which can be especially problematic in older patients. Exacerbation of congestive heart failure can also be seen with verapamil, especially with concomitant beta-blocker therapy. *Combinations of verapamil and beta blockers should be used only with*

TABLE 39-4 Adverse Effects of the Calcium Antagonists

| | Overall % | Head-ache | Dizzi-ness | GI | Flush-ing | Paras-thesia | Decreased SA and/or AV con-duction | CHF | Hypo-tension | Pedal edema | Worsen-ing of angina |
|---|---|---|---|---|---|---|---|---|---|---|---|
| Diltiazem | ≈5 | + | + | + | + | 0 | 3+ | + | + | + | 0 |
| Diltiazem SR | ≈5 | + | + | + | + | 0 | 3+ | + | + | + | 0 |
| Verapamil | 8 | + | + | 3+ | 0 | 0 | 3+ | 2+ | + | + | 0 |
| Verapamil SR | ≈8 | + | + | 3+ | 0 | 0 | 3+ | 2+ | + | + | 0 |
| Amlodipine | ≈15 | 2+ | + | + | + | + | 0 | 0 | + | 2+ | 0 |
| Isradipine | ≈15 | 2+ | 2+ | + | + | + | 0 | 0 | + | 2+ | 0 |
| Nifedipine | ≈20 | 3+ | 3+ | + | 3+ | + | 0 | + | + | 2+ | + |
| Nifedipine-GITS | ≈10 | + | + | + | + | + | 0 | + | + | + | 0 |
| Nicardipine | ≈20 | 3+ | 3+ | + | 3+ | + | 0 | 0 | + | 2+ | + |
| Nitrendipine | ≈20 | 2+ | + | + | 2+ | + | 0 | + | + | + | + |

Note: GI = gastrointestinal; SA = sinoatrial node; AV = atrioventricular node; CHF = congestive heart failure; 0 = no report; + = rare; 2+ = occasional; 3+ = frequent.

Source: Frishman WH et al: Calcium-channel blockers in systemic hypertension. Med Clin North Am 72:488, 1988. Reproduced with permission from the publisher and authors.

*extreme caution.* Diltiazem can cause headache and gastrointestinal complaints in addition to cardiovascular side effects. The calcium antagonists have the potential for exacerbating heart failure.

## DRUG WITHDRAWAL AND OVERDOSE

Although serious problems have been reported with abrupt withdrawal of beta blockers, current experience with the calcium antagonists does not suggest any rebound or overshoot phenomenon. There may be a return of symptoms, however, when therapy is discontinued.

The effects seen with calcium-antagonist overdosage are those expected, based on the physiological action of the drugs. Hypotension, heart block, and left ventricular dysfunction are among the major complications.

## DRUG INTERACTIONS

A number of drug interactions have been reported with the available calcium antagonists. Both nifedipine and verapamil have been reported to increase serum digoxin levels. Verapamil has been reported to increase serum digoxin levels by as much as 70 percent, by decreasing renal and nonrenal clearance as well as the volume of distribution. Nifedipine causes smaller increases. Verapamil bioavailability is decreased by rifampin. The latter causes an increase in first-pass hepatic metabolism. Verapamil and diltiazem may have additive effects on AV conduction. Combinations of beta blockers with nifedipine or verapamil have been studied in patients with angina pectoris; care must be taken with these combinations because of the potential for impairment of left ventricular function, especially in patients with abnormal function at baseline.

## CONCLUSION

Although calcium antagonists are linked by the common trait of inhibition of calcium transport into the cell, their mechanisms of action differ. This results in different actions at the various target organs; these differences allow the clinician to select the agent most appropriate to a given clinical situation.

## SUGGESTED READING

Frishman WH, Lazar E: Calcium channel blockers in patients with both hypertension and angina pectoris. *J Cardiovasc Pharmacol* 12(suppl 6):S69–74, 1988.

Frishman WH, Sonnenblick EH: Calcium channel blockers, in Hurst JW et al (eds): *The Heart,* 7th ed. New York, McGraw-Hill, Chap 97, 1731–1748, 1990.

Frishman WH, Stroh JA, Greenberg S, et al: Calcium channel blockers in systemic hypertension. *Med Clin North Am* 72(2):449–499, 1989.

Skolnick AE, Frishman WH: Calcium-channel blockers in myocardial infarction. *Arch Intern Med* 149(7):1669–1677, 1989.

Strom JA, Frishman WH, Klein NA, et al: Non-invasive assessment of left ventricular size and performance in patients with coronary artery disease treated with oral verapamil and propranolol, in Packer M, Frishman WH (eds): *Clinical Pharmacology of the Calcium-Entry Blocking Drugs.* Norwalk, Appleton-Century-Crofts, p 129, 1984.

Weiner DA: Calcium channel blockers. *Med Clin North Am* 72(1):83–115, 1988.

## 40 | Digitalis

*Frank I. Marcus, M.D.*

The term *digitalis* is used to designate the entire class of cardiac glycosides. The most commonly used cardiac glycoside is *digoxin*.

## PHARMACOKINETICS OF DIGOXIN

### Bioavailability

Digoxin is about 70-percent absorbed when given in tablet form, but is almost completely absorbed when given as an encapsulated liquid concentrate (Lanoxicaps).

### Protein Binding and Metabolism

About 20 to 30 percent of digoxin is protein-bound. The highest concentration is found in the kidney, the next highest in cardiac muscle. The concentration of digoxin in skeletal muscle is less; but since skeletal muscle represents approximately 40 percent of the body's weight, digoxin is distributed principally to this tissue. About 60 percent of digoxin is excreted in the urine, mostly in unchanged form.

## FACTORS THAT INFLUENCE DIGOXIN PHARMACOKINETICS

### Bioavailability

In fewer than 10 percent of subjects, digoxin may undergo extensive biotransformation, by intestinal bacteria, into dihydrometabolites that are much less potent. These patients may require higher-than-usual doses of digoxin to obtain therapeutic serum concentrations of the drug. This type of metabolism may be suspected if a patient requires a high maintenance dose. Prescription of the highly bioavailable capsule form can minimize metabolic inactivation by bacteria, presumably by permitting complete absorption in the more proximal portions of the gut. Abrupt changes in gut flora, such as may occur with antibiotic treatment, can markedly enhance digoxin absorption and cause digitalis toxicity.

### Infants and Children

Infants and children require larger doses of digoxin, as calculated on the basis of body weight or surface area, than do adults to achieve similar serum concentrations of digoxin. This may be due in part to the more rapid elimination half-life of digoxin in children. (This short half-life is not found in neonates.) Infants and children appear to tolerate higher serum concentrations of digoxin without developing tachyarrhythmias, but atrioventricular dissociation or heart block may occur at these higher serum concentrations.

### Elderly Patients

The loading dose and maintenance dose of digoxin need to be reduced in the elderly. This is due to a decrease in the apparent volume of distribution—principally a function of decreased skeletal muscle mass, as well as an age-related decrease in the renal clearance of digoxin.

### Obesity

The dosage of digoxin should be calculated on the basis of *lean body mass* rather than on total body weight, since the concentration of digoxin in fatty tissue is quite low.

### Renal Failure

Impaired kidney function is the most important condition that influences digoxin pharmacokinetics, since digoxin is excreted primarily by the kidneys. Patients with renal failure have a decrease in digoxin clearance, with a consequent increase in the drug's elimination half-life; they require smaller doses. Further, there is a 35- to 50-percent decrease in the apparent volume of distribution of digoxin in subjects with severe renal insufficiency. Thus a smaller-than-usual loading dose should be given to any patient with severe renal insufficiency.

### Hepatic Failure

The pharmacokinetics of digoxin are not significantly altered in patients with acute hepatitis, nor in patients with chronic liver disease due to alcoholic cirrhosis.

### Hypo- and Hyperthyroidism

Serum digoxin levels are lower in patients with hyperthyroidism, and higher in hypothyroid patients, than in euthyroid patients.

## PHARMACOLOGICAL ACTIONS

By its inotropic effect, digitalis improves the circulation in patients with heart failure. This inotropic effect can be demonstrated in both normal and abnormal myocardium. Digitalis also has a parasympathetic effect and causes a diminution of the sympathetic effect on the heart. Finally, it has direct arterial vasoconstrictive action.

## Inotropic Effect

The inotropic effects of digitalis glycosides result from binding to, and inhibition of, Na-K-ATPase of various tissues, including the heart. The glycoside-induced inhibition of Na-K-ATPase produces a chain of events that makes more calcium available to contractile elements, thus enhancing the force of myocardial contraction.

## Enhancement of Parasympathetic Activity

This effect is due to enhanced sensitivity of the arterial baroreceptor reflex: efferent signals are augmented, resulting in increased vagal, and decreased sympathetic, efferent activity. Digitalis also acts centrally to enhance efferent vagal signals. In addition, digitalis may increase the sensitivity of cardiac fibers to the actions of acetylcholine. These parasympathomimetic effects are primarily responsible for the therapeutic efficacy of digitalis in the treatment of supraventricular arrhythmias.

## Diminution of Sympathetic Activity

Through sensitization of the baroreceptor reflexes, digitalis causes a decrease in efferent sympathetic activity. This contributes to the slight slowing of sinus rate and prolongation of the AV nodal refractory period.

## Direct Vasoconstrictor Effect

Digitalis induces a state of contraction in isolated human arteries and veins that is not diminished by alpha-adrenoreceptor blockade but is abolished by a calcium antagonist. The vasoconstrictor effects of intravenous digitalis can result in an increase in systemic resistance, which can worsen congestive heart failure—particularly when the digitalis is given as a bolus.

## ELECTROPHYSIOLOGICAL EFFECTS OF DIGITALIS

The most important electrophysiological properties that relate to the use of digitalis for the treatment of supraventricular arrhythmias are indirect. They depend on vagal and antiadrenergic neural mechanisms.

## Sinoatrial Node

The administration of digitalis to patients with ventricular failure often results in a slowing of the sinus rate. This is largely due to the inotropic effect of digitalis. With improvement of ventricular performance there is a decrease in sympathetic tone. Digitalis should be used with caution in patients with sick sinus syndrome, since it may accentuate symptoms by an increase in the duration of sinus pauses. If digitalis is used in these patients, 24-h ambulatory ECG recordings should be done before and after digitalis administration to determine whether the drug is having an adverse effect.

## Atrium and Atrioventricular (AV) Node

Therapeutic concentrations of digitalis have a predominant vagal action that results in a shortening of the atrial effective refractory period and acceleration of conduction. Digitalis causes a prolongation of conduction and an increase in the refractory periods of the AV node. These effects are predominantly due to the vagal and antiadrenergic influence of digitalis. The cardiac glycosides increase the effective refractory periods of both the fast and slow AV nodal pathways in the anterograde direction. The effect of digitalis on retrograde conduction in the AV node and on the refractory period of VA conduction is variable.

## Purkinje Fibers, Ventricular Muscle, and Accessory Pathways

In therapeutic concentrations digitalis shortens the effective refractory period in the ventricle. It has a variable effect on the anterograde effective refractory period of the accessory pathway in the Wolff-Parkinson-White syndrome. The retrograde effective refractory period of the accessory pathway generally is not affected by digitalis.

## USES OF DIGITALIS

Digitalis has two major uses. One is in the treatment of congestive heart failure; the other is in the treatment and prevention of supraventricular arrhythmias.

## Treatment of Congestive Heart Failure (See Chapter 1)

The signs and symptoms of acute severe congestive heart failure are most rapidly relieved by intravenous diuretic therapy. However, when intravenous digoxin is given to patients treated with diuretics and/or systemic vasodilators, the left ventricular ejection fraction and cardiac index may increase. This may be accompanied by a decrease in mean pulmonary capillary wedge pressure. Therefore, administration of digoxin can further improve cardiac function in patients with persistence of abnormal hemodynamic variables after diuretic and/or vasodilator treatment for congestive heart failure. The effect of digoxin in combination with the ACE inhibitor captopril has been evaluated in patients with severe heart failure. This combination was found to have an additive beneficial effect on cardiac function at rest and during exercise. Recently there have been reports of multicenter trials comparing treatment with digoxin to placebo and/or an ace inhibitor (captopril or enalapril) or the phosphodiesterase inhibitor milrinone in patients with congestive heart failure in sinus rhythm. In the studies in which digoxin was compared with placebo, digoxin was shown to be effective in markedly reducing the frequency of decompensation from heart failure and increasing the exercise time. In one study, patients treated with digoxin had an increase in left ventricular ejection fraction. Also, patients assigned to the placebo and maintained on a diuretic alone had significantly more episodes of manifest heart failure, as evidenced by visits to the emergency room or hospitalization for heart failure, than the digoxin-treated group. In none of the trials with ACE inhibitors or milrinone were these drugs found to be superior to digoxin for the treatment of heart failure. Hence the place of digitalis in the treatment of heart failure seems assured. One must, however, be alert to the fact that an appreciable number of patients with signs and symptoms of heart failure may have circulatory failure because of isolated diastolic dysfunction; digitalis is not likely to help these patients. They may be identified by normal left ventricular ejection fraction in the presence of congestive heart failure.

### Possible Enhanced Mortality in Patients on Chronic Digitalis Therapy After Myocardial Infarction

Although it has been reported that there is an increase in mortality associated with digoxin therapy after myocardial infarction, even after adjustment for major cardiac covariants such as left ventricular ejection fraction and ventricular ectopic beat frequency, this finding has not been confirmed. However, the possibility of increased mortality associated with digitalis after acute myocardial infarction should cause the physician to evaluate carefully the need for digitalis therapy, particularly within the first year after mycardial infarction.

### TREATMENT OF ARRHYTHMIAS (See Chapter 3)

#### Paroxysmal Supraventricular Tachycardia

Most paroxysmal supraventricular tachycardias (PSVTs) in adults are due to reentry involving the AV node or a pathway adjacent to it. Digitalis may prevent supraventricular tachycardia by lengthening the effective and functional refractory period of the AV node and AV nodal transmission time. This effect is primarily on the anterograde limb of the circuit. By this effect digitalis can terminate paroxysmal AV nodal reentrant tachycardia. Digitalis, alone or in combination with beta blockers or calcium antagonists, is useful in preventing recurrences of PSVT.

## Atrial Fibrillation or Flutter

Digoxin does not appear to convert recent-onset atrial fibrillation in patients without heart failure; nor does digoxin alone prevent recurrence of atrial fibrillation in most patients with paroxysmal atrial fibrillation. However, it is useful in decreasing the ventricular rate at rest and during moderate exercise, through two pharmacological actions: (1) it increases the refractory period of the AV node; and (2) it shortens the refractory period of the atrial myocardium through both direct and indirect effects. A decrease in the refractory period of the atrial myocardium results in more atrial impulses reaching the AV junction in a given length of time. This results in a greater degree of concealed conduction in the AV node and, thus, in a slower ventricular rate. Digitalis is the only drug that causes an increase in the refractory period of the AV node as well as an increase in concealed conduction within the AV node. Therefore, digitalis is useful for the treatment of patients with sustained atrial fibrillation. Addition of the calcium antagonist diltiazem or verapamil, or beta-blocking agents, may be useful when the ventricular rate is difficult to control by digitalis alone.

## Multifocal Atrial Tachycardia

Digitalis generally is not effective either in abolishing this rhythm or in slowing the ventricular response. In addition, since this arrhythmia is usually associated with severe obstructive pulmonary disease, a condition in which there is increased sensitivity to digitalis toxicity, digitalis should be avoided for the treatment of multifocal atrial tachycardia unless there is concomitant congestive heart failure.

## Arrhythmias in Wolff-Parkinson-White (WPW) Syndrome

Patients with WPW syndrome may have a narrow-complex regular tachycardia known as *orthodromic reciprocating tachycardia* or *orthodromic circus movement tachycardia*. This arrhythmia is characterized by anterograde conduction through the AV node and retrograde conduction by the accessory pathway. Digitalis is useful in a minority of patients who have this type of tachycardia; and its action is entirely by its effects on the AV node. Rarely the reentrant circuit travels in the opposite direction, with anterograde conduction over the accessory pathway and retrograde conduction over the AV node. This is referred to as *antidromic circus movement tachycardia.* Atrial fibrillation or atrial flutter may develop in patients with WPW syndrome and may be hazardous if there is a rapid ventricular rate. Since the electrical impulses are conducted anterogradely over the accessory pathway, the QRS complexes are wide, and the rhythm is irregular. A rapid ventricular response can lead to ventricular fibrillation. Digitalis can increase the ventricular rate through the accessory pathway and may actually precipitate ventricular fibrillation and sudden death. Most of these patients have short RR intervals (220 ms or less) during atrial fibrillation before digitalis is given. For this reason, it is suggested that digitalis not be used in patients with WPW syndrome. If it must be used, an electrophysiological study should be performed before institution of long-term therapy.

## DIGOXIN DOSING

The usual oral maintenance dose in adults is 0.25 mg. In some younger patients, particularly those who have a large lean body mass, the dose may be 0.5 mg. The maintenance dose is 0.125 mg daily in the elderly or in patients with severe renal insufficiency. The dose of digoxin in the *encapsulated gel* form (Lanoxicaps), which has greater bioavailability, ranges from 0.1 to 0.4 mg per day. The average oral loading dose of digoxin ranges from 1.25 to 1.5 mg given in divided doses over a 24-h period. The oral loading dose for Lanoxicaps is 0.8 to 1.2 mg. *Intravenous doses* are approximately 70 percent of the recommended oral doses for the tablet form.

## DRUG INTERACTIONS WITH DIGOXIN

Serum levels of digoxin can be altered by coadministration of other medicines (Table 40-1). There are two broad categories of interactions: (1) those due to drugs that alter the absorption of digoxin, and (2) those due to drugs that primarily interfere with its elimination. Interactions of the first type usually reduce the serum concentration of digoxin by a modest degree. The second type of interaction can cause a marked increase in serum concentration of digoxin and can result in digoxin toxicity. For patients receiving drugs that may interact with digoxin there should be an appropriate alteration in dosage.

## DIGITALIS TOXICITY

Intoxication with digitalis continues to be a complication of therapy, because of its narrow toxic/therapeutic ratio. The signs and symptoms of digitalis toxicity are well known and include anorexia, fatigue, visual disturbances, and confusion.

In general, the therapeutic serum concentration of digoxin in adults is 1.0 to 2.0 ng/ml. Serum levels of digoxin are helpful in confirming the clinical suspicion of digitalis toxicity, especially if the serum digoxin level is greater than 3.0 ng/ml. If the serum digoxin level is less than 1.5 ng/ml in a patient who does not have hypokalemia and who has been thought to have digoxin toxicity, another explanation for the patient's symptoms should be sought.

Digitalis-induced arrhythmias may be due to the drug's parasympathomimetic effects on the heart and to the effects related to enhanced ectopy. Signs of increased vagal effect include sinus bradycardia, SA exit block, and AV nodal block, usually of the Wenckebach type. Examples of digitalis-induced ectopy include premature atrial contraction, junctional tachycardia, and ventricular ectopic activity. Death, if it occurs, may be due to ventricular tachycardia and/or ventricular fibrillation. Ectopy may combine with signs of excessive vagal effects to produce the ECG pattern of atrial tachycardia with AV block, or of junctional tachycardia with AV block.

*Treatment* of digitalis toxicity depends on the seriousness of the arrhythmia. Correction of hypokalemia, together with cessation of digitalis, may be all that is needed to control digitalis-induced tachyarrhythmia. However, digitalis-induced severe bradycardia or complete heart block may require temporary pacemaker insertion. Atrial, junctional, or ventricular tachycardia may be treated with antiarrhythmic drugs. *Lidocaine* and *procainamide* can be used to treat digitalis-induced ventricular ectopy. Intravenous *diphenylhydantoin* can also be used. In general, quinidine should be avoided since it may raise serum digoxin levels. Beta blockers should be avoided for most patients with heart failure. Anecdotal case reports indicate that amiodarone, bretylium, and intravenous magnesium can suppress life-threatening arrhythmias due to digitalis intoxication. Administration of digoxin-specific Fab fragments has been extraordinarily successful in the treatment of digitalis intoxication manifested by serious arrhythmias. The Fab fragments can rapidly reverse digoxin-induced toxicity. The glycoside is bound to the Fab fragments and eliminated by the renal route. The major concern in using Fab fragments for non-life-threatening arrhythmias is that there is a potential for anaphylaxis if the patient requires a second administration of the antibody fragments. Administration of activated charcoal is an ancillary treatment for massive digoxin overdose.

TABLE 40-1 Pharmacokinetic Interactions with Digoxin

| Interfering drugs | Mean magnitude of interaction, %* | Mechanism of interaction | Suggested dose adjustments |
|---|---|---|---|
| *Drugs that alter absorption or bioavailability of digoxin* | | | |
| Antacid; bran | −25 | Unknown; ? adsorption of digoxin | Give digoxin 1–2 h before antacid or bran |
| Kaolin-pectin (Kaopectate) | −20 to −30 | Adsorption of digoxin | Give digoxin 1–2 h before kaolin-pectin |
| Cholestyramine (Questran) | −30 | Physical binding to resin | Avoid by dosing cholestyramine bid, 8 h from digoxin administration |
| Metoclopramide (Reglan) | −25 | ↓ Bioavailability by ↑ intestinal motility | (?) Administer digoxin as elixir or as Lanoxicaps |
| Propantheline (Pro-Banthine) | +25 | ↑ Bioavailability by ↓ intestinal motility | (?) Administer digoxin as elixir or as Lanoxicaps |
| Sulfasalazine (Azulfidine) | −20 | ↓ Bioavailability | |
| Erythromycin or tetracycline† | +43 to +150 | ↑ Bioavailability due to inactivation of gut flora | Measure serum digoxin level during coadministration of these antibiotics with digoxin |
| Neomycin | −28 | ↓ Bioavailability | Measure serum digoxin levels |
| Cancer chemotherapy | −50 | ↓ Bioavailability due to damage to intestinal mucosa | Measure serum digoxin levels |

| Drugs that interfere with elimination of digoxin | | | |
|---|---|---|---|
| Amiodarone (Cordarone) | +100 | ↓ In renal and total body clearance of digoxin | Reduce digoxin dose by one-half |
| Indomethacin (Indocin)‡ | +50 | ↓ Glomerular filtration | Reduce digoxin dose by one-fourth to one-half |
| Propafenone (Rhythmol) | +20 to +80 | ↓ Nonrenal clearance of digoxin | Reduce digoxin dose by one-fourth to one-half |
| Quinidine | +100 | ↑ (?) Absorption Vol. of distribution<br>↓ Renal and total body clearance of digoxin | Reduce digoxin dose by one-half |
| Quinine | +75 | ↓ Renal clearance of digoxin | Reduce digoxin dose by one-half |
| Verapamil | +75 | ↓ Renal and total body clearance of digoxin | Reduce digoxin dose by one-half |

\* For single-dose studies, the magnitude of the anticipated change in serum digoxin concentration was estimated from pharmacokinetic data, particularly the change in total body clearance.

† Expected to occur in 10% of patients—those who have substantial conversion of digoxin to dihydro-derivatives in the gut.

‡ Interaction only in premature infants.

## SUGGESTED READING

Antman EM, Smith TW: Current concepts in the use of digitalis. *Adv Intern Med* 34:425–454, 1989.

Marcus FI: Pharmacokinetic interactions between digoxin and other drugs. *J Am Coll Cardiol* 5:82A–90A, 1985.

Marcus FI, Huang SK: Digitalis, in Hurst JW et al (eds): *The Heart,* 7th ed. New York, McGraw-Hill, Chap 98, pp 1748–1761, 1990.

Smith TW: Digitalis: Mechanisms of action and clinical use. *N Engl J Med* 318:358–365, 1988.

Smith TW (ed): *Digitalis Glycosides.* Orlando, Grune and Stratton, 1986.

## 41 | Nonglycosidic Cardiotonic Agents

*Thierry H. LeJemtel, M.D.      Edmund H. Sonnenblick, M.D.*

Inotropic stimulation of the heart by a nonglycosidic cardiotonic agent may be indicated in two clinical situations which, from a pathophysiological point of view, differ greatly. In acute heart failure complicating myocardial infarction or coronary bypass surgery, the residual non-infarcted or stunned myocardium and the peripheral circulation are normally responsive to hormonal and metabolic alterations. The major aims of therapy are to increase cardiac output and reduce left ventricular filling pressure without exacerbating myocardial ischemia and tachycardia. In chronic end-stage heart failure, myocardial inotropic reserve is limited, and peripheral arterial resistance is increased and, to a certain extent, fixed. The profound abnormalities of the peripheral circulation are responsible for the symptoms of congestive heart failure and contribute to further reduction in left ventricular performance. Thus, the aim of therapy for chronic congestive heart failure is to reverse the abnormalities of the peripheral circulation without increasing pathological damage or inducing further ventricular arrhythmias.

Nonglycosidic cardiotonic agents can be classified in two major groups. The first includes the *catecholamines* (norepinephrine, dopamine) and their derivatives (dobutamine, isoproterenol). They are available only for parenteral use. The second group are the new specific *type-III phosphodiesterase inhibitors*. Some of these agents may, in addition, increase the affinity of the regulatory site of troponin C for $Ca^{2+}$, which may contribute to their positive inotropic effects. These newer inotropic agents, which are orally active, also produce direct peripheral arterial and venous vasodilatation, which in certain instances may be the predominant factor in improving cardiac performance. Thus specific phosphodiesterase inhibition, which leads to increased cyclic AMP levels in the cells, enhances contractility of the cardiac myocyte and relaxes the vascular smooth muscle. The prototype of the newer inotropic agents is *amrinone,* which, like dobutamine, is available only for parenteral use.

## CATECHOLAMINES AND THEIR DERIVATIVES

Dopamine is a naturally-occurring precursor of norepinephrine, and norepinephrine itself may be used to increase myocardial contractility. However, both dopamine in high doses and norepinephrine constrict the peripheral arterioles; this limits both drugs' usefulness. *Dobutamine,* which is a synthesized catecholamine derivative without vasoconstrictor activity, has become the most widely used parenteral inotropic agent. Endogenous catecholamines and dobutamine have different physiological actions that derive from their relative specificities for alpha- and beta-adrenoceptors (Table 41-1). Alpha receptors include alpha$_1$ receptors, which are post-synaptic and are located in the vascular smooth muscle or the myocardium. The smooth-muscle alpha$_1$ receptors are responsible for vasoconstriction. The alpha$_2$ receptors are mostly pre-synaptic and are responsible for reducing norepinephrine release in the peripheral nerve terminals and reducing sympathetic outflow in the central nervous system.

Beta-adrenergic receptors consist of beta$_1$ receptors, which are located in the myocardium and are responsible for positive inotropic, chronotropic, and dromotropic responses; and beta$_2$ receptors, which are located in the smooth muscles and mediate vasodilatation. Beta$_2$ receptors may also be located in the sinoatrial node, and may be responsible for positive chronotropy. In addition, there are specific dopaminergic receptors in the renal and mesenteric vascular beds that are responsible for arterial vasodilatation.

## Dobutamine

The synthesis of dobutamine resulted from systematic modification of the chemical structure of isoproterenol. It is generally accepted that dobutamine produces a potent positive inotropic action that is mediated through direct stimulation of beta$_1$-adrenergic receptors in the myocardium, which in turn increase cyclic AMP. Unlike dopamine, dobutamine does not stimulate the heart indirectly by releasing norepinephrine from the nerve endings. Dobutamine's relative lack of positive chronotropic effect is not well understood; it may result from specific stimulation of beta$_1$ receptors and/or alpha$_1$-myocardial receptors. Whatever its exact mechanism of action, dobutamine is the cardiotonic agent that exerts the most

TABLE 41-1  Receptor Activity of Sympathomimetic Amines

|  | $\alpha_1$ | $\beta_1$ | $\beta_2$ | Dopaminergic |
|---|---|---|---|---|
| Norepinephrine | 4 + | 4 + | 0 | 0 |
| Epinephrine | 4 + | 4 + | 2 + | 0 |
| Dopamine | 4 + | 2 + | + | 4 + |
| Isoproterenol | 0 | 4 + | 4 + | 0 |
| Dobutamine | 3 + | 4 + | 2 + | 0 |

potent inotropic action while producing limited effects on heart rate and blood pressure. The administration of dobutamine to patients with acute myocardial infarction and left ventricular dysfunction is safe and most often improves cardiac performance without obviously worsening myocardial ischemia. The rate of infusion of dobutamine should start at 2 μg/kg/min and be titrated upward to obtain maximal cardiac output while reducing left ventricular filling pressure, if these measurements are available. If not, heart rate and blood pressure should be closely monitored to prevent tachycardia and major changes in blood pressure. The most serious side effect of dobutamine is the precipitation of ventricular tachycardia, which may necessitate dose reduction or discontinuation of the drug. In chronic congestive heart failure, administration of dobutamine is useful either during acute decompensation or for intermittent inotropic support; this requires short-term hospitalization or use of a small portable infusion pump on an outpatient basis. Although patients with severe congestive heart failure have decreased density and affinity of myocardial beta-adrenergic receptors, most of them experience a hemodynamic and clinical improvement after administration of dobutamine. The fate of the beta receptors and their coupling with adenylate cyclase during long-term administration of dobutamine is unknown. The mechanisms of the prolonged clinical benefits of dobutamine after discontinuation of the infusion are also unknown. Concomitant infusion of dopamine at a dose of 1 to 2 μg/kg/min is useful to obtain dopaminergic renal arterial dilatation, thereby increasing renal blood flow and sodium excretion.

## PHOSPHODIESTERASE INHIBITORS

### Amrinone (Inocor)

At present, the parenteral form of amrinone is the only nonglycosidic, non-catecholamine cardiotonic agent approved by the Food and Drug Administration for use in congestive heart failure. Besides its positive inotropic action, which is at least partly mediated by specific type-III myocardial phosphodiesterase inhibition, amrinone has direct arteriolar and venous vasodilating properties. The peripheral vasodilatation induced by amrinone is also cyclic-AMP–mediated. However, the exact mechanisms by which rising levels of cyclic AMP promote relaxation of the vascular smooth-muscle cells are not fully understood. The arterial vasodilatation appears to occur preferentially in the limbs, and to a lesser extent in the kidneys.

Intravenous amrinone consistently increases cardiac output and reduces left ventricular filling pressure in patients with chronic congestive heart failure, without producing excessive changes in heart rate or systemic blood pressure. The changes in myocardial contractility, as evidenced by the rate of increase of left ventricular pressure, vary from patient to patient. Consequently, in patients experiencing minimal changes in myocardial contractility, arteriolar vasodilatation induced by amrinone contributes substantially to the improvement of left ventricular performance; thus these hemodynamic changes are often accompanied by a decrease in myocardial oxygen requirements.

*Therapy* with amrinone should be initiated with an intravenous bolus ranging from 0.75 to 3.0 mg/kg. This is followed by continuous infusion at a rate ranging from 4 to 10 μg/kg/min. In patients with severe renal insufficiency, the rate of infusion should be reduced to prevent toxic plasma levels of amrinone and potential adverse reactions, such as ventricular tachycardia and hypertension. An important therapeutic application of intravenous amrinone is its concomitant use with dobutamine. This may allow the use of a smaller dose of dobutamine, thus reducing the metabolic cost to the myocardium of increasing left ventricular performance. The beneficial effects of amrinone can also be equated to those of vasodilators. For example, angiotensin-converting enzyme (ACE) inhibitors preferentially benefit the renal circulation, while specific phosphodiesterase inhibition predominantly increases blood flow to the limbs. This argues for combined use of these agents.

*Short-term intravenous administration* of specific phosphodiesterase inhibitors (e.g., amrinone) most often has hemodynamic and clinical benefits in patients with acute and chronic congestive heart failure. The clinical benefits of long-term administration of these new agents in patients with chronic congestive heart failure has not yet been established.

## SUGGESTED READING

Colucci WS, Wright RF, Braunwald E: New positive inotropic agents in the treatment of congestive heart failure: Mechanisms of action and recent clinical developments. *N Engl J Med* 314:290–299, 349–358, 1986.

Colucci WS: Positive inotropic/vasodilator agents. *Cardiol Clin* 7:131–144, 1989.

Goldenberg IF, Cohn JN: New inotropic drugs for heart failure. JAMA 258:493–496, 1987.

LeJemtel TH, Sonnenblick EH: Nonglycosidic cardioactive agents, in Hurst JW et al (eds): *The Heart*, 7th ed. New York, McGraw-Hill, Chap 99, pp 1762–1766, 1990.

Sonnenblick EH, Frishman WH, LeJemtel TH: Dobutamine: A new synthetic cardioactive sympathetic amine. *N Engl J Med* 300:17–22, 1979.

## 42 | Diuretics

*Vera Delaney, M.D., Ph.D.*
*Edmund Bourke, M.D.*

A major consequence of heart failure is enhanced renal reabsorbtion of salt and water. Diuretics counteract this with mobilization and prevention of edema. They are also important in the control of hypertension.

### THIAZIDE DIURETICS AND THEIR COGENERS

These drugs are the mainstay of diuretic therapy. They differ in dose and duration of action (see Table 42-1), but all act predominantly by inhibition of NaCl cotransport in the distal convoluted tubule. The maximal fractional sodium excretion is 10 percent. The cogeners chlorthalidone and metolazone have the longest action, up to 48 h. Metolazone differs from the others in that it does not decrease the glomerular filtration rate (GFR) and is effective with a GFR below 20 ml/min.

Hypokalemia is the most common side effect. It often necessitates $K^+$ supplementation, but iatrogenic hyperkalemia should be avoided. Hyponatremia can be severe in a subset of patients, most often elderly females; generally it occurs within a week of administration and recurs on rechallenge. Contraction alkalosis, volume depletion, hypomagnesemia, hypercalcemia, glucose intolerance, and hyperuricemia may occur. Impotence, acute interstitial nephritis, hyperlipidemia, and lithium toxicity have been reported.

### LOOP DIURETICS

These are the most potent diuretics. Only three are in widespread use in the United States: furosemide, bumetanide, and, less often, ethacrynic acid. Their action has a rapid onset and is short-lived. In urgent settings, they are effective IV within 15 min. Their predominant mechanism of action is to inhibit Na-K-2Cl cotransport in the ascending limb of the loop of Henle. Maximal fractional sodium excretion is 20 percent. They are effective at low GFRs. Following IV use, they also induce venous dilatation, preload reduction, and a decrease in pulmonary congestion. Their action is additive with thiazides.

Severe hyponatremia and glucose intolerance are less common than with thiazides. Volume contraction is more readily induced, as is metabolic alkalosis. The same caution applies to hypokalemia

**333**

TABLE 42-1  Doses and Duration of Action of the Commonly Used Diuretics

| Type of agent | Generic name | Average daily dose (mg) | Duration of action (h) |
|---|---|---|---|
| Loop diuretics* | Ethacrynic acid | 25–150 | 4–6 |
| | Furosemide | 20–160 | 4–6 |
| | Bumetanide | 0.5–3 | 4–6 |
| Mgmt & related drugs | Chlorothiazide | 500–1500 | 6–12 |
| | Benzthiazide | 50–200 | 6–12 |
| | Hydroflumethiazide | 25–50 | 6–12 |
| | Bendroflumethiazide | 2.5–15 | 18–24 |
| | Hydrochlorothiazide | 50–150 | 12–24 |
| | Trichlormethiazide | 2–4 | 18–24 |
| | Methylclothiazide | 5–10 | 18–24 |
| | Polythiazide | 2–8 | 18–24 |
| | Cyclothiazide | 2–6 | 18–24 |
| | Chlorthalidone | 50–100 | 24–48 |
| | Quinethazone | 50–150 | 24–48 |
| | Metolazone* | 2.5–20 | 24–48 |
| Potassium-Ksparing diuretics | Spironolactone | 50–200 | 24 |
| | Triamterene | 100–200 | 6–8 |
| | Amiloride | 5–20 | 12–24 |

*The high doses of loop diuretics and metolazone are required mainly in patients with renal insufficiency.

as with the thiazides. Hypomagnesemia, hyperuricemia, and, rarely, acute interstitial nephritis have been reported. A usually reversible ototoxicity may complicate rapid IV use. These drugs may potentiate aminoglycoside nephrotoxicity. In contrast to the thiazides, they are calciuretic. Their action is impaired by nonsteroidal antiinflammatory agents.

## POTASSIUM-SPARING DIURETICS

These agents—amiloride, triamterene, and spironolactone—are weakly natriuretic, and most often are used as adjuncts. Their predominant action is to block the sodium channels in the cortical collecting tubule. Amiloride and triamterene do this directly. Spironolactone blocks the capacity of aldosterone to increase the activity of sodium channels. Its onset of action is slower than those of the other agents. Blocking sodium channels reduces luminal negativity and reduces $K^+$ movement into the urine, with $K^+$ sparing. Maximal fractional sodium excretion is 2 percent. The action of these drugs is additive to thiazide and loop diuretics; they modulate the kaliuresis of these agents.

They can induce hazardous hyperkalemia when combined with (1) potassium supplements; (2) drugs that may decrease potassium excretion, including nonsteroidals, beta blockers, and ACE inhibitors; or (3) impaired renal function. They may induce mild metabolic acidosis. Neither volume depletion, hyponatremia, hyperuricemia, hypomagnesemia, nor altered calcium or carbohydrate homeostasis is encountered. Gynecomastia, mastodynia, diminished libido, and irregular menses may complicate spironolactone therapy. Triamterene stones and megaloblastosis have been reported with triamterene.

## DIURETICS IN THE MANAGEMENT OF HYPERTENSION

The thiazides are a cornerstone of antihypertensive therapy. The average decrease in blood pressure is 21/10 mmHg, providing adequate control of many cases of mild hypertension. After an initial natriuresis, plasma volume is restored, but peripheral resistance is decreased by an unknown mechanism. These drugs also prevent the salt retention and pseudotolerence seen with some other antihypertensives. Lower doses (e.g., hydrochlorothiazide, 25–50 mg/day) are as effective as higher doses, with less hypokalemia. Furosemide is less effective in mild hypertension but has a role, particularly in chronic renal failure.

## DIURETICS IN THE MANAGEMENT OF CARDIAC FAILURE

In congestive heart failure diuretics act as secondary agents to mobilize edema and relieve dyspnea. A 2-gram sodium diet is recommended. Weight loss is the best proof of diuretic response. A thiazide is the initial drug of choice. Its combination with a potassium-sparing diuretic helps prevent hypokalemia. Secondary aldosteronism is not important in mild failure but may play a role in advanced cases, where addition of spironolactone may help. Overly vigorous diuresis decreases plasma volume and leads to prerenal azotemia. When intrinsic renal failure is present, loop diuretics are required, with increased doses in advanced cases.

In acute pulmonary edema, IV furosemide decreases cardiac preload and pulmonary congestion. This antedates natriuresis and may be mediated by a vasodilatory prostaglandin.

## DIURETICS IN REFRACTORY EDEMA

Refractory edema is present if an edematous patient is not losing weight on twice the conventional doses of loop diuretics, provided he or she is recumbent (to optimize renal hemodynamics) and the following are excluded: (1) surreptitious salt intake (if the urinary sodium exceeds 100meq/day without weight loss, intake is too high); (2) drugs that promote $Na^+$ retention (e.g., steroids, nonsteroidals, estrogens, and some antihypertensives); and (3) hypokalemia (this implies that the diuretic is blocking $Na^+$ reabsorbtion with increased delivery to the cortical collecting tubule, where its subsequent retention promotes potassium secretion, replacing the intended natriuresis). Addition of a potassium-sparing diuretic may reverse such refractoriness.

An edematous intestine may cause refractoriness, circumvented by IV diuretics. Intravenous albumin in refractory nephrotic or cirrhotic edema may restore diuretic responsiveness. Based on their sites of action, 24-h urinary $Na^+$ and $K^+$ excretions are helpful in deciding the choice, dose, and combination of diuretics to use. Furosemide, which acts on the ascending limb, plus metolazone, which acts on the distal convoluted tubule, plus spironolactone, which acts on the cortical collecting tubule, may be very effective when none of these drugs is effective alone. Such combinations should be used stepwise, to prevent dangerous overdiuresis. Finally, peritoneal dialysis or hemofiltration may restore diuretic responsiveness in some patients.

## SUGGESTED READING

Delaney V, Bourke E: Diuretics, in Hurst JW et al (eds): *The Heart,* 7th ed. New York, McGraw-Hill, Chap 100, pp 1767–1780, 1990.

Puschett JB, Greenberg A (eds): *Diuretics: II Chemistry, Pharmacology and Clinical Applications.* New York, Elsevier, 1987.

Lant AF: Diuretic drugs: Progress in clinical pharmacology. *Drugs* 31(suppl 4):40–55, 1986.

Sica DA, Gehr T: Diuretics in congestive heart failure. *Cardiol Clin* 7:87–97, 1989.

Anticoagulants, Antiplatelet Drugs, and Thrombolytic Agents

R. Verhaeghe, M.D.
M. Verstraete, M.D.

## HEPARIN

### Pharmacology

Heparin consists of a mixture of sulphated polysaccharides (molecular weight from 6000 to 30,000); by complexing with antithrombin III, it becomes a potent inhibitor of serine proteases, particularly of thrombin and factor Xa. Its short half-life (90 min) varies widely (extremes: 23 and 360 min) and is dose-dependent. Clearance is enhanced in pulmonary embolism and retarded in hepatic and renal failure. Heparin is administered intravenously or subcutaneously, is not absorbed orally, does not cross the placental barrier, and is not excreted in breast milk.

Low-molecular-weight (LMW) heparin refers to all fractions of heparin with a molecular weight below 8000. Many characteristics, including molecular size and affinity for antithrombin III, vary between available preparations of LMW heparins. Their biological half-life is longer than that of unfractionated heparin.

With "therapeutic" heparinization, the desired range of activated partial thromboplastin time (PTT) is 1.5 to 2.5 times control.

### Adverse Effects and Their Treatment

Bleeding is the major complication; its incidence is higher in women ($\times 2$) and increases with age ($\times 3$ over 60 years), underlying morbidity ($\times 4$), and alcoholism ($\times 7$). LMW heparins are associated with less bleeding. Thrombocytopenia occurs in about 1 percent of patients and is reversible after stopping the drug. Prolonged therapy with full doses may lead to osteoporosis (not until after 6 months). Antithrombin III depletion and hyperkalemia are rare.

## ORAL ANTICOAGULANTS

Oral anticoagulants (warfarin was the first synthesized) are vitamin K antagonists. They inhibit the gamma-carboxylation of glutamic acid residues in the $NH_2$-terminal end of factors II, VIII, IX, and X and of proteins C and S; in this way they hamper the binding of these proteins, via calcium ions, to phospholipids. Coumarin

**337**

derivatives are well absorbed and bind strongly to plasma proteins (90 to 99 percent). The plasma half-life (36 h for warfarin), and consequently the duration of action, depends on the derivative used. Individual sensitivity to oral anticoagulants varies with a factor of 20 in accordance with the variable rate of coumarin degradation. Thus, dosage schemes are individually adapted to the result of the prothrombin time (PT). Lack of standardization in the performance and reporting of this sample assay led the WHO to propose the *International Normalized Ratio* (INR) defined as the PT ratio that would be obtained if the WHO international reference preparation were used to perform the assay.

The therapeutic range for prophylaxis of recurrent venous thromboembolism is an INR of 2.0 to 3.0 (1.2 to 1.5 times the control PT with most rabbit-brain thromboplastins). For arterial thromboembolism, the desired INR lies between 3.0 and 4.5 (1.5 to 2.0 times control PT with most rabbit thromboplastins).

### Adverse Effects and Their Treatment

Bleeding may arise from either a proper dose (but in conjunction with a predisposing factor) or an overdose. Many drugs either potentiate (e.g., phenylbutazone, clofibrate, sulfinpyrazone) or antagonize (e.g., barbiturates, phenytoin, cholestyramine) the effect of coumarins. Oral vitamin $K_1$ (1 to 2 mg) corrects an overdose of coumarins to prevent bleeding. Extensive prolonged hemorrhage may necessitate injection of vitamin $K_1$ (6 to 10 mg daily IV or IM); plasma or a concentrate of the prothrombin complex is reserved for bleeding in vital organs. Skin necrosis is occasionally observed with high initial doses of coumarins, especially in patients with low levels of proteins C and S.

### PLATELET-INHIBITING DRUGS

#### Pharmacology

Numerous drugs affect platelet function, but encouraging clinical results have been obtained mainly with aspirin alone and, on a smaller scale, with ticlopidine. Aspirin inactivates cyclooxygenase in platelets and endothelial cells. Cyclooxygenase is a key enzyme in prostaglandin synthesis. Platelets, in contrast to endothelial cells, are unable to replenish cyclooxygenase during their lifespan; thus the formation of vasoconstricting and platelet-aggregating thromboxane $A_2$ ($TXA_2$) is blocked. Higher doses are required to inhibit cyclooxygenase in endothelial cells than in platelets. A daily dose of 50 mg of aspirin inhibits 80 to 98 percent of platelet $TXA_2$ production and changes platelet function and bleeding time to the same extent as a 10-fold excess dose of the drug. Low-dose aspirin has only trivial effects on vascular, gastric, and renal cyclooxygenase activity.

Ticlopidine is a thienopyridine that inhibits ADP-induced aggregation and prolongs the bleeding time; it probably modifies the ADP receptor in platelets and inhibits the fibrinogen binding to the glycoprotein IIb-IIIa on the platelet membrane.

### Adverse Effects and Their Treatment

Gastrointestinal discomfort is a frequent complaint with regular aspirin intake; it is less frequent with buffered or enteric-coated aspirin. Gastrointestinal bleeding is observed in 1 percent per year of patients on regular aspirin. Allergic reactions are uncommon but can be severe.

Liver dysfunction and reversible granulocytopenia have been reported within 3 months after the start of ticlopidine intake.

### CLINICAL APPLICATIONS OF HEPARIN, ORAL ANTICOAGULANTS, AND ASPIRIN
#### Prevention of Arterial Thromboembolism in Cardiac Disorders

Coumarins are recommended in patients with atrial fibrillation (AF) associated with valvular disease or hyperthyroidism. In the latter case, they can be stopped 1 month after return to a euthyroid state with a normal sinus rhythm. Anticoagulants can also be considered in AF associated with cardiomyopathy or with cardiac failure. Coumarins should be started 3 weeks before elective cardioversion for AF that has been present for more than 2 days, and should be continued until a normal sinus rhythm has been maintained for at least 4 weeks. The evidence favoring the use of anticoagulants in patients with idiopathic or lone AF is still too scant to recommend their use in this condition.

Coumarins are recommended in all patients with mitral valve disease *and* AF *or* after a first embolic episode. Aortic valve disease without concomitant mitral disease or AF seldom causes embolism; therefore anticoagulants are not advised in such cases. Asymptomatic mitral valve prolapse or mitral annular calcification is not treated, but any patient with an unexplained transient ischemic attack (TIA) is given aspirin (150 to 300 mg daily or every other day); recurrent TIAs under aspirin require long-term coumarins (without aspirin). Patients with artificial heart valves are maintained on lifelong oral anticoagulation. Recent valvular prostheses are less thrombogenic than older designs, and thromboembolism is less frequent with aortic than with mitral or tricuspid valve prostheses. Anticoagulant treatment may be discontinued 3 months after surgery in a patient with a biological valve prosthesis if he or she has no history of thromboembolism, no atrial thrombus was visualized at surgery, and no AF, cardiomegaly, or heart failure is present.

Coumarin derivatives pass the placental barrier and can be teratogenic (chondrodysplasia in early pregnancy). Heparin is therefore preferred in the first trimester of pregnancy. It can replace coumarins again after the thirty-sixth week to avoid intracranial hemorrhage in the neonate during delivery. Heparin is continued during breast feeding since, unlike coumarins, it does not pass into the mother's milk.

### Coronary Disease

Heparin and aspirin (325 mg/day) have been shown separately to reduce the incidence of myocardial infarction in patients with unstable angina. In the early phase of a myocardial infarction, subcutaneous low-dose unfractionated or LMW heparin may be considered in patients with increased risk of venous thromboembolism. Full-dose heparins followed by oral anticoagulants may prevent arterial thromboembolism in patients with large transmural infarctions and extensive wall motion defects, which predispose to mural thrombus formation, until improved ventricular contraction facilitates spontaneous fragmentation and lysis.

Long-term aspirin (325 mg/day) is prescribed to reduce the likelihood of vascular death or nonfatal vascular events after a myocardial infarction; many cardiologists are reluctant to use oral anticoagulants for the same purpose because of the uncertain risk/benefit ratio. Primary prevention of myocardial infarction with antithrombotic drugs is a much more debatable issue. Current evidence does not warrant the prescription of lifelong aspirin for all middle-aged men; selective prescribing of aspirin to patients at higher risk of myocardial infarction is a more reasonable approach, provided that care is taken to exclude patients at higher risk of bleeding.

Post-angioplasty rethrombosis is usually prevented with heparin (bolus of 100 U/kg at start of catheterization, followed by infusion of 15 U/kg/h for 24 to 48 h) or empiric administration of aspirin (100 to 300 mg/day for 6 months). A trial comparing warfarin and aspirin (325 mg/day) showed no significant difference between the two drugs in the incidence of restenosis at 9 months.

Early occlusion of aortocoronary bypass grafts is prevented by a combination of dipyridamole (started 2 days before surgery) and aspirin (started 7 h after surgery). The same combination alone has little effect on late reocclusion. Aspirin alone (325 mg/day) started before surgery may also prevent early reocclusion.

## Cerebrovascular and Peripheral Vascular Disorders

Long-term aspirin (325 mg daily) or ticlopidine (250 mg twice daily) in a patient with a TIA or a mild stroke reduces the risk of vascular death or nonfatal vascular event by about 25 percent. Oral anticoagulants are used only to prevent recurrent cerebral emboli of cardiac origin (see "Prevention of Arterial Thrombo-embolism in Cardiac Disorders," above).

Long-term aspirin or ticlopidine can also reduce the occlusion rate in stenotic peripheral arteries and retard atherosclerotic plaque progression. Current evidence to support long-term use of coumarins in arterial disease of the legs is not convincing. Heparin followed by coumarins is used after an acute episode of peripheral embolism unless the source of the embolism can be eradicated.

## Venous Thromboembolism

The most effective prevention of deep-vein thrombosis (DVT) and pulmonary embolism (PE) is with oral anticoagulants and heparin. Injection of a small dose of heparin (5000 IU two or three times daily) is the more popular approach. The protective effect is further increased by simultaneous injection of dihydroergotamine (0.5 mg), but this practice can lead to vasospasm and peripheral ischemia. Patients with arterial disease of the legs, acrocyanosis, or hyperthyroidism, and pregnant women appear more vulnerable to this side effect. A single daily injection of LMW heparin can replace the repeated injections of unfractionated heparin.

A continuous IV infusion of heparin for 5 to 10 days, followed by oral anticoagulants for 2 to 3 months, is the treatment of choice for DVT in most patients. Heparin can be interrupted only after the INR has reached the preset range. Subcutaneous heparin in a comparable therapeutic dose is an alternative scheme. Higher doses of heparin are frequently required in PE to reach the same therapeutic PTT range; in the same condition, oral anticoagulants may be continued for 3 to 6 months. Recurrent thromboembolism requires long-term, and eventually life-long, anticoagulation, especially if factors predisposing to thrombosis are involved.

## THROMBOLYTIC AGENTS

### Pharmacology

Thrombolytic agents activate plasminogen either directly (urokinase, saruplase, alteplase) or indirectly (streptokinase, anistreplase). Urokinase is a two-chain molecule, while saruplase is a one-chain molecule. Alteplase and saruplase induce a relatively fibrin-specific thrombolysis. Streptokinase forms a complex with circulating plasminogen *in vivo;* anistreplase is a complex of streptokinase and human plasminogen in which the catalytic site is blocked by acylation. The half-life of saruplase and alteplase is about 5 min; that of urokinase is about 15 min. Streptokinase has an initial rapid clearance of about 15 min followed by a slower inactivation phase of about 40 min. The biological half-life of anistreplase is also about 90 min. Streptokinase and anistreplase are immunogenic in human beings.

The optimal doses of streptokinase and urokinase are not well established. In addition, there is a poor correlation between the laboratory parameters of the hemostatic system and both the thrombolytic efficacy of the drugs and the incidence of bleeding. Examples of recent intravenous dosage schemes in patients with acute myocardial infarction are: (1) streptokinase 1.5 million units over 60 min, (2) urokinase 1.5 million units as a bolus followed by 1.5 million units over 90 min, (3) alteplase 100 mg over 3 to 6 h (most often a bolus of 6 to 10 mg followed by 50 mg over the first hour and 40 mg over the next 2 h), and (4) anistreplase in a bolus of 30 mg (or units) over 2 to 5 min.

### Adverse Effects and Their Treatment

Bleeding is the main adverse effect of any thrombolytic agent. Serious bleeding requires immediate cessation of therapy, reversal of the hypocoagulable state with plasma or plasma concentrates, and, eventually, infusion of an antifibrinolytic agent (e.g., tranexamic acid 3 to 6 g/24 h). Intracranial bleeding is observed in up to 1 percent of patients. Streptokinase and anistreplase are associated with a variable degree of anaphylaxis; a second infusion may result in an antigen-antibody reaction with serious anaphylaxis.

### Clinical Indications

The main indication for thrombolytic therapy is the acute phase of a myocardial infarction (first 4 to 6 h). Early coronary reperfusion rates vary from 40 to 80 percent in different trials, depending on a number of variables. Early reperfusion is associated with improved left ventricular function and reduced mortality. The advantage of adding aspirin is well demonstrated, but there is no certainty whether heparin prevents early reocclusion and recurrent infarction.

Other indications are PE and DVT. Thrombolytic agents produce a better resolution of massive PE and a better improvement of cardiopulmonary hemodynamics than heparin alone. Lysis is achieved 3 to 4 times more often with thrombolytic agents in recent DVT than with heparin, but bleeding is also 3 times more frequent. The late beneficial effect of thrombolysis on venous function and on the postthrombotic syndrome is not well established. Specialized centers use local low-dose thrombolytic therapy in patients with occluded peripheral arteries and surgical grafts.

## SUGGESTED READING

Collen D, Verstraete M: Anticoagulants, platelet-controlling drugs, and thrombolytic agents, in Hurst JW et al (eds): *The Heart*, 7th ed. New York, McGraw-Hill, Chap 101, pp 1781–1787, 1990.

Collen D, Lijnen HR, Todd PA: Tissue-type plasminogen activator. A preliminary review of its pharmacology and therapeutic use in acute myocardial infarction. *Drugs* 37:25–49, 1989.

Dalen JE, Hirsh J (eds): 2d ACCP Conference on Antithrombotic Therapy. *Chest* 95 (suppl): 15–1695, 1989.

Furberg CD: Secondary prevention trials after acute myocardial infarction. *Am J Cardiol* 60:28A–32A, 1987.

Hirsh J, Deykin D, Poller L: Therapeutic range for oral anticoagulant therapy. *Arch Intern Med* 146:466, 1986.

International Committee for Standardization in Haematology and International Committee on Thrombosis and Haemostasis: ICSH/ICTH recommendations for reporting prothrombin time in oral anticoagulant control. *J Clin Pathol* 38:133–134, 1985.

Monk JP, Heel RC: Anisoylated plasminogen streptokinase activator complex (APSAC). A review of its mechanism of action, clinical pharmacology and therapeutic use in acute myocardial infarction. *Drugs* 34:25–49, 1987.

Salzman E: Low-molecular-weight heparin. Is small beautiful? *N Engl J Med* 315:857–859, 1986.

The Steering Committee of the Physicians' Health Study Research Group: Preliminary report: findings from the aspirin component of the ongoing physician's health study. *N Engl J Med* 318:262–264, 1988.

Stein B, Fuster V, Israel DH, et al: Platelet inhibitor agents in cardiovascular disease: an update. *J Am Coll Cardiol* 14:813–836, 1989.

Tiefenbrunn AJ, Sobel BE: The impact of coronary thrombolysis on myocardial infarction. *Fibrinolysis* 3:1–15, 1989.

Verstraete M, Collen D: Thrombolytic therapy in the eighties. *Blood* 67:1529–1541, 1986.

## 44 | Diagnosis and Management of Hyperlipidemia

*Scott M. Grundy, M.D., Ph.D.*

## DEFINITIONS

### Hypercholesterolemia

*Serum Cholesterol*

- Desirable serum cholesterol: less than 200 mg/dl.
- Borderline high serum cholesterol: 200 to 239 mg/dl.
- High serum cholesterol: 240 mg/dl or higher.

*Low-Density Lipoprotein (LDL) Cholesterol*

- Desirable LDL cholesterol: less than 130 mg/dl.
- Borderline high-risk LDL cholesterol: 130 to 159 mg/dl.
- High-risk LDL cholesterol: 160 mg/dl or higher.

### Hypertriglyceridemia

- Normal serum triglyceride: less than 250 mg/dl.
- Borderline hypertriglyceridemia: 250 to 500 mg/dl.
- Distinct hypertriglyceridemia: over 500 mg/dl.

### Mixed Hyperlipidemia

- Serum cholesterol over 240 mg/dl and serum triglyceride between 250 and 500 mg/dl.

### Hypoalphalipoproteinemia (Low High-Density Lipoprotein [HDL] Cholesterol)

- Serum HDL cholesterol less than 35 mg/dl.

### Coronary Heart Disease (CHD) Risk Factors

- Established CHD (exclusive of high-risk LDL cholesterol).
- Other forms of atherosclerotic disease.
- Premature CHD in first-degree relatives (before age 60).
- Cigarette smoking.
- Hypertension.
- Diabetes mellitus.
- Hypoalphalipoproteinemia (low HDL cholesterol).
- Obesity (over 130 percent desirable weight).
- Male sex.

## CAUSES OF DYSLIPIDEMIA

### Causes of Hypercholesterolemia

*Dietary Causes*

- Excess dietary saturated fatty acids.
- Excess dietary cholesterol.
- Excess caloric intake (obesity).

*Genetic Causes*

- Familial hypercholesterolemia (deficiency of LDL receptors).
- Familial combined hyperlipidemia.
- Polygenic hypercholesterolemia (multiple genetic defects occurring alone or in combination).

*Secondary Causes*

- Nephrotic syndrome.
- Hypothyroidism.
- Diabetes mellitus.
- Obstructive liver disease.
- Dysproteinemias (multiple myeloma, macroglobulinemia).

### Causes of Hypertriglyceridemia

- Genetic deficiency of lipoprotein lipase or apolipoprotein C-II.
- Familial hypertriglyceridemia.
- Obesity.
- Excessive alcohol intake.
- Diabetes mellitus.
- Beta-adrenergic blocking agents.

### Causes of Hypoalphalipoproteinemia

- Cigarette smoking.
- Obesity.
- Lack of exercise.
- Non-insulin-dependent diabetes mellitus.
- Hypertriglyceridemia.
- Beta-adrenergic blocking agents.
- Genetic disorders of HDL metabolism.

## MANAGEMENT OF HYPERCHOLESTEROLEMIA

### Detection of High Serum Cholesterol

All adults over age 20 should be tested for serum total cholesterol. If a person has a desirable level (less than 200 mg/dl), the test should be repeated in 5 years and no therapy is required. If the serum cholesterol is borderline high and the patient has fewer than two other CHD risk factors, one of which can be male sex, the patient should be advised to follow a serum cholesterol–lowering diet, but follow-up management is not required. The total cholesterol level should be retested in 1 year. If the level is borderline high and the patient has two other CHD risk factors, a lipoprotein analysis is indicated. This includes measurement of total cholesterol (TC), fasting triglycerides (TG), and HDL cholesterol (HDL-C); the LDL cholesterol (LDL-C) is calculated indirectly (LDL-C = TC − HDL-C − TG/5). If the total cholesterol exceeds 240 mg/dl, a lipoprotein analysis is indicated.

## Goals of Therapy

For a patient with elevated LDL cholesterol level (borderline high-risk, or high-risk) and fewer than two other risk factors (one of which can be male sex), the minimal goal for LDL cholesterol is a level below 160 mg/dl. If two or more CHD risk factors are present, the minimal goal is less than 130 mg/dl.

## Dietary Therapy

The essential aim of a serum cholesterol–lowering diet is to decrease intakes of saturated fatty acids, cholesterol, and total calories (if the patient is obese). The first step of dietary therapy is to reduce saturated fatty acids to less than 10 percent of total calories, total fat to 30 percent or less of total calories, and cholesterol to less than 300 mg per day. This can be achieved by reducing intakes of dairy fats (whole milk, ice cream, cheese, and cream), fatty meats, baked goods, eggs, and organ meats. After starting the Step One diet, the patient should be tested for lipoproteins at 6 weeks and at 3 months to determine whether the goals of therapy have been obtained. If not, the patient should proceed to the Step Two diet, which further reduces saturated fatty acids to less than 7 percent and cholesterol intake to less than 200 mg per day. This second step of dietary therapy should be continued for another 3 months. If the goals of therapy are not achieved, consideration can be given to the use of cholesterol-lowering drugs. If the goals are obtained, the patient should be continued on the Step Two diet indefinitely.

## Drug Therapy

The drugs of first choice for treatment of high LDL levels are bile acid sequestrants and nicotinic acid. The HMG-CoA reductase inhibitors (e.g., lovastatin) are more potent, but their efficacy and safety have not been proven. Gemfibrozil and probucol have less cholesterol-lowering potential and are second-choice drugs for high LDL cholesterol levels. For severe hypercholesterolemia, the use of drugs in combination (e.g., bile acid sequestrants and lovastatin [or nicotinic acid]) can be highly effective. The essential features of each drug (or class of drugs) will be reviewed briefly:

*Bile acid sequestrants* include cholestyramine and colestipol. These drugs bind bile acids in the intestinal tract and prevent their reabsorption by the intestine. This increases conversion of cholesterol into bile acids in the liver, which reduces hepatic content of cholesterol and thereby increases the activity of LDL receptors. Cholestyramine, 8 g twice daily, or colestipol, 10 g twice daily, reduces LDL cholesterol by 20 to 25 percent. At half these doses, reductions of 15 to 20 percent are common; such doses usually are better tolerated. The major side effects are constipation and various other gastrointestinal complaints. Sequestrants can interfere with absorption of acidic drugs, and they can raise triglyceride levels. Their use as a single drug cannot be recommended in patients with definite hypertriglyceridemia.

*Nicotinic acid* inhibits hepatic production of lipoproteins and reduces VLDL and LDL cholesterol, and raises HDL cholesterol. Therapeutic doses are 1000 to 1500 mg three times daily. Side effects include flushing and itching of the skin, gastric distress, abnormalities in liver function, hyperuricemia, and glucose intolerance. Flushing and gastric distress can be minimized by starting in low doses and gradually increasing the dose. (Aspirin may also reduce flushing.) This drug is especially valuable to hypercholesterolemic patients who have borderline hypertriglyceridemia or low HDL cholesterol.

*HMG-CoA reductase inhibitors* partially block the synthesis of cholesterol in the liver, and thereby increase LDL receptor activity. They lower both LDL and VLDL cholesterol levels. The starting dose is 20 mg per day; this can be doubled for severe hypercholesterolemia. LDL cholesterol levels are reduced by 30 to 40 percent. The major side effect is myopathy, which typically occurs in one of three forms: muscle pain and weakness, moderately elevated creatine levels, or both. Rarely a patient develops severe myopathy with myoglobinuria and even acute renal failure. (This is most likely to occur with concomitant use of cyclosporine, gemfibrozil, or nicotinic acid; these combinations should be avoided if possible.) The use of these drugs with bile acid sequestrants, which can be highly effective in severe hypercholesterolemia, does not increase risk for myopathy.

*Gemfibrozil* is a fibric acid and resembles other drugs in this class—clofibrate, fenofibrate, and bezafibrate. The dose of gemfibrozil is 600 mg twice daily. Although these drugs potentially lower triglyceride levels, they also cause a 10- to 20-percent reduction in LDL cholesterol levels in patients with hypercholesterolemia. The major side effects are gastric distress, myopathy, and cholesterol gallstones. Gemfibrozil was shown to reduce the rate of CHD in hypercholesterolemic patients in the Helsinki Heart Study.

*Probucol* lowers LDL cholesterol by enhancing its clearance from plasma, by an unknown mechanism. The dose is 500 mg twice daily. The drugs generally is well tolerated; its side effects are mostly gastrointestinal. It lowers LDL cholesterol about 15 percent. Probucol has not yet been shown to be effective or safe in a major clinical trial.

## MANAGEMENT OF HYPERTRIGLYCERIDEMIA

For patients with borderline hypertriglyceridemia, dietary therapy should be tried first. This includes weight reduction and decreased intakes of alcohol and carbohydrates. For many patients drug therapy will not be required; but if it is deemed necessary, nicotinic acid and gemfibrozil are effective triglyceride-lowering drugs. When serum triglycerides exceed 500 mg/dl, patients are at risk for acute pancreatitis; if the triglyceride level cannot be driven below 500 mg/dl by use of diet, drug therapy is indicated for prevention of pancreatitis.

## MANAGEMENT OF MIXED HYPERLIPIDEMIA

Elevations of both cholesterol and triglycerides in the same patient call for dietary therapy as discussed above. If drug therapy is needed, nicotinic acid is the drug of choice. Bile acid sequestrants with gemfibrozil, or lovastatin alone, are alternatives.

## MANAGEMENT OF HYPOALPHALIPOPROTEINEMIA

First-line therapy for low HDL cholesterol is to remove causes (smoking, obesity, lack of exercise, uncontrolled diabetes, hypertriglyceridemia, and beta-adrenergic blocking agents). If the patient has a high-risk LDL cholesterol level, LDL-lowering drugs (e.g., lovastatin) can be considered. Treatment of low HDL cholesterol in the absence of known causes and other risk factors may not be justified; but in their presence, nicotinic acid, lovastatin, or gemfibrozil can be considered.

## SUGGESTED READING

Blum CB, Levy RI: Current therapy for hypercholesterolemia. *JAMA* 261:3582–3587, 1989.

Brown MS, Goldstein JR: Receptor-mediated pathway for cholesterol homeostasis. *Science* 232:34–47, 1986.

Consensus Development Conference: Lowering blood cholesterol to prevent heart disease. *JAMA* 253:2080–2086, 1985.

Consensus Development Conference: Treatment of hypertriglyceridemia. *JAMA* 251:1196–1200.

Expert Panel: Detection, evaluation, and treatment of high blood cholesterol in adults. *Arch Intern Med* 148:36–69, 1988.

Frick MH, Elo O, Haapa K, et al: Helsinki Heart Study: primary-prevention trial with gemfibrozil in middle-aged men with dyslipidemia: safety of treatment, changes in risk factors, and incidence of coronary heart disease. *N Engl J Med* 317:1237–1245, 1987.

Grundy SM: Cholesterol and coronary heart disease. A new era. *JAMA* 256:2849–2858, 1986.

Grundy SM: HMG-CoA reductase inhibitors for treatment of hypercholesterolemia. *N Engl J Med* 319:24–33, 1988.

Grundy SM: Lipid-lowering drugs, in Hurst JW et al (eds): *The Heart,* 7th ed. New York, McGraw-Hill, Chap 104, pp 1798–1802, 1990.

Grundy SM et al: Rationale of the diet-heart statement of the American Heart Association. Report of Nutrition Committee. *Circulation* 65:839A–854A, 1982.

Grundy SM, Vega GL: Fibric acids: Effects on lipids and lipoprotein metabolism. *Am J Med* 83(suppl 5B):9–19, 1987.

Lipid Research Clinics Program: The Lipid Research Clinics Coronary Primary Prevention Trial results: I. Reduction in the incidence of coronary heart disease. *JAMA* 251:351–364, 1984, and II. The relationship of reduction in incidence of coronary heart disease to cholesterol lowering. *JAMA* 251:365–374, 1984.

# Index